STUDY GUIDE
MOSBY'S PHARMACOLOGY IN NURSING

22 EDITION

LEDA MCKENRY, PHD, C-APN, FAAN

ED TESSIER, PHARMD, MPH, BCPS

MARYANN HOGAN, RN, MSN

Study Guide prepared by

MaryAnn Hogan, RN, MSN
Clinical Assistant Professor
School of Nursing, University of Massachusetts
  Amherst
Amherst, Massachusetts

ELSEVIER
MOSBY

11830 Westline Industrial Drive
St. Louis, Missouri 63146

STUDY GUIDE FOR MOSBY'S PHARMACOLOGY IN NURSING

ISBN-13: 978-0-323-03126-4
ISBN-10: 0-323-03126-9

Previous edition copyrighted 2001

ISBN-13: 978-0-323-03126-4
ISBN-10: 0-323-03126-9

Acquisitions Editor: Kristin Geen
Associate Developmental Editor: Jamie Horn
Editorial Assistant: Rebecca Williams
Publishing Services Manager: Debbie Vogel
Senior Project Manager: Jodi Willard
Cover Design: Amy Buxton

Printed in the United States of America

Last digit is the print number: 9 8 7 6 5 4 3 2 1

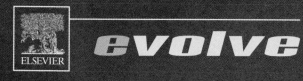

1 Orientation to Pharmacology

1. Complete the following puzzle.

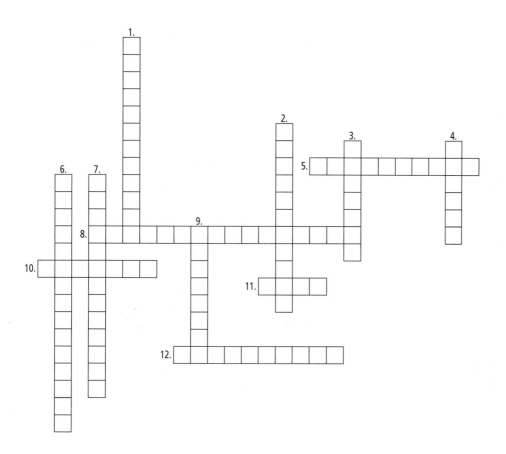

Across

5. The officially approved therapeutic purposes of a drug
8. How a drug is absorbed, distributed, associated with tissue, biotransformed or metabolized, and excreted
10. A simple, informative, and unique nonproprietary name for a drug based on pharmacologic and/or chemical relationships
11. Any substance used in the diagnosis, cure, treatment, or prevention of a disease or condition
12. The type of medicine that is evidence-based

Down

1. Contains descriptions, recipes, strengths, standards of purity, and dosage forms for drugs
2. Another label for the brand name or trade name of a drug
3. A type of nontherapeutic effect that may be experienced when a drug is administered
4. The size, frequency, and number of doses of a therapeutic agent
6. Another name for a drug that can be obtained over-the-counter
7. A type of therapy that includes herbal preparations, acupuncture, aromatherapy, and therapeutic touch
9. A name for a drug that includes a precise description of the chemical composition and molecular structure of a drug

2. _____ is a science that studies the effects of drugs within a living system.

3. In the fifth century BC, _____ advanced the idea that disease resulted from natural causes and could be understood only through a study of natural laws.

4. A _____ contains descriptions, recipes, strengths, standards of purity, and dosage forms for all authorized drugs available within a country.

5. A _____ is any substance used in the diagnosis, cure, treatment, or prevention of a disease or condition.

6. The _____ or _____ name of a drug is based on pharmacologic and/or chemical relationships.

7. A _____ or _____ drug requires that it must be ordered by a physician to be obtained for use.

8. Studying a _____ or _____ drug can help the nurse understand the common characteristics of each drug classification.

9. The officially approved therapeutic purposes of the drug or the conditions for which it is used are known as _____.

10. The _____ step of the nursing process involves gathering data about an individual's experience with medications and allergies and identifying preexisting conditions that might influence the choice of drugs used.

CONNECTING WITH CLIENTS

11. You have an order to administer to a client a medication that you have not heard of before. What should you do before administering the drug?

12. A client has seen several television commercials for drugs that encourage viewers to ask their doctors if the drug is right for them. The client asks you, the nurse, why two names always appear on the screen. How would you respond?

13. You are viewing a client's medication administration record to determine the medications you need to administer this shift. What nursing activities should you include when implementing the plan of care with respect to the drug regimen?

TRAINING FOR TEST TAKING

14. The nurse needs to review key adverse effects and nursing considerations of a medication before administering it to a client. Which of the following sources would be most practical for this purpose?
    1. A pharmacopeia
    2. A Physician's Desk Reference
    3. A pharmacology textbook
    4. A nursing drug handbook

15. A client taking prescribed medications asks the nurse how to find the best information about them on the Internet. Which of the following responses by the nurse would be best?
    1. "It is important to use a search engine, which will screen out unreliable websites."
    2. "There is no way to screen websites for reliability, so it is best to visit reputable websites, such as government or health care agencies, and medical/pharmacy school websites for information."
    3. "Depending on the Internet service provider used, a filter can be used to block all unreliable websites. The ones that are left should be fine to look at."
    4. "You cannot assume that any website is absolutely reliable. That is why it is important to also have information in print, such as the teaching sheets we use in the hospital."

16. A nurse who is safeguarding a client while administering medication therapy would do which of the following?
    1. Give half of a scheduled dose when the drug has toxic adverse effects.
    2. Use best judgment possible when interpreting an unclear medication order.
    3. Chart clearly and specifically about observed drug effects.
    4. Ask another nurse about a medication that is unfamiliar.

17. A client asks why an ordered medication has a few letters and numbers imprinted in each tablet. Which of the following responses by the nurse is best?
    1. "Those markings are not generally useful to people taking the medication, but they can be used to identify the drug and manufacturer if needed."
    2. "They represent a type of coding for the clinical use of the drug, such as to treat heart failure or asthma."
    3. "The markings are quality assurance imprints, which help to identify the expiration date and batch number of the drug."
    4. "The letters indicate the manufacturer, whereas the numbers represent a code for the cost of the medication."

18. The nurse who is writing goals for a client's drug therapy is engaged in which step of the nursing process?
    1. Assessment
    2. Diagnosis
    3. Planning
    4. Implementation

2 Legal and Ethical Aspects of Medication Administration

STAYING ON TOP OF TERMINOLOGY

1. Complete the following word search.

FDA   ORDERS
INVESTIGATIONAL   PRESCRIPTION
LEGEND   SAFEGUARDS
LEGISLATION   STANDARDS
NARCOTICS   TOXICITY
NURSING

```
J  L  F  L  M  I  N  V  E  S  T  I  G  A  T  I  O  N  A  L
N  E  K  D  D  J  Q  B  A  J  K  S  R  E  D  R  O  A  L  R
M  G  K  Y  A  F  P  F  T  N  R  M  I  R  M  I  E  R  C  W
Z  E  A  W  S  X  E  O  Y  U  K  K  I  I  T  S  U  C  K  I
B  N  T  P  Q  G  X  M  O  R  T  R  P  A  T  B  N  O  I  D
D  D  Q  P  U  I  A  Z  U  S  J  Q  L  A  G  B  F  T  Z  A
V  Q  M  A  C  W  C  H  T  I  C  S  N  S  Y  N  E  I  J  P
Y  Z  R  I  J  L  M  I  Q  N  I  D  T  U  X  K  C  C  K  E
E  D  T  V  U  B  G  I  D  G  A  M  G  F  M  B  I  S  M  U
S  Y  H  B  V  Q  X  T  E  R  B  P  G  T  R  X  M  Z  W  C
B  I  Z  I  O  A  K  L  D  X  H  S  Q  M  F  P  O  J  N  Y
F  L  T  I  P  R  E  S  C  R  I  P  T  I  O  N  Z  G  M  I
```

FOCUSING ON THE FACTS

2. The _____ was designed to prevent, and provide increased research into, substance abuse and dependence and to provide for treatment and rehabilitation of drug abusers and drug-dependent persons.

3. Controlled substances that are classified as Schedule I have a high potential for _____.

4. The first step of investigating a new substance for possible future use as a drug is accomplished by testing the drug on _____.

5. The _____ is a quantitative measure of the relative safety of a drug; stated technically, it is the ratio of the median lethal dose to the median effective dose.

5

6. A drug that is listed as Pregnancy Category _____ indicates that studies in animals or humans demonstrate fetal abnormalities, or adverse effects reports indicate evidence of fetal risk.

7. The voluntary adverse-reaction reporting program MedWatch was initiated to detect _____ that have not been revealed by previous clinical or pharmaceutical studies.

8. All people who enroll in experimental drug studies must give _____ to participate.

9. A _____ medication order is one that leaves no room for doubt regarding the medication prescribed, its dosage and route, the dosing interval, and the prescriber's name/signature.

10. A nurse who administers medications carefully to assigned clients to ensure client safety and medication effectiveness is operating under the ethical principle of _____.

CONNECTING WITH CLIENTS

11. As you are selecting a dose of a prescribed medication for a client, you note that a few of the unit dose tablets have a brownish tinge to them, although all of the others are the usual shade of pink. What should you do?

12. You are working in a major medical center that participates in drug research. You are asked to administer a drug to a client that is in Phase III of clinical investigation. What are your expectations about the status of this drug?

13. You are caring for a pregnant client who has an order for a medication that is listed as Pregnancy Category C. What does this mean to you?

14. The nurse is reading manufacturer's information about a new drug released in the past month that has been ordered for an assigned client. The nurse is confident that the new drug has met rigorous standards in development, as mandated in which of the following pieces of legislation?
    1. Kefauver Harris Amendment, 1962
    2. Orphan Drug Act, 1983
    3. Durham-Humphrey Amendment of 1952
    4. Controlled Substances Act of 1970

15. A client brings to the pain clinic visit a prescription bottle for an analgesic that states "no refills." While reading the rest of the label, the nurse anticipates that the medication belongs to which of the following controlled substance groups?
    1. Schedule I
    2. Schedule II
    3. Schedule III
    4. Schedule IV

16. A day shift nurse reporting to work notes that the assignment sheet has "narcotics count" written in the section of the sheet for "additional duties." The nurse plans to do which of the following based on this assignment?
    1. Count all controlled substances with the pharmacist whenever new doses are delivered to the nursing unit.
    2. Count the controlled substances at the beginning of the work shift and verify this with the pharmacy records.
    3. Count the controlled substances at the end of the work shift with the evening supervisor.
    4. Count controlled substances at the beginning and end of the work shift with another nurse.

17. The nurse making rounds at the beginning of the work shift notes that a client's bag of IV fluid has small black specks floating in the bag. Which of the following actions should the nurse take first?
    1. Write an incident report.
    2. Call the pharmacy.
    3. Hang a new bag of solution.
    4. Send the bag of solution to the risk management department.

18. The physician has ordered a drug for a client that is listed as pregnancy category A. Which of the following actions should the nurse take?
    1. Administer the ordered dose.
    2. Question the dose, because it should be half-strength.
    3. Question the dose if the client is in the third trimester.
    4. Refuse to give the dose.

19. The nurse is caring for a client who is eligible to receive an investigational drug. The nurse anticipates that which of the following individuals will obtain informed written consent?
    1. The nursing supervisor
    2. The physician
    3. The researcher
    4. A representative from the FDA

20. The nurse is transcribing a new drug order for a client who has renal insufficiency. The nurse notes that the order contains the usual dose, and is aware that the drug is excreted by the kidneys. Which of the following actions should the nurse take?
    1. Transcribe the order as usual, because the dosage is normal.
    2. Clarify the order with the prescriber.
    3. Delay the start time for 24 hours so this can be discussed during rounds.
    4. Write an incident report.

Chapter **2** **Legal and Ethical Aspects of Medication Administration**

3 Principles of Drug Action

STAYING ON TOP OF TERMINOLOGY

1. Complete the following puzzle

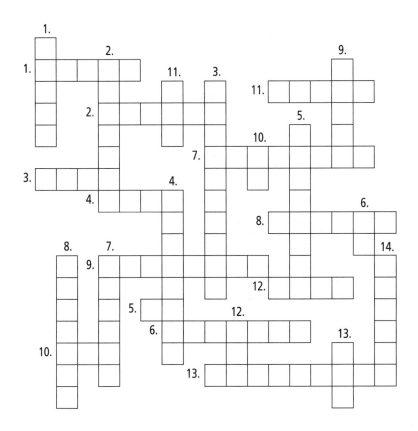

Across

1. A way to administer medications
2. Liquid part of the blood
3. A factor affecting the dose of medications for a child
4. Area in which inhalants are absorbed
5. The abbreviation for therapeutic index
6. A form in which a drug can be taken orally
7. Objective and subjective effects of a drug
8. Environment that increases the absorption of aspirin
9. Movement of a drug in the body is called pharmaco- _____
10. Factor affecting the effects of a drug
11. Organic substance insoluble in water
12. Fundamental unit of all living organisms
13. Term for process of ridding the body of a drug

Down

1. Another term for medications
2. Route in which medications are applied to the skin
3. Adverse reaction produced unintentionally
4. Factors we are born with that can affect drug effects
5. Smallest amount of a substance that can exist alone
6. Abbreviation for route in which a drug is instilled into muscle
7. Organ that can eliminate drugs
8. Organ that aids in absorption of a drug
9. Various places in which drugs can be injected
10. Abbreviation for route in which a drug is instilled into tissue
11. Abbreviation for aspirin
12. Factor affecting the metabolism of a drug
13. Form in which a drug can be applied to the skin
14. Pharmacodynamics of a drug

FOCUSING ON THE FACTS

2. Drugs only modify existing _____ of a tissue or body organ.

3. _____ is the study of drug concentrations during the processes of absorption, distribution, biotransformation, and excretion.

4. A drug that moves from a region of higher concentration to a region of lower concentration is participating in the process known as _____ transport.

5. The initial, temporary large dose of a drug that is given to rapidly effect a therapeutic drug response is the _____ dose.

6. A client with arthritis who cannot tolerate regular aspirin because of gastrointestinal irritation would purchase the medication in an _____-coated form.

7. A client who is about to begin allergy testing would receive injection of potential allergens by the _____ route.

8. An orally administered drug may be given in larger amounts than needed in the circulation to compensate for the _____ effect exerted by the liver.

9. After filtration in the kidney, _____-soluble compounds fail to be reabsorbed by the tubular nephron and are then eliminated from the body.

10. The half-life of a drug may be lengthened in the presence of disease in the _____ or the _____.

CONNECTING WITH CLIENTS

11. You are assigned to a client with chronic obstructive pulmonary disease (COPD) who is taking a β-adrenergic blocker for hypertension. She asks, "If this drug is so good for my blood pressure, how can it interfere with my breathing once in a while?" How would you respond?

12. You are administering oral medications to a client with diabetes mellitus who has gastroparesis as a complication of the disease. What would you do during administration to increase the likelihood that proper absorption will take place?

13. While administering a new ophthalmic medication to a client, he asks why you are "pressing between my nose and my eye." How would you respond?

TRAINING FOR TEST TAKING

14. A client who took an excessive dose of morphine sulfate has received naloxone (Narcan) as an antidote. The nurse understands that best explanation for this drug's effectiveness lies in the principle that drug-receptor binding may be:
    1. Reversible
    2. Graded
    3. Selective
    4. Antagonistic

15. A client who was previously stable has gone into shock. Based on principles of drug absorption, the nurse expects to administer medications by which route at this time?
    1. Subcutaneous
    2. Intramuscular
    3. Intravenous
    4. Intratracheal

16. A client has a dose of warfarin (Coumadin) ordered for 4 PM. Based on knowledge of what happens to this drug during distribution, the nurse checks the recent results for which of the following serum laboratory values?
    1. Albumin
    2. Hematocrit
    3. White blood cells
    4. Platelets

17. A client with a seizure disorder is receiving phenytoin (Dilantin) 100 mg orally three times per day. The medication administration record lists the dosage times as 8 AM, 4 PM, and 12 AM. The nurse who transcribes a new order for a serum Dilantin level would arrange for the phlebotomist to draw the blood sample the following day at which of the following times?
    1. Just prior to the 4 PM dose.
    2. One hour after the 8 AM dose.
    3. Just after the midnight dose.
    4. Just prior to the 8 AM dose.

18. The nurse would report which of the following client findings to the health care provider as a potential adverse effect of a drug that the client has been receiving for the last 48 hours?
    1. Dizziness on standing
    2. Skin rash
    3. Dry mouth
    4. Loss of appetite

19. A client who just received the first dose of an IV antibiotic is starting to develop signs of an anaphylactic reaction. The nurse should ensure that which of the following medications is readily available for immediate use?
    1. ranitidine (Zantac)
    2. digoxin (Lanoxin)
    3. epinephrine (Adrenalin Chloride)
    4. acetylcysteine (Mucomyst)

20. The nurse needs to administer a once daily medication that is known to be irritating to the gastrointestinal tract. The nurse should administer this drug at which of the following times to minimize this adverse effect?
    1. With breakfast
    2. Thirty minutes before lunch
    3. Just before supper
    4. At bedtime

4 | Medication Errors

STAYING ON TOP OF TERMINOLOGY

1. Match the definition on the right with the appropriate word on the left.

_____ Adverse drug event
_____ Medical erroran
_____ Medication error
_____ Medication reconciliation

a. A process that consists of identifying accurate list of all client medications and using it to ensure that the client receives the correct medications
b. Includes errors in prescribing, dispensing, administration, or monitoring
c. A negative or untoward response to a medication
d. The failure to complete a planned aim in the manner intended or using the wrong plan to achieve an aim

FOCUSING ON THE FACTS

2. Computerized physician order entry systems may reduce medication errors by targeting the first step of the medication process, which is _____.

3. A medication error made in the pharmacy would be considered to be an error of _____.

4. An advantage to the use of machine readable bar codes on medications is that this will likely reduce the rate of medication _____.

5. It is common to correctly identify a client before administering medications by checking the client's _____ and _____.

6. When preparing a medication to be administered to a client, the medication should be compared to the order for a total of _____ times.

7. Never chart a medication as being given until it has been _____.

8. When a client is receiving a first dose of an intravenous medication, such as an antibiotic, it is safe practice to remain with the client for _____ minutes after administration to watch for immediate adverse effects.

9. After making a medication error, a nurse should expect to complete a(n) _____ report.

10. A first step within a health care institution to reduce medication errors is to eliminate a culture of _____.

CONNECTING WITH CLIENTS

11. You are receiving in transfer from the postanesthesia care unit a client who had surgery earlier in the day. How would you perform medication reconciliation for this client?

12. You have just drawn up a dose of insulin to give to an assigned client. What additional steps should you take to ensure that a medication error would not be made?

13. You are handing a dose of a medication to a client, when the client states, "This pill does not look like the usual one that I take." What should you do?

TRAINING FOR TEST TAKING

14. The nurse receives telephone orders for medications for a client newly admitted to the nursing unit. Which of the following entries on the order sheet by the nurse upholds the Joint Commission for Accreditation of Healthcare Organizations (JCAHO) guidelines for use of abbreviations in medical records?
    1. Digoxin 0.250 mg PO daily
    2. Lisinopril 25 mg PO QD
    3. Regular insulin 6 U every 6 hours
    4. Lasix 20 mg IV twice daily

15. The nurse considering employment in a hospital learns that it uses computerized physician order entry. The nurse recognizes that this system is likely to have a primary benefit for the client by reducing or eliminating which of the following factors?
    1. Need to clarify unclear orders
    2. Risk of drug interactions
    3. Need for telephone orders
    4. Transcription errors

16. A client has a new order for cefazolin to be given to a client. The pharmacy technician delivers cephalexin. Which of the following actions should the nurse take?
    1. Administer the dose because the medications are interchangeable.
    2. Check for client allergy to cephalexin before administering the dose.
    3. Contact the pharmacy to have the dose replaced.
    4. Make a new entry into the drug name column of the medication administration record.

17. The nurse concludes that safe medication practices are being upheld if the physician orders that which client medication may be kept at the bedside for use as needed?
    1. nitroglycerin (Nitrostat)
    2. digoxin (Lanoxin)
    3. famotidine (Pepcid)
    4. furosemide (Lasix)

18. The nurse has just drawn into a syringe a dose of medication to be given by the intravenous route. Which of the following actions should the nurse take next?
    1. Have two other nurses check the dose.
    2. Label the syringe with the medication name and dose.
    3. Discard the medication vial.
    4. Chart the dose on the medication administration record.

19. A nursing assistant tells the nurse administering medications to a client that a physician who was paged is on the telephone. The nurse should do which of the following as the best action after hearing this information?
    1. Ask the nursing assistant to remain with the client until the medications are taken.
    2. Take the medications out of the room and take the telephone call.
    3. Remain with the client until the medications are swallowed.
    4. Ask the client to be sure to take all the medications.

20. A client is being discharged to home following a hospital stay. What should the nurse do with the remaining medications previously sent to the unit by the pharmacy for this client?
    1. Send them home with the client.
    2. Place them in the stock medication area on the nursing unit.
    3. Discard them in a safe manner by flushing them in the toilet.
    4. Return them to the pharmacy.

5 The Nursing Process and Pharmacology

1. Match the letter for the step of the nursing process on the right to the corresponding nursing activities on the left. Note that each step may be used more than once.

_____ Chief complaint of the client
_____ Checking an identification bracelet
          before drug administration
_____ Nausea related to chemotherapy
_____ Recording secondary effects
_____ Noncompliance with prescribed
          steroid therapy
_____ Monitoring therapeutic response
          to a drug
_____ History of allergy
_____ Behavioral objectives for the client
_____ Instillation of eye drops
_____ Calculating flow rate for oxygen therapy
_____ Vital signs
_____ Observing a client demonstrate proper
          self-medication with insulin

A. Assessment
D. Diagnosis
P. Planning
I. Implementation
E. Evaluation

FOCUSING ON THE FACTS

2. During client assessment, the nurse would assess for a _____ to a drug, which is a condition that would preclude the administration of a drug.

3. "Diphenhydramine 25 mg PO now" would be an example of a _____ medication order.

4. The main pharmacokinetic effect of heavy cigarette smoking is to _____ (raise/lower) drug plasma levels by the induction of microsomal enzyme systems.

5. A drug that is given by the _____ route would be placed under the tongue.

6. When administering an intradermal medication, the nurse would select a small-barrel (1 mL) syringe with a _____- to _____-gauge needle.

7. The nurse selecting a site for intramuscular medication administration would recall that the deltoid muscle can hold up to _____ mL in the average adult.

8. When a client is receiving medications by the intravenous route, the nurse places high priority on assessing the site for signs of leakage, known as _____.

9. To reduce the risk of phlebitis from irritating substances in an intravenous medication, the nurse may consider using an in-line _____ in the intravenous tubing.

10. A common adverse effect of antihypertensive medications is a drop in _____ when moving from a lying to a sitting or standing position.

CONNECTING WITH CLIENTS

11. A client newly admitted to the hospital has a history of heavy alcohol consumption. What general concerns do you have regarding alcohol use and the risk for interactions with prescribed medications?

12. A client who had surgery to repair a fractured arm is at risk for constipation as an adverse effect of drug therapy with oxycodone and acetaminophen (Percocet). The client has no history of other health problems. Within the independent domain of nursing practice, what interventions could you write on the client's care plan to reduce the risk of constipation for this client?

13. A client admitted with pneumonia has a new drug order for an antibiotic. What principles are important to keep in mind when scheduling the doses of this type of drug on the medication administration record?

TRAINING FOR TEST TAKING

14. A client is beginning drug therapy with a medication known to cause blood dyscrasias. The nurse is most interested in reviewing which of the following laboratory test results to determine the client's baseline before administering the first dose?
    1. Serum electrolytes
    2. Liver enzymes
    3. Serum creatinine
    4. Complete blood count

15. A client is taking cholestyramine (Questran) for an elevated cholesterol level. The nurse would assess for which of the following problems that could occur as a result of binding or chelation with this drug?
    1. Deficiency of fat-soluble vitamins
    2. Hyponatremia
    3. Dehydration
    4. Increase in ascorbic acid excretion

16. The nurse learns that a client is not taking a prescribed medication as ordered because of the high cost of the medication. Which of the following nursing diagnoses would be most appropriate for this client?
    1. Ineffective Coping
    2. Noncompliance
    3. Deficient Knowledge
    4. Ineffective Therapeutic Regimen Management

17. The nurse would evaluate that a client taking a central nervous system (CNS) stimulant is experiencing an adverse effect of this type of medication if the client exhibits which of the following symptoms?
    1. Drowsiness
    2. Tremors
    3. Confusion
    4. Dizziness

18. The nurse is administering to a client a medication that is in the form of a troche. The nurse instructs the client to take this medication by do which of the following?
    1. Placing it under the tongue
    2. Chewing it
    3. Letting it dissolve in the mouth
    4. Swallowing it with 8 ounces of water

19. A client has an order for peak and trough drug levels with the 10:00 dose of a medication. For which of the following times should the nurse schedule the trough drug level to be drawn?
    1. 09:30
    2. 10:00
    3. 11:00
    4. 11:30

20. A client has a new order for a daily dose of a diuretic. The nurse would write which of the following on the medication administration record as the best time to give the dose?
    1. 8:00 AM
    2. 1:00 PM
    3. 5:00 PM
    4. 10:00 PM

6 Biocultural Aspects of Drug Therapy

1. Complete the following word search.

AFRICAN   HARMONY
AMERICANS HISPANIC
ASIAN   NATIVE
CULTURE   RELIGION
FOLK   SPIRITUAL
HAITIAN

Y	A	C	U	L	T	U	R	E	Q	N	P
M	M	F	O	L	K	N	N	J	O	S	O
U	E	D	R	B	A	A	Q	I	E	P	X
M	R	L	Z	I	T	S	G	Q	N	I	U
S	I	C	T	I	C	I	H	E	C	R	B
B	C	I	V	A	L	A	G	I	I	I	K
S	A	E	H	E	R	N	N	J	M	T	U
H	N	F	R	M	S	A	G	P	D	U	P
L	S	N	O	G	P	N	K	X	M	A	O
I	I	N	F	S	M	I	Y	M	X	L	Z
W	Y	K	I	E	L	D	K	I	L	N	Y
J	Q	H	Z	E	B	G	J	B	K	M	Z

FOCUSING ON THE FACTS

2. The _____ of a client is a set of learned values, beliefs, customs, and behaviors that influences health beliefs and various practices that relate to pharmacology.

3. One of the goals of Healthy People 2010 is to eliminate health _____ among people of color.

4. A _____ is a Mexican-American folk healer.

5. Although they exist, racial and ethnic disparities in health are unacceptable, particularly because in many case they are associated with worse _____.

6. Many cultural groups avoid _____ medicine until herbal or home remedies are totally ineffective or the illness becomes acute.

7. The _____ study, which examined the effects of untreated syphilis in black males for 40 years, contributed to conspiracy beliefs and negative attitudes toward health care by African Americans.

8. Some Mexican Americans consider health to be the consequence of good _____, whereas others see it as being the result of good _____.

9. The purpose of herbal remedies prepared according to specific prescriptions by Chinese herbalists is to restore the balance of _____ and _____.

10. Culturally, the Native Americans' belief system of being in harmony with _____ is crucial to health maintenance.

CONNECTING WITH CLIENTS

11. A client of the Muslim faith is admitted to the nursing unit. What should you keep in mind regarding the cultural practices of Muslims to develop an appropriate plan of care?

12. You wish to explore with a client the influences of culture on lifestyle and health. Suggest a few opening questions that would be helpful in beginning the discussion.

13. You are working with a Mexican-American client during a clinical rotation. The coassigned staff nurse says, "Mr. M. wouldn't drink his orange juice this morning because he says he cannot take it while he has a 'cold' illness. I told him he has pneumonia, not a cold." How could you explain to the nurse what the client was trying to say?

14. The nurse would question a new order for which of the following types of insulin after learning that the client is of the Jewish faith?
    1. Beef
    2. Pork
    3. Human
    4. Synthetic

15. An African-American client is diagnosed with hypertension. Which of the following antihypertensive drug classes does the nurse anticipate will be most effective for this client based on current literature?
    1. Angiotensin converting enzyme (ACE) inhibitors
    2. Short-acting β-adrenergic blockers
    3. Long-acting calcium channel blockers
    4. Angiotensin II receptor blockers (ARBs)

16. A Mexican-American client comes to the health care clinic in distress. A family member tells the nurse that the client is suffering from "mal ojo." The nurse would question the client about which of the following symptoms?
    1. Abdominal pain and cramping
    2. Depression
    3. Malaise and lethargy
    4. Joint aches and pains

17. A client tells the nurse that she utilizes the services of a Chinese healer, who uses fine needles inserted into the skin to treat the client's chronic pain. The nurse documents that the client uses which of the following therapies?
    1. Moxibustion
    2. Acupuncture
    3. Yin supplementation
    4. Yang supplementation

18. An Asian client who is receiving instructions from the ambulatory care physician nods his head while the physician is speaking. Which of the following actions would be best for the nurse to take before the client leaves the office?
    1. Ask the client to state or explain the instructions given.
    2. Ask the client again if he has any questions.
    3. Document that the client understood the physician's instructions.
    4. Make a note to follow-up by phone in one day to verify understanding.

19. The nurse is taking a health history from a Native American client. The nurse should do which of the following during the interview to deliver culturally appropriate care?
    1. Avoid taking notes during the interview.
    2. Document each response carefully.
    3. Maintain direct eye contact as much as possible.
    4. Keep the interview focused only the questions on the form.

20. A nurse anticipates that a client with which of the following health problems is most at risk for inadequate pharmacotherapy based on genetic variations in response to medication therapy?
    1. Long bone fractures
    2. Renal failure
    3. Glaucoma
    4. Epilepsy

7 Maternal and Child Drug Therapy

STAYING ON TOP OF TERMINOLOGY

1. Match the developmental age labels on the right to the appropriate nursing interventions on the left. Note that some labels will be used more than once.

_____ Perform the procedure swiftly, then comfort	a. Infants
_____ Encourage self-expression and self-care	b. Toddlers
_____ Offer concrete explanation and perform quickly	c. Preschoolers
_____ Explain how medication works	d. School-age children
_____ Make use of magical thinking	e. Adolescents
_____ Allow self-comforting measures	
_____ Use play for expression of feelings	

FOCUSING ON THE FACTS

2. Prescription and over-the-counter (OTC) drugs taken during pregnancy have resulted in fetal drug toxicity and _____ .

3. Drugs crossing the placenta enter the fetal circulation via the _____ .

4. Medications that adversely affect the developing fetus may be lethal or teratogenic, mutagenic (causing genetic mutation), or _____ (causing or accelerating the development of cancer).

5. A major issue regarding the use of drugs in the perinatal period involves the legal and ethical problems associated with drug research experiments during _____ .

6. Excessive maternal intake of alcohol, especially at or near the time of _____ , is associated with fetal alcohol syndrome (FAS).

7. Drug factors that enhance drug excretion into breast milk are nonionization, low molecular weight, _____ solubility, and concentration.

8. A standard medication dosage is nearly nonexistent in pediatrics; medications are usually ordered according to the _____ or _____ of the child.

9. To reduce the risk of aspiration, medications should be administered to children who are in a _____ position.

10. Because infants are nose breathers and nasal congestion will inhibit their sucking, nose drops, if necessary, should be instilled _____ to _____ minutes before feedings.

CONNECTING WITH CLIENTS

11. A breastfeeding client who needs to take a one-time dose of a prescribed medication is advised by the physician to temporarily stop breastfeeding. As the nurse working with this client, what facts do you need to consider to explain this appropriately to the mother?

12. Calculate the following dosages for children using the different rules and the nomogram for determining surface area for children.

Adult dose	Age of child	Weight (lb)	Height (in)	Clark	BSA
Atropine sulfate grain 1/150	18 mo	25	32		
Aminophylline 0.5 g	6 yr	38	42		
Gentamicin 80 mg	22 mo	28	33		

13. A nurse needs to administer a suppository to a child. The medication storage machine supplies only a dose that is twice the ordered dose. The nurse intends to cut the suppository in half. What are your thoughts and what would you suggest to the nurse?

TRAINING FOR TEST TAKING

14. The antenatal clinic nurse would be most concerned about the effects of over-the-counter (OTC) drug use in a client of how many weeks' gestation?
    1. 24
    2. 36
    3. 18
    4. 10

15. The student nurse needs to do a presentation in clinical conference about how physiologic changes during pregnancy that affect the pharmacokinetics of drug action. The student explains that which of the following processes is generally accelerated during pregnancy?
    1. Absorption
    2. Distribution
    3. Biotransformation
    4. Excretion

16. A nurse in the newborn nursery is assigned to four neonates. The nurse would not be concerned about the risk for neonatal withdrawal in the infant of a mother who took which of the following substances?
    1. acetaminophen (Tylenol)
    2. diphenhydramine (Benadryl)
    3. diazepam (Valium)
    4. propoxyphene (Darvon)

17. A client who delivered an infant earlier in the day is planning to bottle-feed the infant. The nurse anticipates that discharge teaching will include physician advice that the infant be given formula that contains which of the following mineral supplements?
    1. Calcium
    2. Sodium
    3. Iron
    4. Zinc

18. A nurse is administering medications to an assigned pediatric client. To enhance cooperation of the child, the nurse allows the child to take the pills from the medication container after noting that the child is at least how old?
    1. 2 years old
    2. 4 years old
    3. 6 years old
    4. 8 years old

19. The nurse needs to administer to a child a medication that has an unpleasant taste. Which of the following foods would be the best choice for the nurse to mix the medication in to disguise the taste?
    1. Milk
    2. Pudding
    3. Cereal
    4. Orange juice

20. The nurse has administered an eye drop to a child. Which of the following actions should the nurse take next?
    1. Allow the child to rub the eyes for better distribution across the eyeball.
    2. Hold pressure on the inner canthus for 30 seconds with a tissue.
    3. Hold the eyelid so that the client cannot blink for 60 seconds.
    4. Ask the client to pretend to "freeze" and not move the head for 30 seconds.

Chapter **7** **Maternal and Child Drug Therapy**

8 Drug Therapy for Older Adults

STAYING ON TOP OF TERMINOLOGY

1. Unscramble the letters for the words below and enter them in the proper places in the scrabble grid from top to bottom.

NUFCONIT, DARCCAI TPUOTOU, DOLOB WLOF, NRISDOUITIBT, VRELI, MALBIUN, PHACAIT.

PTNOBASOIR, CRETNSAIO, NALE SMAS, XCEIETONR, IG YILOIMTT, DYKIEN, TREAW YBDO, LBOSMITEAM, SPAS

TSFIR, KNEICOPMCSOHRA, PCOSMIINOTO, SOSL, HP CGTAISR, CCHMEOOYRT, AFT ROSTSE, SDEECDRAE.

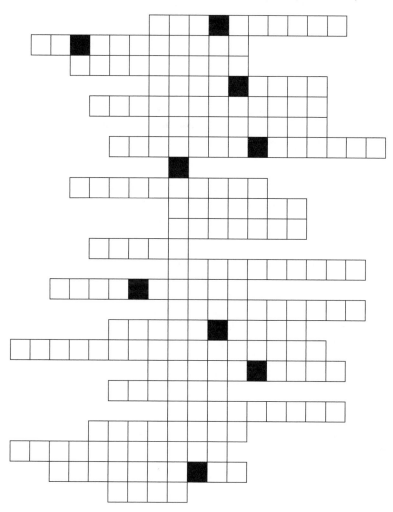

2. The indiscriminate use of numerous medications concurrently is often referred to as _____ .

3. Explicit criteria developed in the early 1990s for determining inappropriate medication use in nursing home residents has become known as the _____ Criteria.

4. Decreased serum _____ for highly protein-bound drugs may lead to increased amounts of free drug in the circulation of older adult clients.

5. Disorders common to older adults, such as heart failure (HF), may impair liver function and influence _____ by decreasing the metabolism of drugs and increasing the risk of drug accumulation and toxicity.

6. Older adults are perceived to have a greater sensitivity to drugs, especially to medications that act on the _____ system.

7. Behavioral and mental changes are very common symptoms of medication _____ , and therefore the nurse should constantly compare the client's current function with his or her past performance.

8. The potential for drug-induced adverse effects declines if the prescriber titrates slowly to the therapeutic effect, the "start _____ , go _____ " approach.

9. Suspect _____ as the cause whenever there is a change in an older adult's behavior, particularly restlessness, irritability, and confusion.

10. The potent medications available to treat older adults often have a narrow _____ between effectiveness and toxicity.

CONNECTING WITH CLIENTS

11. You are assigned to a group of three older adult clients who have medications ordered for this morning. What general physiologic factors in the older adult would you consider that affect pharmacokinetics for these clients?

12. What factors are you concerned about that could complicate drug therapy in the older adult client?

13. What actions can you take to reduce or eliminate potentially adverse risk factors associated with various drug regimens used for older adult clients?

14. What steps should you take to educate the older adult client about medication administration?

TRAINING FOR TEST TAKING

15. The nurse is explaining to an older adult client how changes in physiology affect medication effectiveness. Which of the following examples should the nurse use to describe age-related changes in medication distribution?
    1. Gastric pH is increased
    2. Total body water is decreased
    3. Cytochrome P 450 enzyme system activity is decreased
    4. Renal function is decreased

16. The home health nurse is trying to verify whether a confused older adult client is at risk for polypharmacy because of multiple prescribers. Which of the following methods is likely to be most accurate in gathering this data?
    1. Questioning the client
    2. Consulting with the primary care provider
    3. Asking the client's children
    4. Checking the prescription labels

17. An older adult client indicates that he likes to take an over-the-counter (OTC) sleep aid containing diphenhydramine (Benadryl) as an ingredient. The nurse explains that this medication may not be the best choice for the client for which of the following reasons?
    1. It is expensive and may lead to noncompliance.
    2. It could cause confusion as an adverse effect.
    3. It may be cleared more rapidly than intended via the kidneys.
    4. It should only be used when the client also has allergies.

18. The nurse assesses that there is an increased risk for gastrointestinal bleeding in the older adult client taking which of the following medications?
    1. acetaminophen (Tylenol)
    2. oxybutynin (Ditropan)
    3. naprosyn (Aleve)
    4. diazepam (Valium)

19. The home care nurse is reviewing the older adult client's medications during a routine visit. The nurse notes that two of the six medication containers are duplicates and also have an expiration date that has passed. Which of the following actions is a priority of the nurse?
    1. Ask the client for permission to discard the expired medications.
    2. Put the expired medications into the bottles with unexpired ones for cost effectiveness.
    3. Ask the client why duplicate medications are in the home.
    4. Instruct the client to use the expired medications first because most can be used for a short period after the expiration date.

20. Which of the following strategies would be most helpful for the nurse to use when administering medications to an older adult client?
    1. Offer the medication with very small sips of water.
    2. Allow the client to tip the head back to swallow.
    3. Position the client upright.
    4. Allow the client to take all pills at one time to enhance swallowing.

Substance Misuse and Abuse

STAYING ON TOP OF TERMINOLOGY

1. Complete the following puzzle.

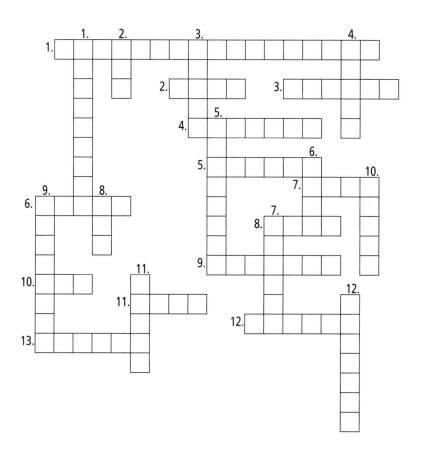

Across

1. Emotional reliance on a drug
2. Initials for federal agency that monitors data on drug abuse
3. Indiscriminate use of drugs
4. Many _____ remedies contain alcohol
5. Sign of drug intoxication with barbiturates
6. Amphetamines are often called pep _____
7. Possible result of acute overdose of opioids
8. Alcoholic beverage often abused by teenagers
9. Related to the belladonna alkaloids
10. Phencyclidine
11. Person can do this if he or she stops abusing
12. Frequently abused over-the-counter (OTC) drug
13. Pinpoint pupil

Down

1. Combination of heroin and cocaine
2. Few drugs without these effects are abused
3. Severe toxicity can lead to this
4. Form of cannabis
5. Often abused by young athletes
6. Adverse effect of steroid use by females
7. An alcoholic beverage
8. A hallucinogenic drug
9. Continuing erections
10. Drug use leading to dependence
11. Effect of intravenous (IV) injection of amphetamines
12. Effect of cocaine

2. _____ dependence is a physiologic state of adaptation to a drug or alcohol in which tolerance to drug effects and development of a withdrawal syndrome in abstinence is usually present.

3. _____ dependence is the emotional state of craving a drug for either its positive reinforcing effects or to avoid the negative effects of withdrawal.

4. Many agencies and most states have _____ of, and active rehabilitation programs for, impaired health care professionals.

5. _____ is a legal term that refers to the ability to guarantee the identity and integrity of the specimen from collection through to reporting of the test results.

6. Although all drugs have some abuse potential, the more commonly abused chemically active substances are the _____ and _____, which are found in coffee, tea, chocolate, and colas.

7. In the late 1990s, law enforcement agencies noted a new trend of involving the use of drugs to facilitate robbery or sexual assault by drugging victims, called _____.

8. The _____ are usually abused because they produce mood elevation, reduction of fatigue, and a sense of increased alertness.

9. Synthetic cannabinoids are available as Schedule II drugs to treat cancer chemotherapy–induced _____ and _____ that is unresponsive to standard therapies.

10. Management of _____ dependence should include gradual drug withdrawal; if the individual is dependent on a short-acting drug, a switch to a long-acting one is recommended for the withdrawal process.

CONNECTING WITH CLIENTS

11. While working in the emergency department, you have been designated as a specimen collector for a nurse who is being evaluated for substance use. What are your responsibilities in this role?

12. While working as an occupational health nurse, you suspect that a worker is abusing one or more substances. What signs or characteristics should you observe for to confirm your suspicions?

13. A client with a history of alcohol abuse underwent emergency surgery. What signs of withdrawal need to be assessed for in this client, and what is the time frame?

TRAINING FOR TEST TAKING

14. A client who went through alcohol withdrawal has been given a prescription for disulfiram (Antabuse). The nurse teaching the client about physiologic effects of drinking alcohol when taking this drug would include which of the following?
    1. Hypertension
    2. Flushing of the face and neck
    3. Respiratory depression
    4. Bradycardia

15. A client is brought into the emergency department with an overdose of cocaine. Which of the following organ systems does the nurse assess as a priority because of risk for complications?
    1. Respiratory
    2. Neurologic
    3. Cardiovascular
    4. Renal

16. A client is brought to the emergency department by friends while experiencing a "bad trip" after taking lysergic acid diethylamide or lysergide (LSD). The crisis intervention nurse prepares to implement which of the following standard treatments for this problem?
    1. "Talk down" the client in a quiet, calm environment.
    2. Seek a PRN order for chlorpromazine (Thorazine).
    3. Apply soft leather restraints for the client's safety.
    4. Place the client in protective isolation.

17. The nurse who is using the CAGE questionnaire as a short assessment of risk for alcohol abuse would ask the client which of the following questions?
    1. "Have you ever felt that you are becoming careless about your drinking?"
    2. "Have you ever felt annoyed by criticism of your drinking?"
    3. "Have you had increasing difficulty with 'getting high' while drinking?"
    4. "Have you ever had an epileptic seizure induced by drinking?"

18. The pediatric clinic nurse is reviewing the laboratory test results of a teenage male who reportedly is abusing anabolic steroids. Which laboratory test result alteration does the nurse determine is characteristic of this problem?
    1. Decreased hemoglobin
    2. Increased high density lipoproteins
    3. Decreased blood glucose levels
    4. Increased liver enzymes

19. The nurse would obtain which of the following medications from the emergency resuscitation (code) cart for possible use in a client admitted with narcotic (opioid) overdose?
    1. naloxone (Narcan)
    2. nalbuphine (Nubain)
    3. norepinephrine (Levophed)
    4. naprosyn (Aleve)

20. The emergency triage nurse notes that a client under the influence of a drug is exhibiting signs of central nervous system excitation. The nurse determines that this client's symptoms are consistent with use of which of the following substances?
    1. Alcohol
    2. Morphine
    3. Amphetamines
    4. Barbiturates

STAYING ON TOP OF TERMINOLOGY

1. Complete the following word search.

ASSESSMENT
BARRIERS
COMPLIANCE
DEVELOPMENTAL
ERIKSON
EVALUATION
HEARING
IMPLEMENTATION
LANGUAGE
LEARNING

MEMORY
MONITORING
NURSING
PERCEPTION
PLANNING
READINESS
TEACHING
THOUGHT
VERBS
VISION

```
T  G  J  O  U  P  L  A  N  N  I  N  G  A
H  H  N  X  T  X  U  X  Y  K  R  K  N  L
L  N  O  I  T  P  E  C  R  E  P  K  I  K
M  V  N  U  R  S  I  N  G  S  J  R  H  O
R  P  F  O  G  O  D  R  T  O  B  X  C  Z
R  A  T  P  O  H  T  D  D  W  Q  R  A  A
L  N  N  O  K  W  T  I  F  W  Z  E  E  P
A  S  S  E  S  S  M  E  N  T  C  D  T  V
N  B  A  R  R  I  E  R  S  O  G  H  R  J
O  H  C  W  M  P  L  Q  M  L  M  T  E  D
I  D  E  V  E  L  O  P  M  E  N  T  A  L
T  B  F  A  B  B  L  B  R  A  H  P  D  A
A  Y  M  V  R  I  S  I  C  R  S  N  I  N
U  J  J  E  A  I  K  V  N  N  O  Z  N  G
L  G  X  N  M  S  N  U  X  I  P  B  E  U
A  R  C  U  O  O  Q  G  S  N  E  B  S  A
V  E  Q  N  A  L  R  I  U  G  Y  S  S  G
E  D  E  U  N  Q  V  Y  M  O  M  W  U  E
I  M  P  L  E  M  E  N  T  A  T  I  O  N
```

2. The Joint Commission for the Accreditation of Healthcare Organizations (JCAHO) requires evidence in the client's clinical record regarding client and family education regarding _____, _____, and _____ _____.

3. Client education is a process that helps people to learn and incorporate health-related _____ into everyday life.

4. To set realistic goals for client teaching related to medication therapy, the nurse needs to first perform an accurate client _____.

5. The client's meaning or perception of the illness experience is very influential in determining the client's participation in the _____, _____.

6. If at all possible, the nurse should avoid using _____ or _____ as interpreters because the shared information sometimes includes sensitive material.

7. A _____ assessment should be conducted on every client to elicit the client's beliefs, values, and attitudes about health, illness, medications, and the client role in health management.

8. The nurse should attempt to modify the medication teaching plan for clients who have _____ and _____ sensory impairments.

9. A nurse who wants to use _____ _____ as a teaching approach for a client unable to express a learning need would be to mention an idea to the client, allow time to pass so the client has time to think about the idea, then reintroduce the idea.

10. _____ is the final step in the process of client teaching for the self-administration of medications.

CONNECTING WITH CLIENTS

11. Because of the shortened length of hospital stays and imposed time limits on office visits under HMOs, a current trend is to relegate counseling about proper medication administration to the community pharmacist. What are some disadvantages to this trend from both client and health care provider perspectives?

12. You are observing a nurse who assesses if the client has memory or concentration problems before beginning medication teaching. What would you expect the nurse to do if the client does have a cognitive impairment that could interfere with retention of medication information?

13. Your client needs to begin taking medication therapy for a chronic health condition. What three nursing diagnoses should you consider as possibly being appropriate for this client either currently or in the near future?

TRAINING FOR TEST TAKING

14. The nurse is working with a client to increase compliance with taking medication therapy. Which of the following approaches by the nurse is most likely to be helpful?
    1. Encourage the client to have all medication prescriptions filled by the same pharmacy.
    2. Assess the client's knowledge of what adverse effects should be reported to the health care provider.
    3. Write out a list of specific times to take medications after taking into consideration the client's personal schedule.
    4. Determine the client's level of understanding about the seriousness of the health problem.

15. A client is scheduled to take a 10-day course of antibiotics (twice daily dosing) for an infection. At a follow-up visit on day 3, the nurse would place highest priority on assessing this client for which of the following risks to medication compliance?
    1. The medication is too costly.
    2. The client has started to feel better.
    3. The medication adverse effects are too severe.
    4. The medication schedule is complex.

16. The nurse has four clients who need instruction about medications that will be taken at home following hospital discharge. The nurse determines that which client should receive instructions first?
    1. A client who is scheduled for discharge within 3 hours.
    2. A client who has postoperative pain rated a "5" and had medication 2 hours ago.
    3. A client who is having difficulty adjusting to the medical diagnosis being treated.
    4. A client who is nervous about being discharged to home.

17. An older adult client who has a hearing impairment needs to begin taking sodium warfarin (Coumadin) for anticoagulation. When conducting medication teaching, the nurse uses which of the following supplemental aids as a priority for this client?
    1. A videotape
    2. A pill box
    3. A magnifying glass
    4. A set of written instructions

18. The nurse is counseling a client who is having difficulty remembering to take a prescribed medication ordered every morning. Which of the following suggestions should the nurse give initially?
    1. Keep the medication where it can be associated with a daily activity, such as brushing the teeth.
    2. Buy a notebook to record when doses are taken.
    3. Purchase a pill box to keep track of when doses are actually taken.
    4. Use a calendar to track medication compliance.

19. Which of the following is the best goal for a client who is learning about a newly ordered medication to treat hypertension?
    1. Understands how medication controls blood pressure.
    2. States the adverse effects that indicate a need to call the physician.
    3. Knows the action and common adverse effects of the medication.
    4. Is motivated to comply with medication therapy.

Chapter **10** **Client Education for Self-Administration of Medication**

20. The nurse who wishes to use "therapeutic seeding" when teaching a client about a prescribed medication would most likely say which of the following on the client's second visit?
    1. "Do you have any concerns about your medication?"
    2. "Write down any questions you think of and we will talk about them at your next visit."
    3. "Often clients worry about the adverse effects of this medication. Do you have any concerns about taking it?"
    4. "Here is a booklet designed to teach you about the medication. Call the office if you have any questions between now and your next visit."

11 Over-the-Counter Medications

STAYING ON TOP OF TERMINOLOGY

1. Match Erickson's stage of development to tasks to be accomplished.

_____ Infant
_____ Toddler
_____ Preschooler
_____ Adolescent
_____ Middle-age adult
_____ Older adult

a. Identity versus role confusion
b. Trust versus mistrust
c. Generativity versus stagnation
d. Initiative versus guilt
e. Autonomy versus shame
f. Integrity versus despair

FOCUSING ON THE FACTS

2. The new _____ _____ label uses simple language and an easy-to-read format to help people compare and select over-the-counter (OTC) medicines and follow dosage instructions.

3. The _____ regulates and makes decisions about the safety and effectiveness of a drug and its classification as prescription or OTC.

4. Prescription drugs can be changed to OTC status based on expert findings that the medication is _____ and _____ for general public use.

5. All solid-dose medications (tablets and capsules) should be taken with _____ ounces of water.

6. The antacids primarily consist of _____, _____ and/or _____ salts and serve to directly increase gastric pH.

7. The _____ blockers are antagonists at the parietal cell of the gastric mucosa and reduce gastric acidity.

8. The most common OTC antitussive agent is _____, which is administered orally and has an onset of action between 15 and 30 minutes and works for up to 6 hours.

9. In OTC preparations the only expectorant with evidence of safety and effectiveness is _____.

10. Clients should be educated that the use of _____ as an OTC contraceptive product does not protect against sexually transmitted infections, including HIV.

CONNECTING WITH CLIENTS

11. A client tells you that she uses aspirin routinely to manage pain of osteoarthritis. What important points would you want to include in a discussion about the over-the-counter (OTC) use of aspirin?

12. A client is considering the use of decongestants for the relief of allergy symptoms. About what adverse effects should you counsel the client?

13. A client with a mild gastrointestinal disorder asks the nurse about the occasional use of antidiarrheal agents. In explaining the action of adsorbent antidiarrheals, what information would the nurse include?

TRAINING FOR TEST TAKING

14. The nurse would place highest priority on teaching which of the following clients about precautions for over-the-counter (OTC) drug use?
    1. A pregnant client
    2. A client with diabetes mellitus
    3. A client on a low-sodium diet
    4. A client who has alcoholism

15. The nurse would be most concerned about the risk of hepatotoxicity in the client who uses which of the following regimens for use of acetaminophen (Tylenol) as an analgesic for mild chronic pain?
    1. One 500-mg tablet 3 times per day and at bedtime
    2. Two 325-mg tablets every 6 hours
    3. Two 325-mg tablets every 4 hours while awake, including bedtime
    4. Two 500-mg tablets 4 times per day and at bedtime

16. A client is using a magnesium-based antacid for relief of mild chronic heartburn. The nurse explains to the client that which of the following is the most common adverse effect that may be expected with the use of this type of medication?
    1. Constipation
    2. Diarrhea
    3. Oral candidiasis
    4. Abdominal pain

17. The mother of a 6-week-old infant calls the clinic nurse to ask the best way to control the infant's new onset constipation before seeking advice about medication. Which of the following items would the nurse suggest?
    1. Add bran to the infant's formula or pumped breast milk
    2. Stop formula or breast milk use and give electrolyte-only solutions such as Pedialyte
    3. Give the infant malt soup extract
    4. Begin to add a strained fruit or vegetable to the diet

18. Which of the following words of advice about over-the-counter (OTC) drugs should the nurse provide to an older adult client who is already taking three prescription drugs for various health problems?
    1. Select an OTC drug that contains several ingredients, so that it can target more than one problem at a time.
    2. OTC medications are routinely safe to use for 6 months after the expiration date.
    3. Ensure that the primary care provider is aware of all medications being taken.
    4. Follow the directions on the package of OTC drugs as often as possible.

19. Which of the following clients who are taking nonsteroidal antiinflammatory drugs should be referred immediately to the health care provider for further follow-up?
    1. A client who has had pain for 5 days.
    2. A client who has had a fever for 2 days.
    3. A client whose site of injury is painful but shows no signs of inflammation.
    4. A client who has developed abdominal pain.

20. The nurse advises a client who has intermittent insomnia that she should avoid over-the-counter (OTC) products for premenstrual syndrome that contain which of the following ingredients?
    1. Acetaminophen
    2. Caffeine
    3. Pamabrom
    4. Pyrilamine

12 Complementary and Alternative Pharmacology

1. Match the therapeutic effects to the herbal remedies.

_____ Prevents liver damage	a. Astragalus
_____ Active against intestinal parasites	b. Echinacea
_____ Increases cells in bone marrow	c. Feverfew
_____ Promotes sleep	d. Garlic
_____ Stimulates interferon production	e. Ginger
_____ Decreases serum cholesterol	f. Ginseng root
_____ Effective for osteoarthritis	g. Green tea
_____ Has multiple pharmacologic actions	h. Hawthorne
including antitumor activity	i. Milk thistle
_____ Relieves headache	j. Chondroitin
_____ Increases cardiac contractility	k. Valerian

FOCUSING ON THE FACTS

2. _____ and _____ therapies are considered to encompass all health systems, modalities, and practices that are not intrinsic to the politically dominant health system.

3. Under the law, manufacturers of _____ _____ are responsible for ensuring safety of their products before they go to market and are also responsible for determining that the claims on their labels are accurate and truthful.

4. _____ is a system of therapeutics based on the theory that "like cures like"—if a large amount of medicine produced symptoms of a disease, then a small amount may reduce those symptoms.

5. _____ is an herb that is recommended to stimulate digestion and to relieve nausea and aches and pains.

6. _____ _____ is a dietary supplement that has been proven useful in moderately improving urinary symptoms in clients with benign prostatic hyperplasia.

7. Because reports from poison control centers and reports to the U.S. FDA indicated increasing life-threatening events associated with _____, the FDA issued a regulation in early 2003 prohibiting its sale in the United States.

8. In laboratory tests, _____ increased the number of immune system cells and developing cells in bone marrow and lymphatic tissue, and seemed to speed their development into immunocompetent cells.

9. One of the dose-dependent therapeutic actions of _____ includes inhibition of platelet aggregation, which reduces the clotting tendency of blood and may prevent heart attack and stroke.

10. The combination of St. John's wort with other antidepressants can lead to the potentially fatal _____ _____.

CONNECTING WITH CLIENTS

11. A client who is pregnant asks you about the use of ginger during pregnancy for relief of nausea and vomiting because of morning sickness. She asks specifically whether this is safe to use. How should you respond based on current evidence?

12. A client reports being diagnosed with osteoarthritis of the knee. What dietary supplement(s) could you recommend and why?

13. A client has been told by several friends that valerian is a helpful therapy for insomnia. What cautions would you share with the client regarding safety and efficacy of valerian?

TRAINING FOR TEST TAKING

14. The nurse could comfortably recommend *gingko biloba* as a complementary or alternative therapy for which of the following client complaints based on the strength of research evidence?
    1. Intermittent claudication
    2. Recent memory loss
    3. Joint inflammation
    4. Failing eyesight

15. A client reports taking feverfew for the treatment of migraine headaches. The nurse explains to the client that feverfew:
    1. Has a clearly documented benefit for this health problem.
    2. Poses no safety risks but has no clearly documented benefit.
    3. Has had no studies to evaluate its effectiveness.
    4. Is a potent and dangerous substance and its use should be avoided.

16. A client reports using an herbal supplement for self-treatment of mild depression. The nurse questions the client directly about the use of which of the following supplements?
    1. Valerian
    2. Red yeast rice
    3. St. John's wort
    4. Ginseng

17. A client states that a friend recommended the use of lobelia to help stop smoking. The nurse would share that which health problem in the client's health history contraindicates the use of lobelia?
    1. Urinary retention
    2. Frequent respiratory infections
    3. Hypertension
    4. Headaches

18. A client reports using a dietary supplement to enhance the function of the liver. The nurse anticipates that the client will report taking which of the following substances?
    1. Milk thistle
    2. Chaparral
    3. Garlic
    4. Feverfew

19. A client reports during history-taking that a favorite beverage is green tea. The nurse then asks the client about prescribed use of which of the following medications, whose action could be antagonized by an ingredient in green tea?
    1. psyllium (Metamucil)
    2. ascorbic acid (Vitamin C)
    3. lisinopril (Prinivil)
    4. sodium warfarin (Coumadin)

20. The nurse is taking a medication history from a client who will undergo an elective surgical procedure in 1 month. The client reports using herbal supplements. The nurse explains that the client should stop taking these products for how long prior to surgery?
    1. 2 to 3 days
    2. 1 week
    3. 2 to 3 weeks
    4. 1 month

Chapter **12** **Complementary and Alternative Pharmacology**

Overview of the Central Nervous System

STAYING ON TOP OF TERMINOLOGY

1. On the drawing below, identify and label the following:

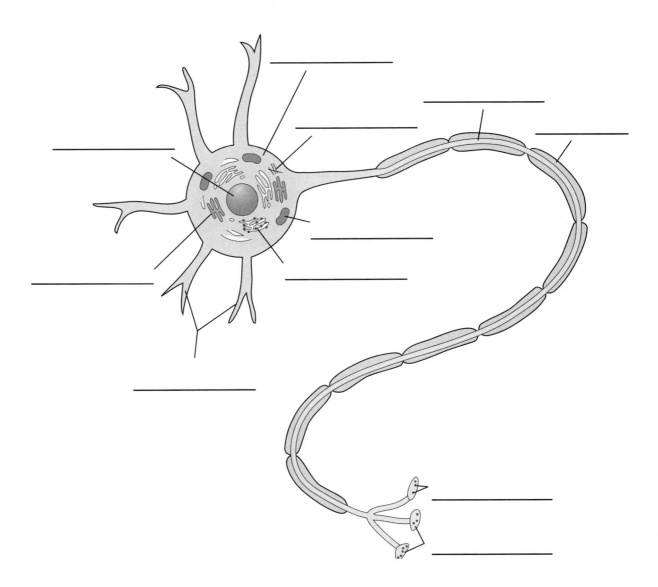

1. Synaptic vesicles
2. Cell body
3. Mitochondria
4. Golgi complex
5. Nerve terminals
6. Dendrites

7. Axon
8. Nucleus
9. Rough endoplasmic reticulum
10. Nissl body
11. Myelin

2.   The blood-brain barrier is a covering of _____ (called _____), that encircle the _____.

3.   The extrapyramidal system is the _____; it affects _____, _____, and _____.

4.   The primary functions of the reticular activating system are _____, _____, and _____.

5.   The best known chemical transmitter of nerve impulses is _____.

6.   Endorphins suppress _____.

7.   An increase in catecholamines and serotonin causes _____.

8.   The _____ controls memory storage and motor functions.

9.   The _____ registers such sensations as pain and temperature.

10. The hypothalamus is a major link between the _____ and the _____.

11. The midbrain, pons, and medulla oblongata comprise the _____.

12. The two major cell types in the CNS are _____ and _____.

13. The three catecholamines that exert an effect on the CNS are _____, _____, and _____.

14 Analgesics

STAYING ON TOP OF TERMINOLOGY

1. Label the opioids that bind with the receptors shown:

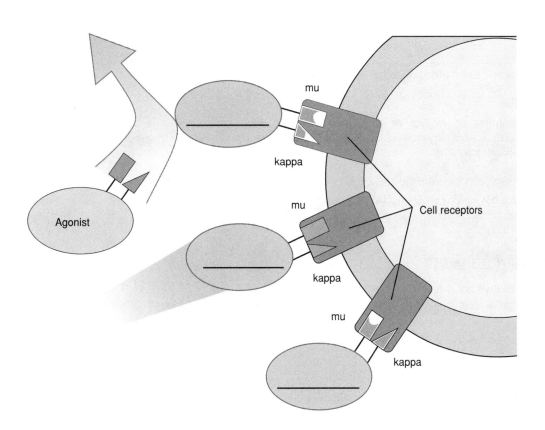

FOCUSING ON THE FACTS

2. According to Margo McCaffery, _____ is whatever the person experiencing the sensation says it is, existing whenever s/he says it does.

3. _____ pain, the presence of severe discomfort or an uncomfortable sensation, lasting from one second to less than six months has a sudden onset and usually subsides with treatment.

4. _____ pain, in which a dysfunction in the central or peripheral nervous system affects nerve conduction in a negative way, often involves neural super-sensitivity.

5. Nociceptive pain typically presents as a throbbing, aching pain observed after trauma to _____, _____, or _____.

6. Each person perceives and reacts to pain differently on the basis of _____, _____, and _____ influences.

7. The _____ with analgesics of clients in pain continues to be well-documented in the literature.

8. Physiologic responses to acute pain generated by the _____ _____ _____ include sweating, pallor, restlessness, agitation and/or increased blood pressure, pulse, or respirations.

9. Acute treatment of respiratory depression with an opioid antagonist such as _____ is required when decreased or shallow opioid-induced respirations are life-threatening.

10. Meperidine has experienced a decline in popularity as an opioid analgesic because it is metabolized in the liver to _____, a CNS neurotoxic metabolite.

CONNECTING WITH CLIENTS

11. A postoperative client has been prescribed morphine sulfate for relief of incisional pain. For what serious adverse effects of this drug would you assess this client?

12. A client has been admitted to the hospital with aspirin overdose. What is the recommended treatment that should be provided to this client?

13. A client with a history of chronic pain is being transferred to the nursing unit. Assuming the appropriate medical orders are written, what three steps of pain management would you need to recall to treat pain according to its severity?

14. The nurse has an order to administer an opioid analgesic to a client who was admitted via the emergency department following a motor vehicle accident. The nurse would use special care when administering this type of drug if the client has a history of which of the following health problems?
    1. Chronic obstructive pulmonary disease
    2. Migraine headaches
    3. Urinary frequency
    4. Back pain

15. An older adult client receiving home health care services has been prescribed acetaminophen with codeine (Tylenol #3) for mild pain following a dental procedure. For which of the following common adverse effects would the home care nurse assess this client at the next routine visit?
    1. Abdominal cramping
    2. Constipation
    3. Shortness of breath
    4. Fatigue following minimal exertion

16. A client has a new physician order to use a fentanyl (Sublimaze) transdermal patch for treatment of chronic pain. Which of the following instructions should the nurse provide to the client regarding this medication?
    1. Cleanse the skin gently with a mild soap and water before application.
    2. Select a clean and dry area on either upper arm to apply the patch.
    3. Hold the patch in place for 10 to 20 seconds to ensure good skin contact.
    4. When removing a used dose, wrap it in a tissue and place it in a wastebasket.

17. A nurse has given instructions regarding use of a patient-controlled analgesia (PCA) pump to an assigned client. Which of the following client statements indicates that the client understands the information presented?
    1. "I can press this button to get pain medication every 2 minutes if I need it."
    2. "I should use the pump whenever my pain level reaches a '7' on a scale of 0 to 10."
    3. "The pump has built-in safety features so that I do not get too much medication."
    4. "It's too bad that there is no way for the pump to keep track of how much medication I actually take."

18. A client with alcohol dependence tells the nurse that he has been taking an oral "antagonist" medication since completing detoxification. The nurse concludes that this client most likely has which of the following medications ordered?
    1. naloxone (Narcan)
    2. naprosyn (Aleve)
    3. nalmefene (Revex)
    4. naltrexone (ReVia)

19. The nurse would caution the client with osteoarthritis who is taking ibuprofen (Motrin) on a regular basis that this medication could lead to which adverse effect over time?
    1. Gastrointestinal bleeding
    2. Dizziness
    3. Increased intraocular pressure
    4. Skeletal muscle weakness

20. An older adult client requires pain medication following a surgical procedure. The nurse would question an order for which of the following medications that is inappropriate for use in older adults?
    1. morphine sulfate (generic)
    2. pentazocine (Talwin)
    3. acetaminophen with codeine (Tylenol #3)
    4. hydromorphone (Dilaudid)

15 Anesthetics

STAYING ON TOP OF TERMINOLOGY

1. Match each physiologic effect to the stage of anesthesia in which it occurs.

_____ Vivid dreams	a. Analgesia
_____ Numbness	b. Excitement
_____ Rapid eye movement	c. Surgical anesthesia
_____ Lowered body temperature	d. Medullary paralysis (toxic stage)
_____ Exaggerated reflexes	
_____ Laughter	
_____ Shallow respiration	
_____ Vasomotor collapse	

FOCUSING ON THE FACTS

2. The two major categories of anesthesia are general and _____ or _____ .

3. The advantage of balanced anesthesia is _____ _____ .

4. Malignant hyperthermia is a dangerous adverse effect of _____ , _____ anesthetics.

5. Dissociative anesthesia produces _____ and _____ but not _____ _____ .

6. _____ _____ , an anesthetic gas, is the most commonly used agent for analgesia during dental surgery, minor surgery, and obstetric procedures.

7. _____ is the only volatile anesthetic agent that sensitizes the myocardium to the effects of catecholamines or sympathomimetic agents.

8. The class of drugs known as _____ are most often used for conscious sedation in which full anesthesia is not required such as during endoscopy, or as a premedication or adjunct in balanced anesthesia.

9. _____ is a rapid-acting nonbarbiturate IV anesthetic (that is often referred to as a dissociative anesthetic) and is a derivative of phencyclidine, a psychotomimetic drug of abuse.

10. The administration of _____ _____ provides surgeons with easier access to and increased visualization of the surgical site and prevents inadvertent client movement during the procedure.

CONNECTING WITH CLIENTS

11. A client who will be undergoing a surgical procedure has had a preoperative visit with the anesthesiologist. The client asks you why anesthesia seems so complicated and why so many drugs are used. What would you consider when formulating a response?

12. A client in the oral surgeon's office is having a tooth extracted using nitrous oxide for anesthesia. What adverse effects would you be concerned about on awakening of the client and how will you promote oxygenation after the procedure?

13. A client has a new order for a one-time dose of a benzodiazepine. What could be the possible reasons this drug would be ordered in this manner?

TRAINING FOR TEST TAKING

14. A client with Parkinson's disease is scheduled for surgery. Prior to receiving anesthesia with halothane, the client should have Levodopa discontinued 6 to 8 hours prior to surgery to reduce the risk of:
    1. Bronchospasm
    2. Laryngeal edema
    3. Cardiac dysrhythmias
    4. Hypotension

15. A nurse working in the postanesthesia care unit would assess the postoperative client who received barbiturates during anesthesia for which most common adverse effect during the recovery period?
    1. Shivering and trembling
    2. Nausea and vomiting
    3. Increased excitability and confusion
    4. Cardiac dysrhythmias and respiratory depression

16. A client is about to receive an intravenous dose of midazolam (Versed) as part of preoperative medication in the preoperative holding area. The nurse explains that an advantage to the use of this drug is which of the following?
    1. A sense of well-being on awakening from surgery.
    2. Amnesic effect to decrease recall of events near the time of administration.
    3. Reduced postoperative pain because of interactive effects with anesthesia.
    4. Reduced risk of respiratory depression in the postanesthesia care unit.

17. A client in the intensive care unit is receiving propofol (Diprivan) by continuous intravenous drip for sedation. The nurse attributes the development of which assessment finding to adverse effects of the drug?
    1. Hypertension
    2. Tachycardia
    3. Constipation
    4. Reduced respiratory rate

18. A client who was intubated and placed on mechanical ventilation is "fighting" the ventilator. Before beginning to administer scheduled medications, including vecuronium (Norcuron), the nurse would ensure that there is an order for which other type of medication?
   1. A benzodiazepine
   2. A cardiac glycoside
   3. A bronchodilator
   4. A gastric pump inhibitor

19. A preoperative client reports a family history of malignant hyperthermia to the anesthesiologist. The nurse reading the preanesthesia report ensures that which of the following medications is readily available for use with this client if needed?
   1. epinephrine (Adrenalin)
   2. aminophylline (Theophylline)
   3. dantrolene sodium (Dantrium)
   4. phenytoin (Dilantin)

20. A client in the emergency room requires sutures following an injury. The nurse would remove the lidocaine solution containing epinephrine from the room to reduce the risk of its accidental use if the client needs sutures in which of the following body areas?
   1. Cheek
   2. Fingertip
   3. Thigh
   4. Abdomen

16 Antianxiety, Sedative, and Hypnotic Drugs

STAYING ON TOP OF TERMINOLOGY

1. Complete the following word search.

AMNESIC   SEDATIVE
ANXIOLYTIC   DIAZEPAM
ANXIETY   FLUMAZENIL
HYPNOTIC   LORAZEPAM
INSOMNIA   ZOLPIDEM

```
M  T  P  Z  O  L  P  I  D  E  M  I  T  H
A  S  D  A  N  X  O  L  A  Z  I  C  Y  L
P  M  A  S  E  D  I  A  F  L  U  P  S  A
E  D  N  I  V  I  N  S  O  M  N  I  A  N
Z  A  X  E  H  Y  P  L  O  O  A  Z  E  P
A  Z  I  N  S  E  Z  A  T  P  I  I  D  E
R  O  O  L  R  I  P  I  L  U  M  A  M  I
O  L  L  F  L  U  C  P  I  D  A  M  A  S
L  O  Y  D  I  A  I  D  E  N  I  L  P  I
H  I  T  L  O  R  A  N  X  O  T  I  E  A
D  L  I  N  E  Z  A  M  U  L  F  A  Z  I
N  O  C  D  A  T  Y  T  E  I  X  N  A  L
A  N  Z  E  P  N  O  D  E  M  A  T  I  I
S  E  D  A  T  I  V  E  F  L  A  Z  D  M
```

FOCUSING ON THE FACTS

2. Antianxiety or anxiolytic agents are used to _____ _____.

3. Sedatives and hypnotics are _____ drugs. The major difference between them is the degree of _____ induced.

4. REM (rapid eye movement) sleep is also referred to as _____ or _____ sleep.

5. Insomnia is a frequent concern of _____.

6. Some general pharmacologic properties of _____ include muscle relaxant, antianxiety, antiseizure, and hypnotic effects.

7. The _____ and the _____ are the sites of cytochrome P450 metabolism for either the active drug or the metabolite dosage forms of the benzodiazepines.

8. _____ is indicated for the treatment of benzodiazepine overdose or to reverse the sedative effects of benzodiazepines following surgical or diagnostic procedures.

9. Zolpidem is used for the short-term treatment of _____.

10. _____ is indicated for the treatment of anxiety disorders, and is considered to be equivalent in efficacy to the benzodiazepines, with usually less sedation.

CONNECTING WITH CLIENTS

11. What data would you consider it necessary to collect from a client receiving sedatives/hypnotics during the assessment phase of the nursing process?

12. In addition to the standard nursing care plan for a client receiving an antianxiety drug, what special considerations would you be aware of when the client is a child?

13. A young adult client reports at a routine physical examination that she has been experiencing increased incidences of insomnia. What are nonpharmacologic approaches would you suggest to the client to try to resolve insomnia?

14. An older adult client has a history of liver disease. The nurse anticipates that which of the following antianxiety medications would be most appropriately ordered for this client?
    1. lorazepam (Ativan)
    2. chlordiazepoxide (Librium)
    3. diazepam (Valium)
    4. flurazepam (Dalmane)

15. The nurse interprets that a client is experiencing a paradoxical reaction to a benzodiazepine after noting that the client is exhibiting which manifestation?
    1. Hiccups
    2. Headache
    3. Hallucinations
    4. Blurred vision

16. After reading the client's history and physical report, the nurse concludes that a benzodiazepine has been ordered for treatment of which of the following client health problems?
    1. Parkinson's disease
    2. Anxiety disorder
    3. Narcolepsy
    4. Chronic pain

17. A client with generalized anxiety disorder also has a history of substance abuse. The nurse concludes that which of the following medications has indications for long-term use that are consistent with the needs of this client?
    1. hydroxyzine (Vistaril)
    2. temazepam (Restoril)
    3. chloral hydrate (Noctec)
    4. buspirone (BuSpar)

18. The nurse would monitor a client receiving PRN doses of hydroxyzine (Vistaril) for which of the following adverse effects of therapy?
    1. Photophobia
    2. Excessive salivation
    3. Sedation
    4. Diarrhea

19. The nurse is assigned to the care of a client who is scheduled to have an electroencephalogram performed. The client tells the nurse that the physician is going to order a sedative before the procedure. The nurse anticipates that the client is referring to which medication that is optimal for this use?
    1. diazepam (Valium)
    2. chloral hydrate (Noctec)
    3. zolpidem tartrate (Ambien)
    4. triazolam (Halcion)

20. The physician has written a prescription for a hypnotic medication as a sleep aid for an older adult client. In providing medication teaching that enhances client safety, the nurse recommends that the client try to limit its use to which of the following frequencies?
    1. Once per week
    2. One to three times per week
    3. Three to four times per week
    4. Five to six times per week

17 Antiepileptic Drugs

STAYING ON TOP OF TERMINOLOGY

1. Complete the following puzzle.

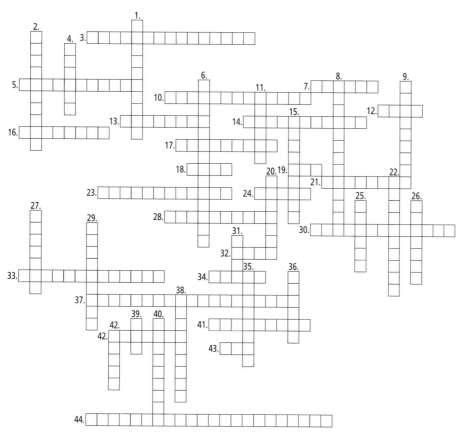

Across

3. Seizures that are undefined in origin (2 words)
5. Antiepileptic drug (AED) indicated as adjunct therapy for the treatment of partial seizures in adults
7. Drug level drawn at a drug's nadir
10. AED indicated for partial onset seizures in adults
12. Valproic _____, a major AED
13. A visual disturbance caused by phenytoin
14. Single AED therapy
16. _____ acid, a major AED
17. A generalized seizure with unaltered consciousness
18. _____ therapy; use of 2 or more AEDs
19. An abbreviation for antiepileptic drugs
21. Divalproex sodium
23. AED used for absence seizures
24. Sustained contractions of large muscle groups
28. An antiepileptic drug used for adjunct therapy
30. A sedative commonly used as an AED before phenytoin
32. What a client may experience before a seizure
33. A major AED
34. A syndrome that may occur with carbamazepine
37. Phenytoin adverse effect common in adolescents (2 words)
41. A major antiepileptic drug
42. _____-Johnson syndrome, an adverse skin reaction to carbamazepine
43. A diagnostic exam for the etiology of seizures (abbreviation)
44. Another diagnostic exam for epilepsy (2 words)

Down

1. AED also used as an analgesic adjuvant
2. A benzodiazepine with antiseizure activity
4. _____ epilepticus
6. Adverse effect of many AEDs
8. An AED that is a pro-drug
9. An AED used for adjunct therapy
11. Various dysrhythmic contractions in the body
15. A γ-aminobutyric acid (GABA) uptake inhibitor used as AED adjunctive therapy
20. A state in which pregnancy is associated with seizures
22. An AED used for adjunct therapy
25. The type of seizure in which the client falls down or drops his head
26. An epileptic episode
27. _____, or nongeneralized seizures
29. Trigeminal _____, an indication for carbamazepine
31. A major inhibitory neurotransmitter
35. The trade name for phenytoin
36. A CNS adverse effect of phenytoin
38. Distressing effect of phenytoin for women
39. A major diagnostic tool in epilepsy (abbreviation)
40. An AED used for Lennox-Gastaut syndrome in children
42. An important concentration to measure for AEDs

2. When recurrent seizures do not have an identifiable cause, this condition is called _____ or _____ epilepsy.

3. Adverse effects of barbiturates affecting the respiratory system are _____, _____, and _____.

4. Hydantoins are not useful in the treatment of _____ seizures.

5. True _____ False _____ Barbiturates are classified as antiepileptic drugs and so are not controlled substances.

6. True _____ False _____ Hydantoins are noted for their lack of drug interactions.

7. Hiccups and headaches are associated with the use of the antiepileptic drug _____.

8. Apnea and laryngospasm are of concern with the client receiving the antiepileptic drug _____.

9. _____ is an antiepileptic and benzodiazepine that can cause ataxia and drowsiness in clients.

10. Client teaching about hirsutism and gingival hyperplasia as adverse drug effects are important when the client begins taking _____.

CONNECTING WITH CLIENTS

11. A 56-year-old client who experienced a head injury and subsequent subdural hematoma has now been diagnosed with epilepsy. Both the client and spouse are upset about this development and look to you for guidance. How would you explain to them what epilepsy is and how antiepileptic drugs will help?

12. A client receiving antiepileptic drug (AED) therapy has a nursing diagnosis of *Risk for Injury related to effects of AED therapy*. What nursing interventions would be appropriate for this client?

13. An older adult client who requires antiepileptic drug (AED) therapy has a history of liver disease. What implications does this have for nursing management of the client?

TRAINING FOR TEST TAKING

14. A client receives an IV dose of an antiepileptic at 0800, 1600, and 2400 each day. The physician orders a serum drug level to be drawn. At which of the following times should the nurse schedule the lab work to be drawn?
    1. 0730
    2. 0900
    3. 1500
    4. 1800

15. A client taking carbamazepine (Tegretol) for 1 month telephones the clinic and reports a sore throat and low-grade fever that started a few days ago. Which of the following responses should the nurse make?
    1. "Can you come in today to be seen by the doctor?"
    2. "Those symptoms can be managed easily by acetaminophen (Tylenol)."
    3. "You may need to take an extra dose of carbamazepine to avoid seizure activity because of the fever."
    4. "If these symptoms persist for another 48 hours, call again and we will schedule you for an evaluation here at the clinic."

16. The nurse is administering phenobarbital (Luminal) by the IV route as ordered to control seizure activity in a client with status epilepticus. To avoid inducing respiratory depression, the nurse injects the medication at a rate no greater than which of the following?
    1. 5 mg/min
    2. 20 mg/min
    3. 60 mg/min
    4. 100 mg/min

17. A 3-year-old client is diagnosed with Lennox-Gastaut syndrome. The nurse anticipates that which of the following antiepileptic drugs may be ordered for this child?
    1. felbamate (Felbatol)
    2. ethosuximide (Zarontin)
    3. phenytoin (Dilantin)
    4. primidone (Mysoline)

18. A client with diabetes mellitus is experiencing neurogenic pain in the legs because of the disorder. The nurse anticipates that which of the following drugs may be ordered for this client?
    1. primidone (Mysoline)
    2. gabapentin (Neurontin)
    3. lamotrigine (Lamictal)
    4. levetiracetam (Keppra)

19. The nurse periodically checks the patellar reflex of the client receiving which of the following antiepileptic medications?
    1. oxcarbazepine (Trileptal)
    2. tiagabine (Gabatril)
    3. magnesium sulfate
    4. phenobarbital (Luminol)

20. A client is beginning antiepileptic drug therapy with oxcarbazepine (Trileptal). The nurse who is teaching the client about the medication includes which of the following points?
    1. "This medication will not cause any drowsiness."
    2. "Dosage may need to be adjusted upward over time because the medication induces its own metabolism."
    3. "This medication may cause the sodium level in your blood to go up."
    4. "You will not need to have serum drug levels drawn for this medication."

18 Central Nervous System Stimulants

STAYING ON TOP OF TERMINOLOGY

1. Complete the following word search.

AMPHETAMINE DEFICIT
ANALEPTIC   CAFFEINE
ANOREXIANT NARCOLEPSY
ATTENTION

N	O	R	A	D	E	F	A	N	I	T
A	M	P	H	E	T	A	M	I	N	E
N	A	R	I	F	O	N	T	R	O	N
R	S	I	S	I	R	A	N	O	R	I
O	N	C	R	C	L	L	O	C	S	T
N	T	N	A	I	X	E	R	O	N	A
A	R	C	O	T	A	P	H	E	T	O
T	A	T	T	E	N	T	I	O	N	L
S	C	A	F	F	E	I	N	E	T	A
Y	S	P	E	L	O	C	R	A	N	S

FOCUSING ON THE FACTS

2. Amphetamines are mainly stimulants of the _____ _____.

3. Attention-deficit disorder (ADD) with hyperactivity is a syndrome characterized by _____, _____, _____, and _____.

4. For clients with narcolepsy, CNS stimulants are useful in controlling _____ and _____.

5. Cataplexy is generalized _____ associated with _____.

6. Hypnagogic illusions are _____ _____.

7. Central nervous system stimulants increase _____ and decrease _____ _____ time.

8. Individual client response to CNS stimulants may be modified by the client's _____ make-up.

9. Acute withdrawal from CNS stimulants typically manifests as feelings of _____ and _____.

10. The exact mechanism of action of anorexiants is unknown, but these agents appear to act on the satiety center in the _____ and _____ areas of the brain.

CONNECTING WITH CLIENTS

11. A client has been prescribed an amphetamine. What important points would be important to include in a client teaching session related to this type of medication?

12. A client will begin taking methylphenidate hydrochloride. About which adverse effects would you teach the client?

13. A client taking a nervous system stimulant also has a history of cardiac disease. For what drug effects would you carefully assess when working with this client?

14. A client has been given a prescription for methylphenidate (Ritalin). The nurse explains that which of the following are the most common adverse effects of this medication?
    1. Nervousness and insomnia
    2. Tachycardias and dysrhythmias
    3. Urticaria or rash
    4. Hypersensitivity reactions

15. A client is taking atomoxetine (Strattera) for treatment of attention deficit hyperactivity disorder (ADHD). The client tells that nurse that he has begun to have "itchy skin" and the nurse notes slight jaundice when observing the client in natural daylight. Which of the following actions should the nurse take at this time?
    1. Recommend the use of an over-the-counter (OTC) anti-itch cream.
    2. Notify the prescriber of these symptoms.
    3. Teach the client to self-assess skin color and report further changes.
    4. Explain to the client that the timing of the doses may need to be adjusted.

16. A client is considering beginning drug therapy with sibutramine (Meridia). Which of the following points would the nurse plan to include in a teaching plan about this medication?
    1. It should be discontinued 1 month before taking an monoamine oxidase (MAO) inhibitor.
    2. Diarrhea is a frequent adverse effect that is dose-related.
    3. It only causes dependence if excessive doses are taken.
    4. It should be used with a reduced calorie diet and other lifestyle modifications.

17. A pediatric clinic nurse is preparing a client taking methylphenidate (Ritalin SR) for an annual physical examination. Which of the following data would be of highest priority for the nurse to gather?
    1. Blood pressure
    2. Temperature
    3. Height and weight
    4. Urine for analysis

18. A client has a history of narcolepsy. The nurse anticipates that which of the following medications will be listed on the client's medication administration record as a standing order?
    1. modafinil (Provigil)
    2. atomoxetine (Strattera)
    3. sibutramine (Meridia)
    4. doxapram (Dopram)

19. An adult client is planning to begin drug therapy with diethylpropion (Tenuate) for the purpose of weight loss. The nurse and client mutually set an optimal weight loss goal of how many pounds per week?
    1. 0.5 to 1
    2. 1 to 2
    3. 3 to 5
    4. 5 to 7

20. The nurse who is reading a client's medical record notes that the client received a single dose of doxapram (Dopram) the previous day. On further reading of the record, the nurse determines that it was ordered for which of the following reasons?
    1. Elevation of blood pressure during a hypotensive episode
    2. Adjunct treatment of seizure activity
    3. General stimulation in myxedema coma
    4. Respiratory stimulation in the postanesthesia care unit

69

19 Psychotherapeutic Drugs

STAYING ON TOP OF TERMINOLOGY

1. Match each drug with its classification.

_____ chlorpromazine   a. MAO inhibitors
_____ Eskalith   b. Tricyclic antidepressants
_____ amitriptyline   c. Phenothiazine derivatives
_____ isocarboxazid   d. Lithium
_____ Prozac
_____ Nardil

FOCUSING ON THE FACTS

2. Nursing management of psychotherapeutic agents focuses on, among other things, monitoring the client's _____ and _____ responses to the medications.

3. Although the exact mechanism of action for the typical antipsychotics is unknown, their major therapeutic effects and adverse effects result from _____ blockade in specific areas of the CNS.

4. Haloperidol is used in the treatment of schizophrenia, psychosis, and for the control of tics associated with _____ syndrome.

5. _____ or _____ drugs are agents that affect cognitive thought processes and affect dopaminergic receptors.

6. The _____ _____ _____Scale, developed by National Institute for Mental Health researchers, has become the standard screening and rating tool for tardive dyskinesia in the United States.

7. Because symptoms of withdrawal may be pronounced for 1-3 weeks after abrupt discontinuation of antidepressants, whenever possible, they should be _____ to avoid or minimize these effects.

8. Pediatric clients with chickenpox, CNS infections, measles, dehydration, gastroenteritis, or other acute illnesses will be at special risk of developing adverse reactions to psychotherapeutic agents and possibly _____ syndrome.

9. The _____ antidepressants may cause increased anxiety in the older client and in those with cardiovascular disease; their use increases the risk of dysrhythmias, tachycardia, stroke, heart failure, and myocardial infarction.

10. Anyone considering the use of an antidepressant in a child or adolescent for any clinical use must balance the risk of increased _____ with the clinical need.

CONNECTING WITH CLIENTS

11. A client will begin taking a monoamine oxidase inhibitor (MAOI). What foods would you teach the client are to be completely avoided while taking MAOI therapy?

12. A client has been taking an antipsychotic drug for approximately one week. Knowing that the drug carries a risk for the adverse effect of neuroleptic malignant syndrome, for what manifestations would you assess this client?

13. A client will begin taking a drug that carries the risk of serotonin syndrome. How would you explain this to the client when providing medication teaching about possible adverse drug effects?

TRAINING FOR TEST TAKING

14. For which of the following clients would the long-acting haloperidol decanoate (Haldol Decanoate) by IM injection be best utilized?
    1. An older adult client who does not have family available for assistance.
    2. A client who is noncompliant with oral therapy.
    3. A young client who forgets to take doses occasionally.
    4. A client who cannot afford the oral dosing form.

15. A young adult client will be starting on antidepressant therapy with fluoxetine hydrochloride (Prozac) 20 mg daily. Which important teaching point would the nurse be sure to share with the client?
    1. "You need to count your pulse rate before getting out of bed in the morning."
    2. "Try taking your medication with breakfast if you experience nausea."
    3. "You may need to reduce your fluids at night because of nocturnal urination."
    4. "You'll have to give up Chianti, nuts, and cheese while you're taking this medication."

16. A female client seems to be fidgety with motor restlessness, and jiggles her legs when asked to sit down. Which medication does the nurse anticipate will be ordered to reduce these manifestations?
    1. olanzapine (Zyprexa)
    2. molindone (Moban)
    3. benztropine (Cogentin)
    4. thioridazine (Mellaril)

17. An older adult client being treated with clozapine (Clozaril) for the last 6 months calls the nurse to cancel a clinic appointment because of flu symptoms including sore throat, fever, and tiredness. Which of the following is the best reply by the nurse?
    1. "Drink plenty of fluids and continue your medication. Let's reschedule your appointment for next week instead."
    2. "It is important to go to the lab and get your blood work done. I'll call ahead so they will know you're coming. Then come in to the clinic to be seen."
    3. "It does sound like the flu. This medication puts people more at risk for flu symptoms, so call me to reschedule when you're feeling better."
    4. "Stop the medication for 2 days and then begin to take it on the third day. Let's also reschedule your regular appointment for 3 days from now."

18. The nurse is assessing a client who recently started taking an antipsychotic medication. Which of the following adverse effects could the nurse expect to observe?
    1. Constipation, decreased sweating, and blurred vision
    2. Increased moisture around the eyes, vomiting, and severe frontal headache
    3. Insomnia, irritability, and muscle weakness
    4. Slurred speech, hand tremors, and severe occipital headache

19. A client taking antidepressant medication says to the nurse, "I've been getting dizzy since I started this drug. Do you think I should stop taking it?" Which response by the nurse is most appropriate?
    1. "Try to change positions slowly and dangle your feet at the side of the bed before getting up. At what time of the day do you take this medication?"
    2. "You'll have to stop driving while taking this drug, and try to take naps during the day to relieve this problem."
    3. "This is very unusual. Stop taking this medicine, and let's call the physician together to see about starting on another medication."
    4. "This medication does not cause dizziness. Have you had a cold or the flu recently?"

20. A client with bipolar disorder is beginning therapy with lithium carbonate (Eskalith). Which of the following would be priority points of client education related to use of this medication?
    1. Moderate amounts of caffeine-containing beverages aid in maintaining lithium levels.
    2. Limit salt intake to avoid concurrent water loss.
    3. Maintain a fluid intake of 2.5 to 3 liters daily.
    4. Lithium levels will need to be drawn every 6 months after dose is stabilized.

Overview of the Autonomic Nervous System

STAYING ON TOP OF TERMINOLOGY

1. Match these terms and definitions commonly associated with the autonomic nervous system.

_____ Conduction	a. From one neuron to another neuron
_____ α_1 sites	b. On the postsynaptic effector cells
_____ Synaptic junction	c. On the presynaptic nerve terminals
_____ Neurohormonal transmission	d. From a neuron to an effector organ
_____ α_2 sites	e. Passage of a nerve impulse across a junction with the use of a chemical
_____ Neuroeffector junction	f. Passage of a nerve impulse along a nerve fiber or muscle fiber

FOCUSING ON THE FACTS

2. The simplest means by which the nervous system responds to environmental change is through the action of the _____.

3. Nerves that contain acetylcholine are called _____, and they are involved in _____.

4. The central nervous system's sensory input and motor output constitute a _____.

5. Muscarinic receptors are located in the _____.

6. Nicotinic receptors appear in the _____.

7. The _____ nervous system functions mainly to conserve energy and restore body resources of the organism, otherwise known as the system of rest and digestion.

8. The _____ nervous system mobilizes the organism during emergency and stress situations, so it is called the "fight or flight" system.

9. The passage of a nerve impulse across a synaptic or neuroeffector junction with the use of a chemical is called _____ transmission.

10. _____ receptors appear in the ganglia of both parasympathetic and sympathetic fibers, the adrenal medulla, and the skeletal (striated) muscle supplied by the somatic motor system.

11. _____ receptors (postganglionic sites) are located in the smooth muscle, cardiac muscle, and glands of the parasympathetic fibers and the effector organs of the cholinergic sympathetic fibers.

12. The catecholamines produced by the sympathetic nervous system include _____ and _____.

13. Once acetylcholine has exerted its effect on the postjunctional sites, the excess amount is inactivated rapidly by the enzyme _____.

Drugs Affecting the Parasympathetic Nervous System and the Neurotransmitter Acetylcholine

21

STAYING ON TOP OF TERMINOLOGY

1. Complete the following word search.

ADRENERGIC
ANTICHOLINERGIC
ANTIMUSCARINIC
ATROPINE
BETHANECHOL
CHOLINERGIC
DIRECT-ACTING
INDIRECT-ACTING

MUSCARINIC
NICOTINE
NICOTINIC
PARASYMPATHOLYTIC
PARASYMPATHOMIMETIC
SYMPATHOLYTIC
SYMPATHOMIMETIC

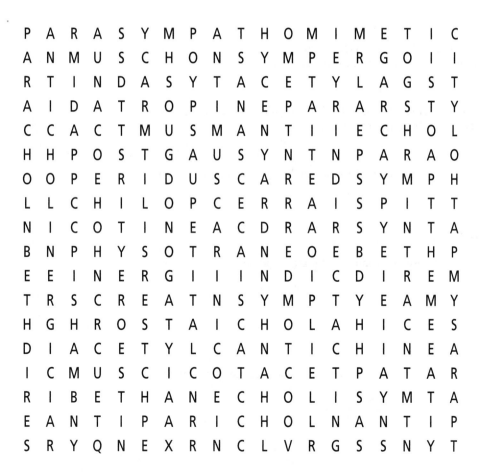

```
P A R A S Y M P A T H O M I M E T I C
A N M U S C H O N S Y M P E R G O I I
R T I N D A S Y T A C E T Y L A G S T
A I D A T R O P I N E P A R A R S T Y
C C A C T M U S M A N T I I E C H O L
H H P O S T G A U S Y N T N P A R A O
O O P E R I D U S C A R E D S Y M P H
L L C H I L O P C E R R A I S P I T T
N I C O T I N E A C D R A R S Y N T A
B N P H Y S O T R A N E O E B E T H P
E E I N E R G I I I N D I C D I R E M
T R S C R E A T N S Y M P T Y E A M Y
H G H R O S T A I C H O L A H I C E S
D I A C E T Y L C A N T I C H I N E A
I C M U S C I C O T A C E T P A T A R
R I B E T H A N E C H O L I S Y M T A
E A N T I P A R I C H O L N A N T I P
S R Y Q N E X R N C L V R G S S N Y T
```

2. Adrenergic blocking drugs block the action of the _____.

3. Cholinergic blocking drugs block the action of the _____.

4. Antimuscarinic drugs block the _____ and are also called _____ drugs.

5. Cholinergic drugs may be obtained from _____ or they may be _____. The two groups of cholinergic drugs available are _____ and _____.

6. The muscarinic effect is the action of _____ at the _____ nerve endings, which is like that of _____.

7. _____ is used to help reduce nicotine symptoms as an aid to smoking cessation.

8. Although not limited to action at the neuromuscular junction, _____ is used to terminate neuromuscular blocking agents in general surgery.

9. A therapeutic uses for a muscarinic agonist includes stimulating the _____ for clients with spinal cord injury.

10. _____ _____ is used for anticholinergic substance toxicity and overdose.

CONNECTING WITH CLIENTS

11. A client has an order for a stat dose of atropine. What are its possible uses and how does it work?

12. What important concepts would you want to teach a client who is taking Nicorette?

13. What steps should a client take in changing a nicotine transdermal patch?

14. A client is taking bethanechol (Urecholine) for urinary retention secondary to spinal cord injury. Knowing the client is at risk for cholinergic overstimulation, the nurse would assess this client for which of the following manifestations?
    1. Hypertension
    2. Nausea and vomiting
    3. Pallor of the skin
    4. Tachycardia

15. The nurse notes that the medication administration record of a client contains neostigmine as an ordered medication. The nurse concludes that this client may have which diagnosis?
    1. Cataracts
    2. Ulcerative colitis
    3. Overactive bladder
    4. Myasthenia gravis

16. A client requires the use of vecuronium (Norcuron) for neuromuscular blockade to aid in tolerating a mechanical ventilator. The nurse questions this newly ordered medication because there is no order for which type of drug that should be ordered concurrently?
    1. An antianxiety agent
    2. A respiratory stimulant
    3. A catecholamine
    4. A gastrointestinal stimulant

17. A client will be receiving an eye medication containing atropine before an eye procedure. The nurse would administer this drug cautiously if the client has a history of which of the following?
    1. Macular degeneration
    2. Detached retina
    3. Angle-closure glaucoma
    4. Cataracts

18. A client in the emergency department has been given an intravenous dose of atropine sulfate. The nurse evaluates the client for which of the following intended therapeutic effects of the drug?
    1. Increased blood pressure
    2. Increased pulse
    3. Increased oxygen saturation
    4. Increased bowel sounds

19. A client has been given instructions to use a scopolamine patch before traveling to reduce or prevent emesis because of motion sickness. For best effect, the nurse teaches the client to apply the patch how long before beginning to travel?
    1. 30 minutes
    2. 1 hour
    3. 2 hours
    4. 4 hours

20. An older adult female client is prescribed tolterodine (Detrol, Detrol LA) for occasional urge incontinence. What client teaching is important with this medication?
    1. Use sugarless hard candy to manage dry mouth.
    2. Begin a bladder training program every hour while awake.
    3. Avoid taking this drug with grapefruit juice.
    4. Do not take this drug with acetaminophen (Tylenol) because of increased liver toxicity.

Chapter **21** **Drugs Affecting the Parasympathetic Nervous System and the Neurotransmitter Acetylcholine**

22 Drugs Affecting the Sympathetic (Adrenergic) Nervous System

STAYING ON TOP OF TERMINOLOGY

1. Match the physiologic response to the receptor stimulated.

_____ Cardiac muscle   a. α_1
_____ Cerebral blood vessels   b. α_2
_____ Bronchial smooth muscle   c. β_1
_____ Liver   d. β_2
_____ Insulin secretion
_____ Adipose tissue
_____ Pupil size
_____ Platelet aggregation

FOCUSING ON THE FACTS

2. Catecholamine produces a significant increase in cardiac contraction, or a positive _____ effect. It also increases heart rate, or a positive _____ effect. An increase in atrioventricular conduction, or a positive _____ effect, also occurs.

3. The α-adrenergic blocking agents fall into three categories: _____, _____, and _____.

4. Direct-acting adrenergic drugs work at _____ receptors as agonists.

5. The indirect-acting adrenergic drugs act indirectly on receptors by first triggering the release of the catecholamines _____ and _____ from their storage sites.

6. Certain physiologic stimuli such as _____ and _____ significantly increase blood levels of catecholamines.

7. Catecholamines have antagonistic effects on _____, and they decrease liver and skeletal muscle glycogen and increase _____ in adipose tissue.

8. Catecholamines _____ bronchial smooth muscle, which can enhance respirations.

9. Catecholamines may produce spontaneous firing of Purkinje fibers, which may cause ventricular _____ and increase the susceptibility of ventricular muscle to _____.

10. As a drug, dopamine is unique in low dosages (0.5 to 2 mcg/kg/min) because it acts mainly on dopaminergic receptors to cause _____ of renal and mesenteric arteries.

CONNECTING WITH CLIENTS

11. A client has just received an intravenous dose of epinephrine. What adverse effects should you be assessing for in this client?

12. An older adult client with polypharmacy from seeing multiple health care providers has a prescription for a β-adrenergic blocking agent. Can you think of three drugs that interact with this type of drug and what physiologic effects would occur?

13. A client with heart failure is receiving intravenous dobutamine (Dobutrex). What adverse effects would you assess for in this client?

TRAINING FOR TEST TAKING

14. A client is receiving dopamine hydrochloride (Intropin) for cardiovascular support following major surgery. The nurse would be most concerned and notify the prescriber if which of the following pieces of assessment data were noted?
    1. Pulse rate 110 beats/min
    2. Systolic blood pressure 114 mm Hg
    3. Urine output 35 mL
    4. Pedal pulses weakly palpable on the right foot

15. A client is receiving dopamine hydrochloride (Intropin). The nurse who is assessing the intravenous site would look for which of the following signs of extravasation?
    1. Warmth
    2. Swelling
    3. Coolness and hardness
    4. Red streak along vein

16. A client is receiving drug therapy with an ergot alkaloid. The clinic nurse evaluates the effectiveness of this drug by asking the client about the status of which of the following health problems?
    1. Nosebleeds
    2. Headaches
    3. Muscle aches
    4. Low blood pressure

17. A client is beginning drug therapy with a β-adrenergic blocker to decrease the risk of experiencing myocardial infarction. The nurse would administer this drug cautiously if the client had which of the following concurrent diagnoses?
    1. Hypertension
    2. Intracranial aneurysm
    3. Pneumonia
    4. Insulin-controlled diabetes mellitus

18. A client with hypertension is started on drug therapy with atenolol (Tenormin). The nurse would teach the client to withhold a dose of the drug and notify the prescriber if the heart rate was irregular or slower than how many beats per minute?
    1. 50
    2. 40
    3. 60
    4. 30

Chapter **22**   **Drugs Affecting the Sympathetic (Adrenergic) Nervous System**

19. A client taking a β-blocking agent whether the drug can be discontinued sometime in the future. An appropriate response would be that this would be the judgment of the prescriber but, if the drug was discontinued, the dose would be tapered down over what period of time?
    1. 2 to 3 days
    2. 4 to 7 days
    3. 1 to 2 weeks
    4. 2 to 4 weeks

20. A client requires the use of a β-blocking agent that is cardioselective in affecting β_1 receptors but not β_2 receptors because of concurrent history of lung disease. Which of the following drugs does the nurse anticipate will be ordered for this client?
    1. carteolol (Cartrol)
    2. atenolol (Tenormin)
    3. nadolol (Corgard)
    4. pindolol (Visken)

Chapter **22** **Drugs Affecting the Sympathetic (Adrenergic) Nervous System**

STAYING ON TOP OF TERMINOLOGY

1. Complete the following word search.

AKATHISIA	DYSTONIA
AKINESIA	LEVODOPA
ANTICHOLINESTERASE	NEOSTIGMINE
BACLOFEN	SELEGILINE
BENZTROPINE	SPASMS
DEMENTIA	SPASTICITY
DESIGNER DRUGS	TOLCAPONE
DONEPEZIL	

```
B  A  C  L  O  F  E  N  A  T  S  P  A  S  M  S  I  D
B  A  C  Y  T  R  N  T  R  O  P  S  I  G  N  E  Y  S
I  N  E  O  S  T  I  G  M  I  N  E  F  E  N  S  T  E
S  A  N  Y  I  C  P  D  O  N  A  D  F  E  T  A  I  K
E  B  E  N  Z  D  O  D  A  K  A  E  S  O  P  T  C  L
L  E  S  T  E  R  R  A  K  A  T  S  N  R  E  D  I  I
E  D  E  M  E  N  T  I  A  D  E  I  N  E  R  D  T  Z
G  E  O  D  O  N  Z  O  F  E  A  G  T  R  O  L  S  E
I  G  R  N  A  W  N  K  A  K  I  N  E  S  I  A  A  P
L  O  S  T  A  Z  E  D  R  U  B  E  B  A  C  I  P  E
I  T  O  L  C  Z  B  A  P  O  N  R  S  E  L  S  S  N
N  S  E  L  E  G  E  T  O  L  C  D  A  N  T  I  S  O
E  N  T  O  L  C  A  P  O  N  E  R  T  I  A  H  E  D
A  K  A  B  E  N  Z  A  I  T  O  U  P  A  N  T  N  E
D  E  A  P  O  D  O  V  E  L  I  G  M  E  N  S  I  C
D  O  N  A  A  N  T  I  A  K  A  S  S  E  L  A  G  I
T  R  O  P  A  K  A  S  K  I  B  C  H  O  L  K  E  N
A  N  T  I  C  H  O  L  I  N  E  S  T  E  R  A  S  E
```

2. _____ _____ is a progressively debilitating disorder of the CNS caused by a degeneration of the dopamine-producing neurons of the substantia nigra, which produces a dopamine/acetylcholine imbalance.

3. _____ _____ is a progressive and presently incurable disease characterized by the loss of, or decrease in, acetylcholine receptors caused by an autoimmune process resulting in skeletal muscle weakness and fatigue.

4. Two classes of drugs used in the treatment of Parkinson's disease are those with central _____ activity and those that affect brain _____ levels.

5. Enhanced CNS effects can occur when anticholinergic agents are given concurrently with _____ and other anticholinergic or other antimuscarinic medications.

6. Because of its method of excretion, a dosage reduction of amantadine (Symmetrel) is recommended for clients with _____ impairment.

7. With the administration of _____, clients with a history of or predisposition to psychiatric disorders may experience symptoms such as insomnia, confusion, and agitation.

8. The most serious effects of myasthenia gravis are _____ and _____; these effects may result in aspiration pneumonia or respiratory failure.

9. The peripheral _____ inhibitors are primarily used to diagnose and treat myasthenia gravis and as an antidote for the curariform effects of tubocurarine (Tubarine) and pancuronium (Pavulon).

10. For dysphagia in a client with myasthenia gravis, the medication should be administered _____ to _____ minutes before meals, with a subsequent rest period mealtime to allow for peak muscle strength for eating.

CONNECTING WITH CLIENTS

11. Can you identify two drugs that interact with anticholinesterase agents and the effect that occurs with each?

12. What are the more frequent adverse effects of the direct-acting skeletal muscle relaxant dantrolene (Dantrium)?

13. What would be appropriate monitoring, intervention, and education strategies for a client receiving baclofen (Lioresal)?

TRAINING FOR TEST TAKING

14. A nurse is caring for a client receiving benztropine (Cogentin) for treatment of Parkinson's disease. The nurse determines that drug therapy is effective after noting which of the following?
    1. Increased ability to sit up and stand
    2. Decrease in systolic and diastolic blood pressure
    3. Decreased temperature and tremors
    4. Increased alertness and cognition

15. A client who has Parkinson's disease is started on carbidopa/levodopa (Sinemet) therapy. When the client asks how long it will take to see a noticeable change in symptoms, the nurse replies that, although client response is variable, improvement is often seen in what timeframe?
    1. 3 to 4 days
    2. 1 to 2 weeks
    3. 2 to 3 weeks
    4. 1 to 2 months

16. The nurse is caring for a client receiving neostigmine (Prostigmin) for treatment of myasthenia gravis. Which medication does the nurse ensure is readily available as an antidote to this medication if toxicity occurs?
    1. Atenolol
    2. Atropine sulfate
    3. Calcium gluconate
    4. Calcium carbonate

17. The nurse anticipates an order for which of the following drugs when a client is undergoing diagnostic evaluation for myasthenia gravis?
    1. ambenonium (Mytelase)
    2. pyridostigmine (Mestinon)
    3. bromocriptine (Parlodel)
    4. edrophonium (Tensilon)

18. A client who is newly diagnosed with Alzheimer's disease also has a history of liver disease. The nurse concludes that which medication will not likely be ordered for this client?
    1. tacrine (Cognex)
    2. rivastigmine (Exelon)
    3. galantamine (Reminyl)
    4. donepezil (Aricept)

19. A client with multiple sclerosis is receiving baclofen (Lioresal). For what adverse drug effects would the nurse assess this client?
    1. Insomnia
    2. Diarrhea
    3. Vertigo
    4. Double vision

20. A client is being started on drug therapy with tizanidine (Zanaflex). What should the nurse include in client teaching about this medication?
    1. The effects of the medication are assisted by small amounts of alcohol.
    2. It is important to change positions slowly.
    3. The drug may cause a slight elevation in blood pressure.
    4. It will have no effect on cognition or judgment.

Chapter **23** **Drugs for Specific Dysfunctions of the Central and Peripheral Nervous Systems**

24 Overview of the Cardiovascular System

1. Complete the following puzzle.

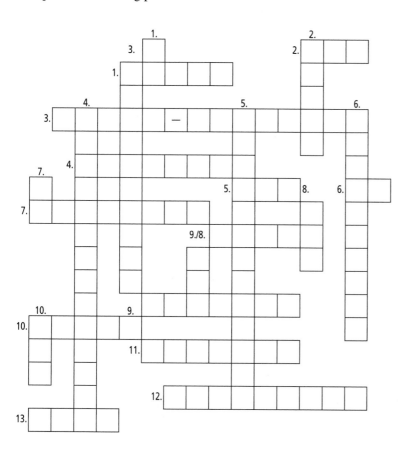

Across

1. Major parasympathetic nerve innervation of the heart
2. Abbreviation for adenosine triphosphatase
3. Name of law pertaining to force of heart contraction
4. Fibers that are part of conduction system of heart
5. Number of ventricles
6. Abbreviation for calcium
7. Term for speed
8. Term for when heart conduction does not occur
9. Term for the period of heart contraction
10. Organ that pumps blood
11. Main cation affecting electrical stimulation of the heart
12. Stimulus that changes the resting membrane
13. Calcium, potassium, and sodium are examples

Down

1. Abbreviation for sodium
2. Top chambers of the heart
3. Chambers that force blood to various parts of the body
4. Term for cardiac contraction recovery
5. Neurotransmitter that stimulates the vagus nerve
6. Digoxin is an example of this classification
7. Node that stimulates the heart to contract
8. Possible abbreviation for electrocardiogram
9. Letters on graph depicting ventricular contraction
10. Part of conduction system of heart

2. Cardiac muscle contraction begins with a rapid change in the _____ _____ of the cell membrane.

3. _____ is the stage in which an electrical impulse results in contraction of the ventricular muscle; it is represented by the QRS complex on the electrocardiogram (ECG).

4. The cells that possess the property of _____, the ability to initiate an impulse, are called pacemaker cells.

5. _____ refers to the ability to transmit an action potential or nerve impulse from cell to cell.

6. Cardiac tissue is nonresponsive to stimulation during the initial phase of systole (contraction) and this phenomenon is known as_____.

7. _____ are graphic representations of electrical currents produced by the heart.

8. The rise in free _____ ion concentration is considered to be the primary event in excitation-contraction coupling that is responsible for increasing muscle tone and vasoconstriction.

9. _____ is the volume of blood expelled by the ventricles of the heart; it is equal to the _____ multiplied by the_____.

10. _____ refers to the strength of the muscular contraction of cardiac tissue and can be adversely affected by a number of factors, including myocardial ischemia or infarction.

11. _____ is a term that refers to the amount of blood entering the ventricle before contraction and affects the stretching of the muscle fiber in the ventricle.

12. _____ is the pressure against which the ventricle is pumping blood and is primarily determined by peripheral vascular resistance (e.g., blood pressure).

25 Agents Used in the Treatment of Heart Failure

STAYING ON TOP OF TERMINOLOGY

1. Complete the following word search.

INAMRINONE
CHF
CHRONOTROPIC
DIGITALIZATION
DIGOXIN
DROMOTROPIC
ECG
FAB
FIBRILLATION

GLYCOSIDE
INOTROPIC
LANOXIN
MILRINONE
NURSING
PACEMAKERS
SERUM
TOXICITY

```
G N C P S F L K O A M R T S Q D W V K X
Y L S E R Z Z L Q W H F O Z X Z H V I K
O S R W E J G K P J A B X W C L B Q L R
O U W V K Y X U A C V L I E R H P E S R
M B P X A H A Y H S Q Z C K R N R Z I U
R Y I O M C X K K C F Z I G J B J Y Z V
J I N E E W J W R M J A T L X Z W Z W V
F H A O C E D X H B G L Y C O S I D E B
G E M Y A H W A L V E C R H D L B M I Y
H N R G P W F Z G Q N P I R J E X C E K
N O I T A L L I R B I F O O Z V C M N O
U N N S O A F D G Z X M U N I X O G I D
R I O U R U V P I N O T R O P I C Y H J
K R N V R U U J M T N A P T X R T D Y Z
T L E S P N N F R D A J E R Y E K T J Q
Q I J J K E X O C O L M B O A I B J Y O
X M Q W U D P Y O N G F A P Z N R O C Q
G M N R R I D I G I T A L I Z A T I O N
W O B R C B D P V Q Q B W C O Z X B Q K
J W W W J B H Y J U Y W J B Y X J Z X W
```

2. _____ _____ is an abnormal condition that reflects altered structure and/or function of the ventricle and most often results in reduced cardiac output.

3. Drugs with a positive _____ effect strengthen or increase the force of myocardial contraction.

4. Drugs with _____ action affect heart rate.

5. A _____ effect refers to drugs that affect conduction velocity through specialized conducting tissues.

6. _____ originally was an herbal remedy derived from the biennial flower foxglove that was used for hundreds of years by common people.

7. Digoxin possesses _____ inotropic action, _____ chronotropic action and _____ dromotropic action.

8. A number of adverse effects are noted with digoxin, most of which are _____ related.

9. Digoxin is ideal for use in atrial fibrillation for slowing the ventricular rate because it increases the _____ _____ of the AV junction and also slows _____ at this site.

10. Digoxin immune Fab is an _____ for severe digoxin toxicity.

CONNECTING WITH CLIENTS

11. What are three factors to assess in a client that may predispose that client to digoxin toxicity?

12. What points of information should be included in client education for a client who is receiving cardiac glycoside therapy?

13. What are some of the adverse effects you would assess for in a client who is receiving inamrinone (Inocor) for treatment of heart failure?

14. The nurse is assigned to the care of a client receiving digoxin. What adverse effects should the nurse assess for during the shift as part of routine care?
   1. Nausea and vomiting
   2. Constipation
   3. Shortened PR interval on cardiac rhythm strip
   4. Increase in pulse of 30 beats from baseline

15. A client with a new diagnosis of heart failure will begin drug therapy with digoxin. When explaining how this drug will help, the nurse would consider including which of the following points of information?
   1. It raises pressure in the veins in the lungs.
   2. Myocardial oxygen demand is raised.
   3. Heart size is often decreased toward normal.
   4. Excess blood is shunted away from the coronary circulation.

16. The nurse working on a cardiac unit is reviewing the results of laboratory studies drawn early in the morning. The nurse would do a further assessment on a client that had which of the following digoxin levels?
   1. 0.8 ng/mL
   2. 1.3 ng/mL
   3. 1.9 ng/mL
   4. 3.0 ng/mL

17. A nurse overhears a physician explain to a client that he will be started on digoxin therapy using rapid digitalization to aid in improving new onset symptoms of heart failure. The nurse anticipates that the first dose of digoxin will be how many milligrams?
   1. 0.625
   2. 0.125
   3. 0.25
   4. 0.5

18. The nurse is working with an older adult client taking digoxin. The nurse would monitor for development of which of the following, which is the earliest sign of digoxin toxicity?
   1. Anorexia
   2. Vomiting
   3. Blue-tinged vision
   4. Abdominal distress

19. The nurse would administer a scheduled dose of digoxin after noting which of the following safe potassium level results from lab work drawn in early morning?
   1. 2.6 mEq/L
   2. 3.4 mEq/L
   3. 4.5 mEq/L
   4. 5.6 mEq/L

20. The nurse would include which of the following points in a teaching plan for a client being discharged to home on digoxin?
   1. Report a weight gain of 4 pounds or more per day.
   2. Report a pulse rate of less than 60 or greater than 110 to the prescriber.
   3. Restrict sodium intake to 4 grams daily.
   4. Take the dose with a high fiber meal.

26 Antidysrhythmics

STAYING ON TOP OF TERMINOLOGY

1. Match the antidysrhythmic drug to its classification.

_____ procainamide	a. Group I-A
_____ mexiletine	b. Group I-B
_____ adenosine	c. Group I-C
_____ quinidine	d. Group I
_____ propranolol	e. Group II
_____ encainide	f. Group III
_____ bretylium	g. Group IV
_____ lidocaine	
_____ sotalol	
_____ moricizine	

FOCUSING ON THE FACTS

2. _____ _____ is an abnormal condition in which the myocardium contracts steadily but at a rate less than 60 beats/min.

3. _____ _____ is an abnormal condition in which the myocardium contracts regularly but at a rate greater than 100 beats/min.

4. A shift in the origin of impulse formation can generate an abnormal pacemaker or an _____ _____, resulting in activation of some part of the heart other than the SA node.

5. _____ phenomenon is the mechanism responsible for initiating ectopic beats and a necessary condition for this to occur is _____ block.

6. Quinidine depresses_____, velocity of _____, and _____ of the heart.

7. Lidocaine should not be administered to clients with _____- _____ syndrome.

8. Procainamide stabilizes the cell membrane by preventing the ready movement of _____ and _____ across this cellular barrier.

9. Antidysrhythmic drugs in Group III prolong the effective _____ period by prolonging the action potential, thus prolonging repolarization.

10. Amiodarone is indicated for life-threatening ventricular _____ and ventricular _____ .

CONNECTING WITH CLIENTS

11. A client who was admitted to the coronary care unit has an intravenous lidocaine drip running. In writing a care plan for this client, what would be the goals for the client while receiving this drug?

12. What hormone is amiodarone structurally related to and how does this drug work?

13. Your client has a new drug order for sotalol (Betapace). What do you recall about this drug and how is it different from other β-adrenergic blocking drugs?

TRAINING FOR TEST TAKING

14. A client with myasthenia gravis requires treatment of ventricular dysrhythmias with an antidysrhythmic drug. The nurse would question a newly written order for which of the following drugs that could worsen the client's myasthenia symptoms?
    1. quinidine gluconate (Quinaglute)
    2. procainamide (Pronestyl)
    3. disopyramide (Norpace)
    4. sotalol (Betapace)

15. A client is receiving procainamide (Pronestyl) by the intravenous route. The nurse should place highest priority on monitoring which of the following vital signs because of adverse drug effects?
    1. Temperature
    2. Pulse
    3. Blood pressure
    4. Respirations

16. The nurse would plan to administer an intravenous dose of lidocaine as per protocol order for a client who develops which of the following cardiac rhythms?
    1. Sinus tachycardia
    2. Ventricular tachycardia
    3. Atrial fibrillation
    4. Atrial flutter

17. A client is receiving an intravenous lidocaine drip after receiving a bolus dose by the IV push route. The nurse exercises caution to ensure that the drug is administered at the proper dose, and does not exceed a dose of how many milligrams per minute?
    1. 1 mg/min
    2. 2 mg/min
    3. 3 mg/min
    4. 4 mg/min

18. The nurse would question an order for acebutolol (Sectral) in a client with which of the following health problems?
    1. Heart failure
    2. Ventricular dysrhythmias
    3. Hypertension
    4. Angina

19. A client has been taking amiodarone (Cordarone) for almost a year for suppression of ventricular dysrhythmias. At the client's regular health visit, the nurse reinforces client teaching about the medication, making special note of what unique adverse effect may occur in some clients after one year of therapy?
    1. Reddened eyes
    2. Hard brittle nails
    3. Blue-gray tinge to the skin
    4. Increased risk of fungal infection

96

20. A nurse who is administering a dose of diltiazem (Cardizem) would avoid using which of the following items on the client's breakfast tray to administer the dose?
    1. Low-fat milk
    2. Grapefruit juice
    3. Regular coffee
    4. Decaffeinated tea

27 Antihypertensives

STAYING ON TOP OF TERMINOLOGY

1. Complete the following word search.

ANGIOTENSIN
BARORECEPTOR
DIURETICS
HYPERTENSION
THIAZIDES
VASODILATORS
CAPTOPRIL

CLONIDINE
HYDRALAZINE
HYDROCHLOROTHIAZIDE
LOSARTAN
NIFEDIPINE
NITROPRUSSIDE
PRAZOSIN

```
E D I Z A I H T O R O L H C O R D Y H
C A N G N B A R O C L O N H Y P I N D
N I F E G H Y D R A T H I S I D U P A
L O S A I C A P T T H I R N I T R S E
P B A R O R E C E P T O R E D A E R N
A R T A T H Y D R O T A R T Z I T N I
C A T E E P R A Z A S O R O P S I A P
L O S A N C L U L P I T S A R T C R I
O T E N S A R I C L O I C A P R S E D
N T I N I A D S I N N C A R T I D I E
I A Z A N O I S N E T R E P Y H A Z F
D A C T S S A R C L H P R I L A P O I
I N D A C L O P R I I T I N G H A R N
N E V A Z Z H Y D R A L A Z I N E E T
E D I L V A S I L A Z T O C A P E Z R
R E C T O R P T E L I R P O T P A C E
E L O S A R T A N I D H Y D R O P R I
C L O P I L I N E W E P R U S C A P W
C A P L O S E D I S S U R P O R T I N
```

2. Vasodilators promote blood flow to the extremities by increasing the lumen of
_____.

3. Calcium channel blockers are used primarily for their _____,
_____, and _____ properties.

4. Calcium channel blockers inhibit the contraction of smooth muscle of the peripheral
arterioles, resulting in widespread reduction in _____ and
_____.

5. Individuals with preexisting diabetes mellitus are at the highest risk for
_____ _____ damage with uncontrolled hypertension.

6. _____ diuretics are recommended as first-line drug therapy for uncomplicated hypertension.

7. The potassium-sparing diuretic agents, such as _____ and
_____, are useful in counteracting the potassium loss induced by other
diuretics.

8. The _____ _____ and the _____ are considered
the drugs of choice for individuals with hypertension and diabetes mellitus.

9. The most serious adverse effects of captopril and other ACE inhibitors are
_____ and acute renal failure.

10. Prazosin is a selective α_1-adrenergic blocking agent that dilates both
_____ and _____.

CONNECTING WITH CLIENTS

11. To which antihypertensive agents do blacks generally respond better?

12. What are some of the special needs of the older adult receiving antihypertensive drug
therapy?

Chapter **27** **Antihypertensives**

13. What is the treatment for bradycardia experienced by a client who accidentally took an overdose of a calcium blocker?

TRAINING FOR TEST TAKING

14. A client diagnosed with hypertension without complications has not achieved blood pressure reduction with diet and exercise. Which of the following types of medications does the clinic nurse anticipate will be ordered as a first-line agent?
    1. A peripheral vasodilator
    2. A thiazide diuretic
    3. A β blocker
    4. A calcium channel blocker

15. A client with hypertension has been prescribed hydrochlorothiazide 25 mg daily. At what time should the ambulatory care nurse recommend the client take the dose each day?
    1. 08:00
    2. 12:00
    3. 16:00
    4. 20:00

16. A hypertensive client is adding atenolol (Tenormin) to the antihypertensive drug regimen. What teaching points about this drug should the nurse share with the client?
    1. Withhold the dose of drug and call prescriber if the pulse rate is less than 60.
    2. Depression and weight gain are unpleasant but benign adverse effects of the drug.
    3. Headaches and nausea are frequent adverse effects of this drug.
    4. Assess personal ability to undertake physical exertion because the drug causes fatigue.

17. A client taking lisinopril (Prinivil) for hypertension is found to have the following drug adverse effects at a regular office visit. Which of these would the nurse consider benign or least important?
    1. Sore throat
    2. Fever
    3. Dry cough
    4. Urine protein of 2+

18. A client is assigned to the care of a client receiving losartan (Cozaar). The nurse would place highest priority in attending to which adverse effect of this drug?
    1. Constipation
    2. Angioedema
    3. Muscle pain
    4. Headache

19. A client is admitted to the emergency department with subarachnoid hemorrhage. From which of the following calcium channel blockers will this client most likely benefit?
    1. isradipine (Dynacirc)
    2. nicardipine (Cardene)
    3. felodipine (Plendil)
    4. nimodipine (Nimotop)

20. The nurse would question an order for nifedipine (Procardia) if the client has which of the following health problems documented on the medical record?
    1. Systolic heart failure
    2. Raynaud's phenomenon
    3. Angina pectoris
    4. Restless legs syndrome

28 Vasodilators and Blood Viscosity–Reducing Agents

STAYING ON TOP OF TERMINOLOGY

1. Match the description on the right to the term on the left.

_____ Angina pectoris
_____ Hemorrheology
_____ Ischemic
_____ Nitrates
_____ nitroglycerin
_____ pentoxifylline

a. A term that refers to tissue in which actual blood supply is less than required and leads to abnormal conditions within the cell or tissue

b. A drug that is used to reduce or prevent the pain of angina, to treat HF, and on rare occasions to treat hypertension

c. A class of drugs that are effective in treating stable angina pectoris because of their dilating effect on the veins and arteries

d. A temporary interference with the flow of blood, oxygen, and nutrients to heart muscle, or intermittent myocardial ischemia

e. A drug that is used as an adjunct to surgery for the treatment of intermittent claudication caused by occlusive arterial disease of the limbs

f. A science that deals with the deformation and flow properties of blood under physiologic and pathophysiologic conditions

FOCUSING ON THE FACTS

2. _____ angina refers to chest pain that occurs with exercise or stress and is relieved by rest; it is often predictable with increased oxygen demand.

3. Myocardial ischemia can usually be detected on the electrocardiogram as ST segment _____, whereas myocardial infarction usually presents as ST segment _____.

4. Drug therapy for angina pectoris is aimed at increasing myocardial oxygen _____, reducing myocardial oxygen _____, and minimizing or removing the _____.

5. The most common adverse effect of nitrates is _____, which is related to _____ of cerebral vessels.

103

6. When clients who have intermittent claudication are walking, they first experience _____ and then _____ and _____ in the muscles.

7. Pentoxifylline restores RBC _____ and lowers blood _____.

8. The most common adverse effects of pentoxifylline are _____, _____, and _____.

9. Epoprostenol (Flolan) directly dilates the pulmonary and systemic arteries and also inhibits _____ aggregation.

10. Pentoxifylline should be used with caution in clients with impaired _____ and _____ function.

CONNECTING WITH CLIENTS

11. What are important client teaching points when administering extended-release nitroglycerin by the buccal route?

12. What would be three therapeutic objectives that you could use to evaluate the use of antianginal agents?

13. What information about the mechanism of action of pentoxifylline would you use when determining how to teach a client about this medication?

TRAINING FOR TEST TAKING

14. A client who recently began using nitroglycerin telephones the clinic nurse to report headache and flushing after each dose. The nurse considers which of the following explanations when responding to the client?
    1. The client needs a larger dose to achieve maximal effectiveness.
    2. This is an expected adverse effect that should diminish or disappear over time.
    3. This indicates an adverse effect and may require substitution of a different drug.
    4. The client may be having an unusual hypersensitivity reaction to the drug.

15. A client enjoys walking 2 miles per day, but tends to get chest pain after the first mile. The nurse should encourage the client to take a dose of which prescribed medication before beginning this activity?
    1. metoprolol (Lopressor)
    2. pentoxifylline (Trental)
    3. papaverine (Pavabid)
    4. nitroglycerin (Nitrostat)

16. A client has recent onset of chest pain and is learning about the use of nitroglycerin sublingual tablets. The nurse evaluates that the client understands proper use after stating to take:
    1. "up to three doses if needed 2 minutes apart and then call 911 if the chest pain isn't gone."
    2. "up to five doses if needed 3 minutes apart and then call 911 if the chest pain isn't gone."
    3. "up to three doses if needed 5 minutes apart and then call 911 if the chest pain isn't gone."
    4. "up to five doses if needed 5 minutes apart and then call 911 if the chest pain isn't gone."

17. A client who has learned the appropriate information about using a transdermal nitroglycerin patch would need further information after stating to:
    1. Remove the patch at bedtime each night.
    2. Apply a fresh patch every morning.
    3. Trim the patch if needed so it fits in nonhairy areas.
    4. Wear the patch while bathing.

18. Which of the following pieces of information would be important to teach a client who has been given a new prescription for sublingual nitroglycerin tablets?
    1. Store the drug in a cool, dark area.
    2. Place the tablets in a small metal pill container for convenient use.
    3. Open a new supply every 12 months.
    4. Drink a cool beverage while the tablet is dissolving under the tongue.

19. The nurse would expect a medication order for pentoxifylline (Trental) to be written for a client who has undergone which of the following surgical procedures?
    1. Carotid endarterectomy
    2. Aortic valve replacement
    3. Femoral popliteal bypass grafting
    4. Vein ligation and stripping

20. The nurse would assess the client taking pentoxifylline for which of the following most frequent adverse effects of the drug?
    1. Dizziness
    2. GI upset
    3. Sedation
    4. Headache

Chapter **28** **Vasodilators and Blood Viscosity–Reducing Agents**

29 Overview of the Blood

STAYING ON TOP OF TERMINOLOGY

1. Complete the following puzzle.

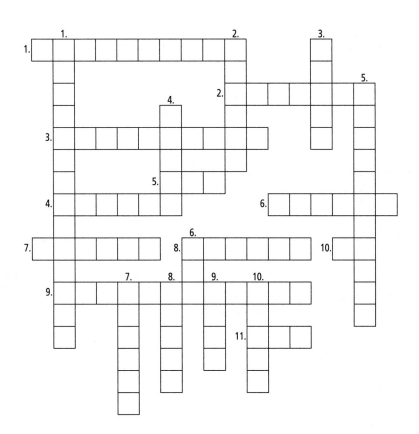

Across
1. Cells that fight infection
2. Protein that helps maintain osmolality
3. Combines with oxygen
4. Liquid portion of the blood
5. Abbreviation for hematocrit
6. Chemical substance involved with clotting
7. Combines with platelets to reinforce clots
8. Disorder caused by decreased hemoglobin
9. Another word for platelets
10. Antigen present on RBC
11. Abbreviation for platelet

Down
1. Hormone produced by kidney
2. Pooling of blood
3. Fluid other than blood that carries leukocytes
4. First letter of the Greek alphabet
5. One type of WBC
6. Types of blood
7. Gas carried by RBCs
8. Fluid that circulates in arteries and veins
9. Must occur to prevent hemorrhage
10. Various blood classifications

2. _____ is the packed cell volume of the red blood cells expressed as a percentage of the total blood volume, or the blood viscosity.

3. Red blood cells (RBCs, erythrocytes) are small and disk shaped cells in the bloodstream that have a life span of approximately _____ days.

4. A person with a hemoglobin count below 10 g/dL is usually diagnosed as having _____.

5. The granular leukocytes are _____, _____, and _____; the nongranular leukocytes are _____ and _____.

6. A normal platelet level in the blood is between _____ and _____/mm³.

7. _____, a plasma protein that is converted to fibrin by thrombin in the presence of calcium ions, is necessary for coagulation.

8. _____ is a process that spontaneously stops the bleeding in damaged blood vessels.

9. The chemical events in the blood coagulation mechanism involve two distinct pathways: the _____ pathway and the _____ pathway.

10. Persons with type A blood can safely receive blood from type _____ and type _____ donors.

11. Type O persons can receive only type O blood; they are called _____ _____ because they can donate blood to anyone.

12. Rh factor is particularly important when an Rh-_____ woman is impregnated by an Rh-_____ man.

30 Antiplatelets, Anticoagulants, Fibrinolytics, and Blood Components

STAYING ON TOP OF TERMINOLOGY

1. Match the drug to the reaction it causes when given with oral anticoagulants.

_____ Androgens	a.	Increases effect of an anticoagulant
_____ Estrogens	b.	Decreases effect of an anticoagulant
_____ vitamin K		
_____ aspirin		
_____ cimetidine		
_____ Oral contraceptives		
_____ meperidine		
_____ Barbiturates		

FOCUSING ON THE FACTS

2. Although anticoagulants are used to treat thrombosis, they do not _____ clots, but prevent the _____ of existing clots.

3. Classic examples of _____ drugs are aspirin and clopidogrel (Plavix).

4. The inhibition of _____ observed with aspirin poses a risk for GI irritation or bleeding and is one of the concerns with its use.

5. Because of the risk for potentially life-threatening _____ _____ suppression, use of ticlopidine is generally limited to clients who have not responded to or tolerated other antiplatelet therapy.

6. The oral anticoagulant most commonly used is _____, which interferes with the production of vitamin K–dependent clotting factors.

7. _____ produces its anticoagulant effect by combining with antithrombin III, a naturally occurring anticlotting factor in the plasma.

8. _____ _____ is the antidote for heparin overdose.

9. Fibrinolytic drugs dissolve clots by converting _____ in the blood to _____.

10. Depending on the individual's size and preexisting blood integrity, an acute whole blood loss of more than _____ mL is manifested by signs of anemia.

109

CONNECTING WITH CLIENTS

11. What symptoms should you assess for in a client receiving a blood transfusion that could indicate a transfusion reaction is occurring?

12. What risks would you be concerned about if a client was receiving a fibrinolytic agent while also receiving an anticoagulant?

13. What are some of the nursing implications for an older adult who is receiving an anti-coagulant drug?

TRAINING FOR TEST TAKING

14. A client is receiving warfarin sodium (Coumadin) for prevention of a thromboembolic event. The nurse determines that the client's latest International Normalized Ratio (INR) result is optimal if which of the following values is noted?
    1. 1.7
    2. 2.5
    3. 3.6
    4. 4.5

15. The nurse is preparing to administer a scheduled dose of heparin (Liquiprin) to a client. Which of the following actions should the nurse take as part of routine procedure?
    1. Use a syringe that has a 20- to 22-gauge, 1-inch needle.
    2. Aspirate before injecting.
    3. Massage the area gently after injection.
    4. Rotate sites on the lower abdomen.

16. A client taking warfarin sodium (Coumadin) who is experiencing small episodes of bleeding visits the urgent care clinic and has an international normal-ized ratio (INR) level drawn. After noting that the level is critically high, what medication should the nurse have readily available for use if ordered?
    1. phytonadione (Mephyton)
    2. protamine sulfate (Protamine)
    3. argatroban (Acova)
    4. aminocaproic acid (Amicar)

17. The nurse advises a client taking anticoagulant ther-apy that which of the following drugs would be best to use for self-treatment of occasional headaches?
    1. ibuprofen (Motrin)
    2. naproxen (Aleve)
    3. acetaminophen (Tylenol)
    4. aspirin (Ecotrin)

18. The nurse would notify the physician prior to begin-ning an intravenous infusion of alteplase (Activase) if which of the following vital signs were measured as part of the admission to the emergency depart-ment?
    1. Temperature 100.8 oral
    2. Blood pressure 194/112 mm Hg
    3. Pulse 104
    4. Oxygen saturation 91%

19. The nurse is preparing to hang a unit of blood on an assigned client. The nurse asks another nurse to monitor the other clients, because the nurse will need to remain with the client receiving the transfusion for at least how long after the unit is hung?
    1. 5 minutes
    2. 10 minutes
    3. 15 minutes
    4. 30 minutes

20. A client who needs a blood transfusion has a history of having a febrile nonhemolytic reaction to a transfusion in the past. The nurse questions the physician about an order for which of the following, which the client should receive to prevent this from occurring with this transfusion?
    1. acetaminophen (Tylenol)
    2. aspirin (Ecotrin)
    3. diphenhydramine (Benadryl)
    4. epinephrine (Adrenalin)

31 Antihyperlipidemic Drugs

1. Complete the following word search.

ATHEROSCLEROSIS HYPERLIPIDEMIA
CHOLESTYRAMINE LIPOPROTEIN
CHYLOMICRONS LOVASTATIN
GEMFIBROZIL NIACIN

```
C H O L E S T Y R A M I N E N
H O Z I L A T H E T C H O L I
Y L I P O L O V A H N I A T A
L S C L E R E M I E L O B A C
O C H O S T Y N I R G E M G H
M I A L I P O P R O T E I N O
I G E M S T R A T S I A C I L
C L I B V A I E R C N I V A E
R O S I S F I B E L I P O C F
O T H E R M I C R E O Z A I I
N I T N O P N I A R C H Y N B
S N I T A T S A V O L O S I L
L E F I L O S T A S N I C H I
G E M F I B R O Z I L P O R P
T E I I P O A T H S S T A R E
H Y P E R L I P I D E M I A M
```

FOCUSING ON THE FACTS

2. Hyperlipidemia is a/an _____ disorder characterized by increased concentrations of _____ and _____ .

3. An important relationship exists between atherosclerosis and _____ .

4. High-density lipoproteins pick up _____ from _____ and carry them to _____.

5. Lipoproteins are _____ bound to _____, which act as carriers; they are classified according to their _____.

6. Low-density lipoproteins contain the major portion of _____ in blood and may be considered the most harmful.

7. Chylomicrons are the _____ particles and least _____ of the lipoproteins; they are produced in _____.

8. The inflammatory process of atherosclerosis appears greatest in _____ and _____ sized arteries.

9. Lipid profiles should be obtained in the fasting state at least every _____ years for all individuals over the age of _____ years.

10. One of the most important adverse effects with the HMG CoA enzyme inhibitor drugs is _____, which is manifested by myalgias, myositis and the risk for rhabdomyolysis.

CONNECTING WITH CLIENTS

11. A client will be receiving a bile acid sequestrant. Can you identify two drugs that interact with bile acid sequestering agents and the effects they produce?

12. A client has a new order for clofibrate. What education strategies would be appropriate for this client?

13. What would be some of the adverse effects that you would assess for in a client receiving an HMG coenzyme A reductase inhibitor (a "statin")?

14. A client is taking lovastatin (Mevacor). The nurse should be sure that the breakfast tray does not contain which of the following beverages?
    1. Grapefruit juice
    2. Orange juice
    3. Coffee
    4. Tea

15. The nurse is due to administer a first dose of pravastatin (Pravachol) to a client. Which laboratory test results should the nurse review to ensure there is no contraindication to giving the drug?
    1. Serum creatinine
    2. Blood glucose
    3. Liver enzymes
    4. Serum electrolytes

16. The nurse explains to a client with high cholesterol levels that which of the following B-complex vitamins has a lipid-lowering effect?
    1. Folic acid
    2. Niacin
    3. Cyanocobalamin
    4. Thiamine

17. The nurse is assessing a client who started taking cholestyramine (Questran) 1 month ago. The nurse inquires whether the client has experienced which of the following most frequent adverse effects of this drug?
    1. Blurred vision
    2. Increased concentration of urine
    3. Muscle weakness
    4. Indigestion or abdominal pain

18. A client will be taking nicotinic acid (Nicobid) as adjunct treatment for hyperlipidemia. The nurse explains to the client that which of the following is an expected adverse effect of the medication?
    1. Warmth and flushing
    2. Excessive tearing and salivation
    3. Constipation alternating with diarrhea
    4. Dizziness and ringing in the ears

19. The nurse needs to schedule medications for a client receiving colestipol (Colestid). If the client will take this medication at 8 AM, the nurse should schedule the other medications to be given no earlier than which time?
    1. 9 AM
    2. 10 AM
    3. 11 AM
    4. 12 noon

20. The ambulatory care nurse anticipates that a client who has just begun taking fenofibrate (TriCor) will have a reduction in which laboratory value at the next scheduled office visit?
    1. Chylomicrons
    2. Triglycerides
    3. Low-density lipoproteins
    4. High-density lipoproteins

32 Overview of the Urinary System

STAYING ON TOP OF TERMINOLOGY

1. Match the function to the site of the nephron in which it occurs.

_____ Sodium reabsorption   a. Proximal tubule
_____ Chloride reabsorption   b. Distal tubule
_____ Glucose reabsorption   c. Descending loop of Henle
_____ Urine concentration   d. Ascending loop of Henle
_____ Aldosterone affects sodium   e. Collecting duct
         reabsorption
_____ Increased potassium secretion
_____ Passive water uptake produces a
         hypertonic filtrate
_____ Passive sodium reabsorption produces
         a hypotonic filtrate
_____ Potassium reabsorbed

FOCUSING ON THE FACTS

2. The urinary system is composed of organs that manufacture and excrete urine from the body: two _____, two _____, the _____, and the _____.

3. The kidneys regulate _____ in the body; they are responsible for the maintenance of body fluids, electrolytes, and acid-base balance.

4. _____ _____ occurs as a result of plasma flowing across a cluster of capillary blood vessels and into the urinary space of the Bowman's capsule.

5. The kidneys excrete metabolic byproducts of the body, especially _____ -type substances such as urea.

6. When ADH is released from the posterior pituitary gland, urine output is_____, and the urine is more _____.

7. As the blood pH becomes more acidic, the kidneys respond by increasing the renal tubule excretion of _____ and _____.

8. A decrease in red blood cells below normal, or tissue hypoxia, stimulates an increased release of _____ from the kidneys.

9. The normal range for blood urea nitrogen (BUN) in the adult is about _____ to _____ mg/dL.

10. The results for _____ may be nonspecific and influenced by a number of diseases, but it is a useful screening tool.

11. _____ _____, which is a widely used test of urine to determine glomerular filtration (GFR), is theoretically reliable but is commonly compromised because of the difficulty of getting a complete 24-hour specimen.

12. _____ of urine can assist the identification of the causative microorganism in a number of conditions, such as cystitis, pyelonephritis, prostatitis and other genitourinary infections.

33 Diuretics

STAYING ON TOP OF TERMINOLOGY

1. Match the diuretic to the site of the nephron it influences to produce therapeutic action.

_____ furosemide   a. Proximal tubule
_____ acetazolamide   b. Distal tubule
_____ hydrochlorothiazide   c. Loop of Henle
_____ spironolactone
_____ Diamox
_____ bumetanide

FOCUSING ON THE FACTS

2. Diuretics are useful in treating _____, _____, _____, and _____. They influence water and _____ balance.

3. Diuretics modify renal function to induce_____, or the loss of body water by _____.

4. _____ diuretics represent the mainstay in the treatment of hypertension.

5. Clinically, among the most frequently used diuretics are those that act in the _____ _____ _____, and are thus referred to as "_____ diuretics."

6. _____ diuretics like mannitol act as diuretics by drawing fluid into the lumen of the renal tubule.

7. _____ _____ diuretics work in the distal tubule and are weak diuretics.

8. The _____ _____ inhibitors like acetazolamide (Diamox) have very specific roles in the management of _____ and short-term management of certain types of _____.

9. The loop diuretics inhibit the reabsorption of _____ and _____ in the renal tubules.

10. Ethacrynic acid (Edecrin) is classified as a loop diuretic, but is rarely used because of a risk for serious _____.

CONNECTING WITH CLIENTS

11. An older adult client who will be beginning therapy with a diuretic drug tells you that she has heard from friends that it is important to take extra potassium in the diet when taking "water pills." In what situations would this not be true?

12. You are assigned to the care of an older adult who is taking a diuretic. What are the signs of dehydration that should be monitored in this client during your shift?

13. You are updating the care plan for a client who is new to diuretic therapy. What goals should you include in the plan of care for this client related to the use of diuretics?

TRAINING FOR TEST TAKING

14. The nurse is assigned to the care of four clients. For which client would the nurse expect mannitol (Osmitrol) to be prescribed?
    1. An older adult with increased intraocular pressure from glaucoma.
    2. A young adult with increased intracranial pressure from a head injury.
    3. An adult who is beginning to develop acute renal failure.
    4. A client who has had mildly progressive renal insufficiency.

15. A client with liver disease complicated by ascites is taking a diuretic. The nurse monitors which of the following is the best indicator of fluid balance for this client?
    1. Lung sounds
    2. Pulse and blood pressure
    3. Abdominal girth
    4. Daily weight

16. A client taking a potassium-wasting diuretic asks the nurse about foods that are naturally high in potassium. Of the following foods that the client enjoys, which one would the nurse encourage as having the highest amount of potassium per serving?
    1. Baked potato with skin
    2. Frozen cooked lima beans
    3. Orange juice
    4. Raw tomato

17. A client will be taking a diuretic medication as a once-daily dose. At which of the following best times should the nurse advise the client to take this medication?
    1. Mid-morning
    2. Late afternoon
    3. At bedtime
    4. On arising in the morning

18. The nurse would advise a client taking which medication to avoid using salt substitutes?
    1. furosemide (Lasix)
    2. bumetanide (Bumex)
    3. spironolactone (Aldactone)
    4. chlorothiazide (Diuril)

19. A client taking hydrochlorothiazide (HCTZ) had a potassium level drawn earlier in the day. The nurse would report which of the following results to the prescriber?
    1. 5.0 mEq/L
    2. 4.3 mEq/L
    3. 3.6 mEq/L
    4. 3.2 mEq/L

20. A client has been newly started on diuretic therapy. As part of client teaching about the medication, the nurse explains that the client should report an overnight weight gain of how many pounds?
    1. 4
    2. 3
    3. 2
    4. 1

34 Uricosuric Drugs

STAYING ON TOP OF TERMINOLOGY

1. Match the definitions on the right to the terms on the left.

_____ allopurinol
_____ colchicine
_____ Gout
_____ Hyperuricemia
_____ Urate nephropathy

a. A disease associated with an inborn error of uric acid metabolism that increases the production or inhibits the excretion of uric acid

b. A complication that results from the formation of uric acid or calcium oxalate calculi in the kidneys

c. Used for treatment and prophylaxis of acute gouty arthritis and treatment of chronic gouty arthritis

d. Decreases uric acid production by inhibiting xanthine oxidase from converting hypoxanthine to xanthine and xanthine to uric acid

e. High levels of uric acid in the blood

FOCUSING ON THE FACTS

2. Gout is a/an _____ disease that manifests itself by attacks of _____, _____, and _____ of joints.

3. The hallmark of gout is _____, or high levels of _____ _____ in the blood.

4. Tophi are _____.

5. Xanthine oxidase is the enzyme necessary to convert _____ to _____ and _____ to _____ _____.

6. Allopurinol inhibits the production of_____ _____.

7. Colchicine decreases _____ and the motility of_____.

8. Low dosages of _____ can interfere with the excretion of uric acid, resulting in an exacerbation of gout.

9. A less-frequent adverse effect of colchicine that can occur when used for chronic therapy is _____.

10. Allopurinol helps to_____, but does not _____, acute episodes of gout.

CONNECTING WITH CLIENTS

11. A client is newly diagnosed with gout and will begin medication therapy. What would you include in a care plan as the treatment goals for gout?

12. A client is taking probenecid but is not diagnosed with gout. What other mechanism of action does this drug have?

13. Develop an educational tool listing drugs that interact with probenecid to give to an older adult.

TRAINING FOR TEST TAKING

14. A client has experienced an acute attack of gout. The home care nurse anticipates that it will take at least how long after initiating colchicine therapy to see reduction in swelling of the affected joint(s)?
    1. 12 hours
    2. 1 day
    3. 2 days
    4. 3 days

15. The client asks the nurse to clarify an explanation provided by the physician regarding the use of colchicine to manage an acute attack of gout. The nurse reinforces that the client may discontinue use of the drug when which of the following occurs?
    1. All signs of joint swelling are gone
    2. Hair starts to fall out
    3. Pain from the attack is resolved
    4. Urine becomes pale and clear

16. A client has just been prescribed allopurinol (Zyloprim) to prevent attacks of gout. To determine the effectiveness of the medication on uric acid levels, which of the following would be the best time to schedule the client to have a uric acid level drawn?
    1. 3 to 5 days
    2. 1 week
    3. 3 weeks
    4. 2 months

17. Which of the following points should be included in medication teaching for a client who is starting drug therapy with allopurinol (Zyloprim)?
    1. Maintain high fluid intake of approximately 80 to 96 ounces daily.
    2. Take allopurinol on an empty stomach.
    3. Each foods that produce acid urine while taking this drug.
    4. Increase intake of B vitamins while taking this drug.

124

18. A client has a new order for probenecid (Benemid). The nurse interprets that this drug is being given to exert which of the following effects?
    1. Reduce inflammation caused by high uric acid levels.
    2. Reduce the pain of gout.
    3. Decrease production of uric acid.
    4. Reduce urate reabsorption in the kidney.

19. The nurse interprets that a client with which of the following health problems is likely to best tolerate drug therapy with probenecid (Benemid)?
    1. History of uric acid renal calculi
    2. Blood dyscrasias
    3. Chronic obstructive pulmonary disease
    4. Severe renal impairment

20. Because of its route of excretion, the nurse would be most careful in administering sulfinpyrazone (Anturane) to a client with which of the following health problems?
    1. Mild cirrhosis
    2. Renal insufficiency
    3. Migraine headaches
    4. Glaucoma

35 Drug Therapy for Renal System Dysfunction

STAYING ON TOP OF TERMINOLOGY

1. Complete the following word search.

ACUTE	EVALUATION
AZOTEMIA	FAILURE
BUN	FLUID
CHRONIC	HEMODIALYSIS
CREATININE	INTERVENTIONS
DIAGNOSIS	KIDNEY
DOSING	NURSING
DRUGS	PERITONEAL
EPOETIN	RENAL
ESRD	WEIGHT

```
A C K S D A X E D Q Q Q R Y Y
S N O I T N E V R E T N I A E
T N W S D T E X Q F H G H H A
O G S Y A N Q J W K G K R P P
R X H L L A E N O T I R E P A
D Q L A N E R Y U K E W T L C
L G N I S R U N G K W B M N U
X R Z D A B K Q N L I F C T X
H Z X O E J R W Z T C I E E J
H N B M U A B F A I L U R E F
H B E E L U C H R O N I C L D
C D S H N M A U D E V D U H C
T R G A E A Z O T E M I A T R
B N X C M S S D P E D A W V E
F A K C P I R O B U B G M S A
O P N X N L E D Y P Y N X G T
Y X B G E T Y Q R D P O G Q I
G S Q V I H R O D U D S R Z N
V M C N D T T V N U G I O A I
V G F R A R E Z D C O S T U N
U X Q N O I T A U L A V E S E
```

FOCUSING ON THE FACTS

2. Acute renal failure, or a rapid _____ in renal function, occurs in approximately _____ % of all hospitalized individuals.

3. Chronic renal failure is an _____ impairment of kidney function.

4. Azotemia is a build-up of _____.

5. End-stage renal disease leads to the need for _____, _____, or _____.

6. In peritoneal dialysis, needed _____ are passed into the bloodstream and _____ are removed, through the processes of _____, _____, and _____.

7. Two laboratory tests used to evaluate renal functioning are _____ and _____.

8. _____ is a procedure in which the blood is shunted from the body through a machine for _____ and _____ and then returned to the client's circulation.

9. In general the range of serum creatinine, which varies with age, is usually between _____ and _____ mg/dL and a normal BUN ranges between _____ and _____ mg/dL.

10. Drugs that are eliminated from the body primarily as _____ drug or as pharmacologically active _____ in the urine typically require dosage adjustment for clients with reduced renal function.

CONNECTING WITH CLIENTS

11. What signs and symptoms would you assess for in a client with chronic renal failure (CRF)?

12. What explanation would the nurse give to a client about why epoetin alfa is given for chronic renal failure (CRF)?

13. What two dosing methods for medications would the nurse anticipate being used for clients with renal insufficiency or impairment?

TRAINING FOR TEST TAKING

14. The nurse would question an order for which of the following types of antibiotics when ordered for a client with worsening renal insufficiency?
    1. Penicillins
    2. Cephalosporins
    3. Macrolides
    4. Aminoglycosides

15. A client with renal failure is taking calcium acetate (PhosLo). The nurse evaluates that the drug is having the anticipated effect if which of the following laboratory test results is noted?
    1. Calcium level less than 11.0 mg/dL
    2. Phosphorus level less than 6.0 mg/dL
    3. Potassium level less than 5.0 mEq/L
    4. Sodium level less than 145 mEq/L

16. The nurse provides anticipatory guidance to a client with renal failure taking calcium acetate (PhosLo) by explaining that which of the following will help to prevent the most frequent adverse drug effect?
    1. Increasing activity and fiber as allowed in the renal diet.
    2. Increasing fluid intake to 2 liters per day.
    3. Decreasing intake of milk and milk products.
    4. Decreasing nighttime driving.

17. Which of the following laboratory test results indicate that a client with end-stage renal disease would specifically benefit from drug therapy with sevelamer (Renagel)?
    1. Potassium level 5.8 mEq/L
    2. Magnesium level 4.9 mg/dL
    3. Calcium level 12.6 mg/dL
    4. Sodium level 154 mEq/L

18. The nurse instructs the nursing assistant to report any elevations in which vital sign in a client with end stage renal disease who is receiving epoetin alfa (Epogen)?
    1. Temperature
    2. Pulse
    3. Respirations
    4. Blood pressure

19. The nurse preparing to administer a dose of epoetin alfa (Epogen) to a client with renal failure would do which of the following to safely give the drug?
    1. Administer it by the IM route.
    2. Shake the vial to mix the contents.
    3. Discard any unused portion.
    4. Mix the dose with injectable iron for additive effects.

20. A client with renal failure who is receiving epoetin alfa (Epogen) has had a sudden rise in hematocrit. The nurse would place highest priority on assessing which of the following body systems for adverse effects?
    1. Neurologic
    2. Respiratory
    3. Gastrointestinal
    4. Genitourinary

36 Overview of the Respiratory System

STAYING ON TOP OF TERMINOLOGY

1. Match the definitions on the right to the terms below.

_____ Bronchial glands
_____ Bronchoconstriction
_____ Bronchodilation
_____ Cellular respiration
_____ Gas transport
_____ Mucokinesis

a. Involves the exchange of gases between the air in the lungs, the blood, and the cell
b. The process of moving mucus along the tracheobronchial tree
c. Involves the use of oxygen in the catabolism of energy-yielding substances for the production of energy
d. Secrete a relatively watery fluid through ducts leading to the surface of the ciliated epithelium
e. Results from relaxation of bronchial smooth muscle
f. A narrowing of the lumen of the bronchial airway.

FOCUSING ON THE FACTS

2. _____, one of the body's regulating systems, helps to maintain physiologic dynamic equilibrium.

3. The most urgent and critical need for maintaining life is a continued, uninterrupted supply of _____.

4. The products of the goblet cells and bronchial glands form the sol-gel film that makes up the _____ _____.

5. The normal adult produces approximately _____ mL of respiratory secretions per day and swallows this material without being aware of it.

6. Activation of the parasympathetics fiber (vagus nerve) of the tracheobronchial tree releases acetylcholine, which results in _____.

7. Most of the adrenergic receptors present in the bronchial smooth muscle are a_2 receptors that are stimulated mainly by _____ released from the adrenal medulla.

8. A xanthine drug such as theophylline may inhibit the action of _____ and prolong dilation of bronchial smooth muscle.

9. The basic rhythm for respiration is initiated and maintained in the medullary _____ area, which is located beneath the lower part of the floor of the _____ _____ in the medial half of the medulla.

10. The humoral regulation of respiration is achieved primarily through changes in the concentrations of _____, _____, or _____ _____ in body fluids.

11. An increase in the _____ _____ tension of the blood directly stimulates the inspiratory and expiratory centers, which increases both the rate and the depth of breathing.

12. The pH of the blood is determined by the ratio of _____ ions to _____ _____.

37 Bronchodilator, Antiasthmatic, and Mucolytic Drugs

STAYING ON TOP OF TERMINOLOGY

1. Match the definition on the right to the appropriate term on the left.

_____ Aerosol therapy
_____ Expectorant
_____ Mucokinetic agent
_____ Mucolytic agent
_____ Mucus
_____ Nebulizer
_____ Sputum
_____ Xanthine derivative

a. Serves to break down mucus
b. A proteinaceous material that has a mucopolysaccharide as its major component
c. An abnormal, viscous secretion that is an excretory production of the lower respiratory tree
d. Promotes the removal of abnormal or excessive respiratory tract secretions by thinning hyperviscous mucus
e. A device for producing a fine spray of water
f. Has central nervous system stimulatory properties, produce diuresis and relax smooth muscle
g. An agent that has mucokinetic and/or mucolytic properties
h. Uses a suspension of fine liquid or solid particles dispersed in a gas or in a solution that is deposited in the respiratory tract

FOCUSING ON THE FACTS

2. Asthma (also referred to as bronchial asthma) may involve bronchial smooth muscle _____, mucosal _____ or _____, and mucus _____.

3. With mild intermittent asthma, attacks occur less than _____ to _____ times weekly or nocturnal asthma symptoms occur less than _____ to _____ times monthly.

4. The xanthine group of drugs includes _____, _____, and _____.

5. Xanthines inhibit mast cell _____ and the release of _____ and other mediators that are responsible for _____.

6. Bronchodilators are used to treat _____.

7. The effectiveness of the _____ depends on their conversion to theophylline.

8. The rate of absorption of oral _____ depends on the dosage form used.

9. Treatments for asthma are based on the severity of the disorder and often include use of _____ agents in addition to bronchodilators.

10. The most commonly used bronchodilators are administered via the _____ route.

CONNECTING WITH CLIENTS

11. You have just received inter-shift report on a client who will be receiving aerosol therapy during the day. What do you recall about the effects of aerosol therapy on the respiratory system?

12. What nursing interventions do you need to implement for a client when acetylcysteine (Mucomyst) is administered for its antidotal use?

13. You are taking care of a client who has a new order for a medication that will be administered via metered dose inhaler. What steps would you teach the client to properly use this method of drug self-administration?

TRAINING FOR TEST TAKING

14. After reviewing the medication administration record for a client with asthma, the nurse concludes that which of the following concurrently ordered medications will likely decrease the effectiveness of albuterol (Proventil)?
    1. isoproterenol (Isuprel)
    2. propranolol (Inderal)
    3. phenelzine (Nardil)
    4. epinephrine (Adrenalin)

15. The nurse is instructing a client with asthma about the use of albuterol (Proventil) by metered dose inhaler. The nurse explains that when used by the inhalation route, the drug should have an effect in how much time?
    1. 30 seconds to 1 minute
    2. 1 to 2 minutes
    3. 3 to 5 minutes
    4. 5 to 15 minutes

16. A client is receiving ipratropium (Atrovent) by inhalation. The nurse expects that the client's medical history will reveal which of the following health problems?
    1. Chronic emphysema
    2. Status asthmaticus
    3. Acute bronchospasm
    4. Acetaminophen overdose

17. A client with asthma utilizes a combination of drugs by inhalation. The nurse teaches the client to rinse the mouth to prevent candidiasis after use of which of the following medications?
    1. terbutaline (Brethine)
    2. metaproterenol (Alupent)
    3. fluticasone (Flovent)
    4. tiotropium (Spiriva HandiHaler)

18. A client has been started on bronchodilator therapy with theophylline (Bronkodyl) by continuous intravenous infusion. The nurse noting the result of the first serum theophylline level would conclude that the drug is being appropriately dosed after reading which test result?
    1. 8 mg/L
    2. 17 mg/L
    3. 24 mg/L
    4. 31 mg/L

19. The nurse notes that a client has an order for dornase alfa (Pulmozyme). The nurse concludes that this client has a diagnosis of which of the following?
    1. Asthma
    2. Chronic bronchitis
    3. Emphysema
    4. Cystic fibrosis

20. A client has an order to take three inhalers at 09:00: ipratropium (Atrovent), albuterol (Proventil), and beclomethasone (Vanceril). Which medication should be used first?
    1. ipratropium
    2. albuterol
    3. beclomethasone
    4. Any; the order is not important

38 Oxygen and Miscellaneous Respiratory Agents

STAYING ON TOP OF TERMINOLOGY

1. Match the definition on the right to the term at the left.

_____ Analeptics	a. Inadequate cellular oxygen
_____ diphenhydramine	b. High carbon dioxide content in the blood
_____ Hypercapnia	c. Passage of light of differing wavelengths through living tissue to analyze differences in absorption
_____ Hypoxemia	
_____ Hypoxia	
_____ Pulse oximetry	d. A broad classification of CNS stimulants
	e. A generic name for an antihistamine
	f. Diminished oxygen tension in the blood

FOCUSING ON THE FACTS

2. Pulse oximetry provides a continuous reading of _____.

3. Of all the tissues affected by _____, or oxygen lack, the _____ is the most susceptible to disruption of normal function and irreversible damage.

4. Individuals with _____ are subject to _____, which is high carbon dioxide content in the blood.

5. Tachypnea is defined as an _____ and may indicate the need for _____.

6. Oxygen is a/an _____, _____, and _____ gas that is essential for _____.

7. Carbon dioxide is a/an _____, _____ gas; when used as a pharmacologic agent it affects _____, _____, and the _____.

8. If an _____ antitussive agent is given with a CNS-_____, a reduced dosage should be used.

9. The rate of oxygen consumption by the kidneys is more than most other tissues and it is primarily used for _____ _____.

10. Exposure to 100% oxygen for a period of 6 hours causes an _____ response with subsequent destruction of the _____ membrane of the respiratory tract.

CONNECTING WITH CLIENTS

11. You learn in inter-shift report that your client will be beginning oxygen therapy. As you wait for report to end, can you recall and identify the seven methods of oxygen administration?

12. What should you include in a teaching plan for a client who will be taking an antihistamine?

13. You learn that an assigned client is being considered for hyperbaric oxygen therapy. For what conditions might this therapy be considered?

TRAINING FOR TEST TAKING

14. The nurse has an order to apply oxygen to a client who suffered smoke inhalation in a fire. The nurse anticipates that which of the following methods of oxygen delivery will be utilized for this client?
1. Simple face mask
2. Ventimask
3. Nonrebreathing mask
4. Nasal cannula

15. A unit secretary asks the nurse why it is so important to be careful of the amount of oxygen given to premature infants. The nurse explains that excessive oxygen could lead to which problem for the infant?
1. Hirschsprung's disease
2. Wilm's tumor
3. Acute renal failure
4. Retrolental fibroplasia

16. Which of the following data assessed by the nurse indicates the most favorable outcome of oxygen therapy for an adult client?
1. Pao_2 of 85 mm Hg
2. $Paco_2$ 48 mm Hg
3. pH 7.33
4. Respiratory rate 22 breaths/min

17. Which of the following points would the nurse include in a teaching plan for the client going home with oxygen therapy ordered?
1. Check the equipment at least once per week.
2. Avoid the use of electrical appliances in the vicinity of the oxygen.
3. Make sure that no one smokes or lights a match within 6 feet of oxygen.
4. Put a small amount of Vaseline around the nose or mouth to prevent drying.

18. The nurse notes that a client is receiving benzonatate (Tessalon Perles). The nurse concludes that the drug is having the anticipated benefit after noting that the client no longer has which manifestation?
    1. Hoarse voice
    2. Adventitious lung sounds
    3. Nonproductive cough
    4. Dry nasal passages

19. The nurse is discussing the effects of diphenhydramine (Benadryl) with a client. About which most frequent adverse effect would the nurse be sure to advise the client?
    1. Excessive mouth watering
    2. Urinary urgency
    3. Diarrhea
    4. Sleepiness

20. A client has a new prescription for fluticasone nasal (Flonase). What instructions should be given to the client regarding self-administration by the nasal route?
    1. Blow the nose before delivering the spray.
    2. Aim the spray toward the nasal septum.
    3. It may take one week before experiencing full benefits.
    4. Avoid the use of any topical decongestants.

39 Overview of the Gastrointestinal Tract

1. Match the disorder/disease to the anatomic site in the GI system.

_____ Gingivitis   a. Mouth
_____ Gastritis   b. Esophagus
_____ Achalasia   c. Stomach
_____ Hepatitis   d. Small intestine
_____ Malabsorption   e. Large intestine
_____ Diabetes   f. Liver
_____ Diverticulitis   g. Gallbladder
_____ Peptic ulcer   h. Pancreas
_____ Colitis
_____ Cholelithiasis
_____ Constipation
_____ Hemorrhoids

FOCUSING ON THE FACTS

2. Food substances entering the alimentary canal undergo _____ and _____ changes called _____.

3. Deglutition is also called _____.

4. Difficulty in swallowing is known as _____.

5. The peristaltic process is the squeezing of the _____ down the _____; it is accomplished by _____.

6. Cholecystitis is _____ of the gallbladder; it is often associated with the presence of _____.

7. The alimentary canal extends from the _____ to the _____.

8. Drugs affecting the GI tract exert their action mainly on _____ and _____ tissues.

9. _____ diseases, _____ deficiencies, and _____ trauma can cause irritation or inflammation of the buccal structures of the mouth.

10. Esophageal disorders are characterized by _____ _____ or _____ and difficulty in _____.

11. The time required for digestion in the stomach depends on the amount of _____ eaten. Normal emptying time is _____ to _____ hours.

12. Biotransformation of drugs in the liver is accomplished by the _____ _____ enzyme system.

Drugs Affecting the Gastrointestinal Tract

STAYING ON TOP OF TERMINOLOGY

1. Match the antiemetic with its proposed site of action.

_____ diazepam	a. Emetic center
_____ diphenidol	b. Chemoreceptor trigger zone
_____ Antihistamines	c. Cerebral cortex
_____ Anticholinergics	d. Peripheral sites
_____ phenothiazine	

FOCUSING ON THE FACTS

2. Treatment of oral candidiasis includes both _____ treatments (nystatin oral rinse, clotrimazole troches or lozenges) and _____ administered antifungals.

3. Xerostomia, or dry mouth, can be caused by a number of conditions, but is often a complication of _____ drug therapy.

4. A number of drugs or foods decrease _____ _____ _____ tone, which worsens symptoms of gastroesophageal reflux disease (GERD).

5. The H$_2$ blockers are somewhat less effective in gastric acid suppression when compared to the _____ _____ inhibitors.

6. Antacids are chemical compounds that buffer or neutralize _____ _____ in the stomach and thereby _____ gastric pH.

7. It has been recommended that all persons with a non–drug-induced _____ ulcer be treated with a combination of _____ and _____ _____ _____ to eradicate *H. pylori*.

8. Antacids that contain magnesium may cause_____, whereas aluminum- and calcium-containing antacids tend to cause _____.

9. Misoprostol, a gastric mucosa–protecting agent, is indicated for the prevention of gastric ulcers associated with the use of _____ _____ _____.

10. Pancrelipase contains the enzymes _____, _____ and _____, and is indicated for clients with _____ _____ and _____ _____.

CONNECTING WITH CLIENTS

11. What information would be important for you to share with a parent who is using a mouthwash containing alcohol?

12. What nursing interventions should you consider implementing for a client who is receiving metoclopramide (Reglan)?

13. What are the most frequent adverse effects of ondansetron that should be assessed in your postoperative client?

TRAINING FOR TEST TAKING

14. A hospitalized client has physician orders to receive antacid therapy and digoxin as part of the medication regimen. If the client needs to take the antacid at 09:00, for what time should the nurse schedule the daily dose of digoxin?
    1. 08:00
    2. 08:30
    3. 09:00
    4. 10:00

15. A hospitalized client who has a duodenal ulcer receives a dietary tray on the nursing unit at 08:00, 12:00, and 17:00. In addition to the bedtime dose, the nurse should schedule the doses of sucralfate (Carafate) on the medication administration record for which of the following optimal times?
    1. 06:00, 10:00, 15:00
    2. 07:00, 11:00, 16:00
    3. 08:00, 12:00, 17:00
    4. 09:00, 13:00, 18:00

16. The nurse is explaining to an adult client the use of a scopolamine (Transderm-Scop) patch. Which of the following instructions should the nurse give the client?
    1. Change the patch every 5 days and apply it to the abdomen.
    2. Change the patch every 5 days and apply it to the upper arm.
    3. Change the patch every 3 days and apply it to the area behind the ear.
    4. Change the patch every 3 days and apply it to any area free of excessive hair.

17. Which of the following would be an appropriate goal of therapy for a client receiving ursodiol (Actigall)?
    1. Remains free of symptoms of gastroesophageal reflux without experiencing adverse drug effects.
    2. Remains free of diarrhea without experiencing adverse drug effects.
    3. Remains free of nausea and vomiting without experiencing adverse drug effects.
    4. Remain free of biliary colic and other abdominal discomfort without experiencing adverse drug effects.

18. A client with inflammatory bowel disease is being considered drug therapy with sulfasalazine (Azulfidine). The nurse would alert the physician if the client reported an allergy to which of the following during the admission history?
    1. Oral sulfonylureas
    2. Acetaminophen
    3. Potassium-sparing diuretics
    4. β-adrenergic blocking agents

19. The nurse has provided medication instructions to a client who will be using diphenoxylate and atropine (Lomotil) for treatment of diarrhea. The client demonstrates proper understanding of the use of this drug if the client states to:
    1. Use the medication until diarrhea and abdominal cramping have completely subsided.
    2. Stop the medication and call the prescriber if diarrhea continues longer than 2 days.
    3. Continue the medication for at least 24 hours after fever is resolved.
    4. Take the medication as needed for diarrhea, up to 6 doses per day.

20. A client with a peptic ulcer requires drug therapy with a H_2 receptor blocker. The client is an older adult who has mild renal insufficiency. The nurse anticipates that the client would probably not be a candidate for which of the following drugs?
    1. cimetidine (Tagamet)
    2. ranitidine (Zantac)
    3. famotidine (Pepcid)
    4. nizatidine (Axid)

41 Overview of the Eye

1. Match the definition on the right to the term at the left.

_____ Accommodation	a.	The anterior covering of the eye
_____ Cataract	b.	Constriction of the pupil
_____ Cornea	c.	Lens opaqueness and loss of transparency
_____ Cycloplegia	d.	Dilation of the pupil
_____ Miosis	e.	A change in the shape of the lens to adjust to variations in distance
_____ Mydriasis	f.	Paralysis of the ciliary muscle

FOCUSING ON THE FACTS

2. The eye is the _____ organ for the sense of _____.

3. The cornea is the _____ covering of the eye; it is normally _____, so it allows_____ to enter the eye.

4. Contraction of the sphincter muscle causes _____ of the pupil, also known as _____.

5. Contraction of the dilator muscle causes _____ of the pupil, also known as _____.

6. Accommodation occurs when the lens changes _____, which ensures that the image on the retina is _____.

7. With age the lens may lose its _____ and become _____; this is known as a _____.

8. _____ stimulation accommodates the eye for near vision.

9. A trabecular meshwork called the _____ of _____ drains the aqueous humor into the venous system of the eye.

10. The retina contains nerve endings plus the _____ and _____ that function as visual sensory receptors.

11. _____, which is bilateral, occurs every few seconds during the waking hours.

12. Tear fluid is lost by evaporation and by draining into the _____ _____ at the inner corners of the upper and lower eyelids.

42 Ophthalmic Drugs

STAYING ON TOP OF TERMINOLOGY

1. Match the definition on the right to the term at the left.

_____ Chalazion
_____ Conjunctivitis
_____ Hordeolum
_____ Keratitis
_____ Uveitis

a. Acute inflammation of the conjunctiva
b. Corneal inflammation caused by bacterial infection
c. Infection of the uveal tract, or vascular layer of the eye
d. Infection of the meibomian (sebaceous) glands of the eyelids.
e. Acute localized infection of the eyelash follicles and glands of the anterior lid margin

FOCUSING ON THE FACTS

2. Glaucoma is characterized by _____; it can lead to _____.

3. Miotics are useful in treating _____ and _____.

4. Anticholinesterase drugs inhibit _____ by _____.

5. Three major types of glaucoma are _____, _____, and _____.

6. Ocular drugs are administered by topical application of a _____ or _____.

7. _____ _____ are not to be worn during eye infections.

8. If two or more family members are using eye medications, each should have a separate vial to prevent_____-_____.

9. Systemic effects of ocular β-adrenergic ophthalmic drugs can be minimized by applying pressure for _____ to _____ seconds over the _____ _____ next to the nose.

10. Prostaglandins agonists are useful in treating glaucoma because they reduce _____ _____ by increasing _____ _____ outflow.

CONNECTING WITH CLIENTS

11. You are caring for a client who is receiving ophthalmic drugs. What are four possible nursing diagnoses that could apply to this client?

12. A pediatric client has an order for an eye ointment. How would you administer this drug?

13. What adverse systemic effects would you assess for in a client receiving a β-blocking antiglaucoma agent?

TRAINING FOR TEST TAKING

14. A client taking ophthalmic medication to treat glaucoma has listened to instructions regarding use of the medication. The nurse evaluates that the client has an appropriate understanding when the client states to use a new bottle every:
    1. 2 weeks.
    2. month.
    3. 3 months.
    4. 6 months.

15. An immunocompromised client has been prescribed sulfacetamide (Sulamyd) for treatment of an eye infection. The home health nurse would assess this client for which of the following less frequent but serious adverse effect of this medication?
    1. Local allergic reaction
    2. Conjunctivitis
    3. Burning sensation with application
    4. Stevens-Johnson syndrome

16. The nurse notes a client drug order for ophthalmic betamethasone (Betnesol). The nurse checks the client's medical record for documentation about which of the following ocular problems?
    1. Bacterial conjunctivitis
    2. Minor corneal abrasion
    3. Allergic inflammation of the anterior eye
    4. Chronic open-angle glaucoma

17. The nurse working with a group of older adults concludes that the client taking which antiglaucoma medication has had the least success in controlling intraocular pressure with first-line drugs?
    1. isoflurophate (Floropryl)
    2. pilocarpine (Pilocar)
    3. timolol (Timoptic)
    4. dipivefrin (Propine)

18. A client taking timolol (Timoptic) needs to reduce the risk of systemic absorption of the drug. The nurse teaches this client to do which of the following?
    1. Move the eyeball inside the closed lid for 1 minute after instillation.
    2. Hold pressure over the inner canthus for 30 second to 1 minute after instillation.
    3. Massage over the upper eyelid for 10 to 15 seconds.
    4. Press upward on the lower conjunctival sac to push excess medication up and out.

19. The nurse would administer a dose of ophthalmic tetracaine (Pontocaine) to which of the following clients?
    1. A client who has glaucoma.
    2. A client who will undergo tonometry.
    3. A client who will have cataract surgery.
    4. A client who has a detached retina.

20. The urgent care nurse would prepare which of the following medications for use in a client who needs diagnostic testing to determine whether there is a foreign body in the eye?
    1. ketotifen fumarate (Zaditor)
    2. levocabastine (Livostin)
    3. fluorescein (Fluorescite)
    4. lodoxamide (Alomide)

43 Overview of the Ear

STAYING ON TOP OF TERMINOLOGY

1. Match the ear disorder to its anatomic site.

_____ Seborrhea   a. External ear
_____ Otosclerosis   b. Middle ear
_____ Otitis media   c. Inner ear
_____ Tympanic perforation
_____ Meniere's disease

FOCUSING ON THE FACTS

2. The tympanic membrane is a/an _____ located between the _____ and _____.

3. The Eustachian tube connects the _____ and the _____; it is usually collapsed except when _____.

4. The auditory ossicles are the _____, _____, and _____; the ossicles amplify and transmit _____.

5. The primary organ of hearing is the _____.

6. The three divisions of the ear are called the _____, _____, and _____ ear.

7. The _____ _____ protects the middle ear from foreign substances and transmits sound to the bones of the middle ear.

8. The _____ _____ of the inner ear consists of the vestibule, cochlea, and semicircular canals.

9. The _____ _____ of the inner ear consists of a series of sacs and tubes within the bony labyrinth.

10. The most common ear disorders include _____ of the ear, _____ accumulation, and various other painful or distressing conditions.

11. The most commonly reported problem of the middle ear is inflammation, known as _____ _____.

12. Genetic diseases or slowly progressive diseases such as _____ or _____ disease may cause hearing deficits.

44 Drugs Affecting the Ear

STAYING ON TOP OF TERMINOLOGY

1. Match the definition on the right to the term at the left.

_____ Cerumen   a. An adverse drug effect on hearing, balance, or both
_____ Ototoxicity   b. Ringing or buzzing sound in the ears
_____ Tinnitus   c. Earwax
_____ Vertigo   d. A feeling that the room is in motion

FOCUSING ON THE FACTS

2. Antibiotic ear preparations are used as _____ agents to treat infections of the _____ _____ _____ surface.

3. Clients often refer to otitis externa as "_____ _____."

4. Before instilling eardrops, assess that the ear canal is clear and not impacted with _____ and that the _____ _____ is intact.

5. Cochlear _____ causes a progressive or continuing hearing loss.

6. Antimicrobial ophthalmic preparations, although less viscous than otic preparations, are also safe to use in the ear if the _____ _____ is intact.

7. Ciprofloxacin is a _____ type of antibacterial effective against gram-negative and some gram-positive pathogens.

8. _____, _____ oil and _____ oil are used as emollients to help relieve itching and burning in the ear.

9. To identify areas for education, assess the client requiring an otic drug for improper _____ or _____ practices that may contribute to the development of infections.

10. Eardrops are more comfortably tolerated if they are _____ (if not contraindicated) before instillation.

11. A client is receiving chloramphenicol. For what adverse effects would you assess this client?

12. How would you administer ear drops to an adult? What would you do differently if the client was a child?

13. What monitoring, intervention, and education would you consider for a client receiving a drug that can cause ototoxicity?

TRAINING FOR TEST TAKING

14. A client requires an otic preparation containing hydrocortisone. The nurse determines that the client understands the action of the medication when the client states that the hydrocortisone will decrease which of the following?
    1. Risk of hearing loss
    2. The density of cerumen
    3. The number of bacteria
    4. Inflammation and pain

15. The nurse would assess a client taking an ototoxic drug for which sign of cochlear damage?
    1. Hearing loss
    2. Vertigo
    3. Ataxia
    4. Headache

16. The pediatric nurse has provided instruction to a parent of a 2-year-old child requiring the use of eardrops. Which statement about manipulating the pinna indicates correct understanding of the procedure for instillation?
    1. Pull the pinna down and back.
    2. Pull the pinna down and forward.
    3. Pull the pinna up and back.
    4. Pull the pinna up and forward.

17. A client has received a prescription for an otic medication to treat an outer ear infection. In addition to specific points about the antibiotic, the nurse would include which piece of general information about otic medications?
    1. Use the drug whenever ear pain occurs.
    2. Lie on the side for 5 minutes after instillation.
    3. Gently massage the area immediately behind the ear before instillation
    4. Expect that symptoms may worsen temporarily for 24 hours.

18. A client telephones the ambulatory clinic reporting irritating amounts of earwax. The nurse initially recommends which of the following over-the-counter (OTC) products?
    1. isopropyl alcohol in glycerin (Swim-Ear Drops)
    2. boric acid and isopropyl alcohol (Auro-Dri Eardrops)
    3. carbamide peroxide and glycerin (E.R.O. Ear Drops, Murine Ear)
    4. hydrocortisone, propylene glycol, alcohol, benzyl benzoate (EarSol-HC Drops)

19. The nurse is most concerned about irreversible hearing loss in a client taking which of the following medications?
    1. aspirin
    2. clarithromycin
    3. furosemide
    4. ethacrynic acid

20. The nurse would place highest priority on assessing for hearing loss or problems with balance in a client receiving which of the following types of antibiotics?
    1. penicillin
    2. cephalosporin
    3. aminoglycoside
    4. sulfonamide

45 Overview of the Endocrine System

STAYING ON TOP OF TERMINOLOGY

1. Fill in the various endocrine glands on the following picture.

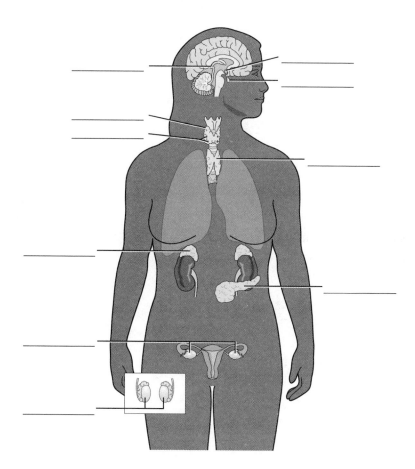

FOCUSING ON THE FACTS

2. _____ are active, natural chemical substances secreted into the blood-stream from the endocrine glands.

3. The major types of hormones are the _____ hormones and the hormones derived from _____ _____.

4. To maintain the internal environment, hormone secretion is controlled by a self-regulating series of events known as _____ _____.

5. The excretion of hormones is primarily via the _____ and, to a lesser extent, the _____.

6. Research in endocrinology has advanced the concept of specific _____ within or on the surface of cells, which has led to knowledge of hormone _____.

7. The central nervous system may play a decisive role in regulating pituitary function to meet environmental demands through activity of the_____.

8. The thyroid gland, one of the most richly vascularized tissues of the body, secretes three hormones essential for the proper regulation of metabolism: _____, _____, and _____.

9. The synthesis of the thyroid hormones and their maintenance in the blood in adequate amounts depend largely on an adequate intake of _____.

10. The primary function of the parathyroid glands is to maintain adequate levels of _____ in the extracellular fluid.

11. The adrenal cortex synthesizes three important classes of hormones: the _____, _____, and _____.

12. _____ is a hormone secreted by the beta cells of the islets of Langerhans in the pancreas in response to increased levels of glucose in the blood.

46 Drugs Affecting the Pituitary

STAYING ON TOP OF TERMINOLOGY

1. Complete the following word search.

ABUSE
ACTH
ALLERGIC
ANTERIOR
CONFUSION
CRH
DIABETES
DWARFISM
ELECTROLYTES
ENDOCRINE
GIGANTISM
GONADOTROPIN
HORMONE

HUMATROPE
INSIPIDUS
LH
NURSING
PITUITARY
POSTERIOR
SOMATOSTATIN
SOMATREM
TRH
TSH
URINE
VASOPRESSIN

```
E  A  A  N  T  E  R  I  O  R  C  C  J  M  R  I  Y  I  H
L  C  M  B  P  R  W  O  S  A  O  D  P  K  I  X  P  L  U
E  T  J  I  U  C  H  Q  L  N  D  I  O  U  N  X  I  M  M
C  H  S  T  E  S  W  L  F  K  W  A  S  L  S  V  T  E  A
T  O  F  T  L  Y  E  U  J  K  A  B  T  S  I  E  U  R  T
R  R  V  N  F  R  S  Q  U  R  R  E  E  O  P  I  I  T  R
O  M  H  P  G  I  U  L  K  I  F  T  R  M  I  X  T  A  O
L  O  R  I  O  I  S  C  R  S  I  E  I  A  D  V  A  M  P
Y  N  C  N  F  M  Z  C  H  J  S  S  O  T  U  R  R  O  E
T  E  N  I  R  C  O  D  N  E  M  J  R  O  S  M  Y  S  F
E  B  S  G  I  G  A  N  T  I  S  M  L  S  L  Z  R  M  X
S  N  U  R  S  I  N  G  O  N  A  D  O  T  R  O  P  I  N
E  N  I  S  S  E  R  P  O  S  A  V  O  A  C  K  J  M  F
K  X  G  R  K  W  U  B  Y  A  N  X  V  T  H  C  W  Q  O
W  E  X  Z  U  S  A  T  T  I  E  J  N  I  R  J  M  X  X
D  I  C  X  D  S  I  C  G  P  V  Y  E  N  A  A  X  M  O
```

FOCUSING ON THE FACTS

2. The anterior pituitary is responsible for secreting hormones that affect _____.

3. _____ and _____ are synthetic derivatives of human growth hormone.

4. The anabolic effects of somatrem result from the indirect effect of other hormones known as _____ or _____-_____ growth factors (IGF-1).

5. The anterior pituitary hormones include _____ hormone, _____, _____, _____-_____ hormone, _____ hormone, and _____.

6. The posterior pituitary hormones are _____ and _____.

7. Growth hormone is also contraindicated in clients with closed _____ or in those with a known sensitivity to _____ _____, such as neonates.

8. One difference between somatostatin and octreotide is that octreotide is a more potent inhibitor of _____ hormone, _____, and _____.

9. The ADH effect of vasopressin is the result of increasing _____ _____ in the _____ _____ of the nephron.

10. In addition to diabetes insipidus, desmopressin is also frequently used for the treatment of _____ _____.

CONNECTING WITH CLIENTS

11. Your client has just begun drug therapy with vasopressin. What adverse drug effects would assess for in this client?

12. You are assigned to a pediatric client who is beginning drug therapy with somatrem. What are the nursing considerations related to monitoring, nursing care, and client education?

13. An adolescent client has been abusing growth hormone to aid in performance during sporting events. In addition to the drug's adverse effects, what risks would you teach this client about this practice?

TRAINING FOR TEST TAKING

14. A child in the endocrine clinic is taking somatrem (Protropin). The nurse would assess this client for which adverse effect that indicates excessive dosing?
    1. Excessive growth rate
    2. Exophthalmus
    3. Hyperglycemia
    4. Hyperthyroidism

15. A client taking pegvisomant (Somavert) would be monitored for its effects on which health problem for which it is prescribed?
    1. Dwarfism
    2. Acromegaly
    3. Diabetes insipidus
    4. Syndrome of inappropriate ADH

16. A client is taking norditropin in the form of the NordiPen delivery system. The client should be instructed by the nurse to take this medication at which of the following times of day?
    1. On awakening
    2. After breakfast
    3. Before supper
    4. Bedtime

17. The nurse in the intensive care unit notes that some doses of vasopressin (Pitressin) have arrived in the unit's pharmacy "in" box. The nurse anticipates that this medication has been ordered for the client with which of the following problems?
    1. Heart failure
    2. Cerebrovascular accident
    3. Active GI bleeding
    4. Hypertensive crisis

18. The nurse concludes that which of the following outcomes for a client receiving vasopressin (Pitressin) would be unrelated to the effects of this drug?
    1. Decreased thirst
    2. Decreased urine specific gravity
    3. Resolution of signs of dehydration
    4. Decreased urine output

19. A physician has prescribed desmopressin (DDAVP) for a child experiencing nocturnal enuresis. The caregiver telephones the clinic and states that the child is complaining of headache and is excessively sleepy. The nurse alerts the physician because the client is most likely experiencing which of the following adverse drug effects?
    1. Hypernatremia
    2. Water intoxication
    3. Dehydration
    4. Hypoglycemia

20. A client has been receiving desmopressin (DDAVP). The nurse evaluates that the client is having the expected effect of therapy if which of the following changes is noted in assessment data?
    1. Pulse rate increased from 70 to 78
    2. Blood pressure decreased from 140/90 to 132/86 mm Hg
    3. Urine output 80 mL/hr decreased from 150 mL/hr
    4. Blood glucose 124mg/dL decreased from 189 mg/dL

STAYING ON TOP OF TERMINOLOGY

1. Match the sign or symptom to the endocrine disorder.

_____ Diarrhea	a.	Hyperthyroidism
_____ Renal stones	b.	Hypothyroidism
_____ Brittle hair	c.	Hyperparathyroidism
_____ Fast reflexes	d.	Hypoparathyroidism
_____ Irritability		
_____ Calcium level decreased		
_____ Ptosis		
_____ Lethargic		
_____ Cold, dry skin		
_____ Bone pain		
_____ Intolerance to heat		

FOCUSING ON THE FACTS

2. Adenomas are tumors often seen in _____ _____.

3. _____ is the most commonly used treatment in North America for hypothyroidism.

4. Iodine is the oldest of the _____ drugs; it inhibits _____.

5. Myxedema is a form of _____.

6. Radioactive iodine, or RAI, is preferred for clients who are poor _____ _____, those with advanced _____ _____, and _____ clients.

7. In idiopathic hypoparathyroidism, serum calcium levels are _____ and serum phosphate levels are _____.

8. In addition to primary hyperparathyroidism, another important etiology of hypercalcemia is the presence of _____ with or without _____ _____.

9. Drugs to treat hypercalcemia include modalities to increase calcium _____ (e.g., hydration, diuretics) and drugs to alter calcium _____ from bone.

10. The primary options for treatment of hyperthyroidism are _____ drugs, _____ , and _____ .

CONNECTING WITH CLIENTS

11. What two medications would you expect to be used to increase serum calcium levels in an assigned client who has hypoparathyroidism?

12. You note that the medication administration record indicates a client is receiving zoledronic acid (Zometa). For what two conditions might this client be receiving this drug?

13. What teaching needs would you expect to address for a client receiving sodium iodide ^{131}I?

TRAINING FOR TEST TAKING

14. A client who has started parenteral drug therapy with calcitonin (Miacalcin) as treatment for hypercalcemia reports nausea and flushing. The nurse takes which of the following actions to assist the client?
    1. Encourage the client to drink increased fluids.
    2. Change the administration time to bedtime.
    3. Encourage increased protein intake in the diet.
    4. Move the client's bed to one near the door rather than the window.

15. A client asks how etidronate (Didronel) is going to lower her calcium level. The nurse considers which of the following explanations when formulating an answer?
    1. It alters absorption of vitamin D in the gastrointestinal tract.
    2. It inhibits absorption of calcium in the gastrointestinal tract.
    3. It indirectly affects calcium by changing the serum phosphorus level.
    4. It inhibits bone resorption by reducing activity of osteoclasts.

16. A client with osteoporosis has been prescribed alendronate (Fosamax). The client indicates understanding of proper use of this medication by stating which of the following?
    1. Take the medication at bedtime.
    2. Take the medication with the first meal of the day.
    3. Sit upright for at least 30 minutes after taking the dose.
    4. Refrain from vigorous exercise for one hour after taking the dose.

17. A client with hypothyroidism has begun treatment with levothyroxine. The nurse explains that which of the following signs indicate an overdosage?
    1. Tachycardia, nervousness, and chest pain
    2. Dry skin, weight gain, and tremors
    3. Bradycardia, sleepiness, and ataxic gait
    4. Constipation, lethargy, and increased sweating

18. A client admitted to the hospital with a history of hypothyroidism and hyperlipidemia is taking levothyroxine (Synthroid) and cholestyramine (Questran). If the standard daily dosage time for levothyroxine is 7am, the nurse should optimally schedule the dose of cholestyramine for which of the following optimal times?
    1. 8 AM
    2. 9 AM
    3. 10 AM
    4. 12 noon

19. A client will be receiving radioactive iodine therapy with sodium iodide 131 (Iodotope). The nurse should explain to the client the need for which of the following interventions during drug therapy?
    1. Triple flushing the toilet
    2. Wearing vinyl gloves during administration
    3. Using disposal meal trays, dishes, and utensils
    4. Limit fluid intake to 1500 mL

20. The nurse teaches the client taking propylthiouracil (Propyl-Thyracil) about which of the following adverse effects of drug therapy?
    1. Diarrhea
    2. Fever
    3. Headaches
    4. Excessive thirst

48 Drugs Affecting the Adrenal Cortex

STAYING ON TOP OF TERMINOLOGY

1. Match the definition on the right with the term to the left.

_____ Circadian rhythm
_____ Corticosteroids
_____ Glucocorticoid
_____ Mineralocorticoid
_____ Septic shock
_____ Ultradian rhythm

a. Are synthesized from cholesterol and stored in the adrenal cortex
b. Usually results from a gram-negative bacteremia that leads to circulatory insufficiency
c. Aldosterone is the main hormone of this type
d. A pattern based on a 24-hour cycle with the repetition of certain physiologic phenomena
e. A periodic or intermittent function with a frequency greater than once every 24 hours
f. Hydrocortisone, or cortisol, is the primary hormone of this type

FOCUSING ON THE FACTS

2. Corticosteroids are adrenocortical _____ that are divided into two classes, _____ and _____ .

3. Circadian rhythm appears to be controlled by the _____-_____ and _____-_____ cycles.

4. _____ is secreted in times of physiologic stress.

5. The glucocorticoids are often administered for their _____ activity.

6. Corticosteroids are synthesized from _____ and stored in the _____ _____ .

7. When exogenous corticosteroids are administered for sustained periods of time (e.g., beyond 10 to 14 days), it leads to the suppression of _____-_____ hormone and _____ hormone.

8. During stress, _____ and _____ are released from the adrenal medulla, and have a synergistic action with the corticosteroids.

169

9. Mineralocorticoids are secreted by the adrenal cortex to increase the rate of _____ reabsorption by the kidneys,

10. Acute withdrawal of chronically administered corticosteroids can lead to acute _____ crisis.

CONNECTING WITH CLIENTS

11. Your client needs to begin drug therapy with a glucocorticoid. What three actions of glucocorticoids are likely to affect this client?

12. What adverse effects would you look for in a client receiving an adrenocorticoid drug on the gastrointestinal, immune, and musculoskeletal systems?

13. What important assessment information would you obtain in a client receiving aminoglutethimide (Cytadren)?

TRAINING FOR TEST TAKING

14. A client has a new order to begin drug therapy with prednisone (Deltasone). The nurse anticipates that the pattern of administration of the daily dose will be which of the following?
    1. All medication will be given as a single dose in the morning
    2. Half of the dose will be given in the morning and half in the evening.
    3. Two-thirds of the dose will be given in the morning and one-third in the evening.
    4. One-third of the dose will be given in the morning and two-thirds in the evening.

15. The nurse assessing for adverse effects of prednisone (Deltasone) would look for which of the following in the client?
    1. Euphoria
    2. Low blood glucose levels
    3. Dehydration
    4. Hypertension

16. The nurse assesses the laboratory test results for a client taking prednisone (Deltasone). Which of the following laboratory results is an expected change based on adverse effects of this medication?
    1. Serum sodium 145 mEq/L
    2. Blood glucose 192 mEq/L
    3. Potassium level 3.5 mEq/L
    4. Blood urea nitrogen 30 mg/dL

17. The nurse providing anticipatory guidance about the adverse effects of glucocorticoids to a female client would explain that this type of drug could cause which of the following?
    1. Sunken eyes
    2. Increased muscle mass
    3. Thickening of torso
    4. Thickened skin

18. A client is just beginning a course of glucocorticoid therapy with dexamethasone (Decadron). The nurse would suggest which of the following dietary adjustments based on knowledge of drug effects?
    1. Add foods high in sodium.
    2. Add foods low in potassium.
    3. Reduce intake of alcohol.
    4. Do not increase current intake of caffeine.

19. A client is receiving aminoglutethimide (Cytadren). The nurse anticipates that the client may have which of the following disorders?
    1. Addison's disease
    2. Adrenal carcinoma
    3. Insufficient ACTH production
    4. Pheochromocytoma

20. A client is taking fludrocortisone (Florinef). The nurse determines that therapy is most effective if the client has which of the following outcomes?
    1. Shows no signs of Addison's disease.
    2. Eats a high sodium diet.
    3. Has minimal fluid volume deficit.
    4. Has normal blood glucose results.

171

Chapter **48** **Drugs Affecting the Adrenal Cortex**

49 Drugs Affecting Conditions of the Pancreas

STAYING ON TOP OF TERMINOLOGY

1. Match the sign or symptom to the blood glucose disorder.

_____ Cold sweating   a. Hyperglycemia
_____ Thirst   b. Hypoglycemia
_____ Polyuria
_____ Pallor
_____ Blurred vision
_____ Anxiety
_____ Fruity breath

FOCUSING ON THE FACTS

2. The two primary hormones released by the pancreas are _____ and _____ .

3. The process in which the liver breaks down and releases its glucose stores is called _____; the production of glucose is called _____ .

4. Diabetes mellitus is a disorder of _____ metabolism that involves an insulin _____, insulin _____, or both.

5. Clients with type 1 diabetes have very little or usually no production of _____ insulin.

6. The age of onset for type 2 diabetes is usually after _____ years, and approximately _____% of the diabetes cases are type 2.

7. The treatment of diabetes mellitus usually includes _____, _____, and, if necessary, _____ .

8. In the absence of insulin, glucose cannot enter the cell, so _____ _____ _____ are used in metabolism, resulting in acidosis and ketosis.

9. The high urine glucose in diabetes mellitus serves as an osmotic diuretic leading to _____ and _____ disturbances.

10. Clients with diabetic ketoacidosis may exhibit _____, _____ respirations (Kussmaul breathing) in an attempt to "blow off" _____ _____.

CONNECTING WITH CLIENTS

11. How would you teach a client with diabetes mellitus who is beginning insulin therapy about intrasite rotation of insulin injection sites?

12. A client with diabetes tends to have recurrent episodes of low blood glucose while the medication regimen is adjusted. What "quick fixes" would you teach the client for mild hypoglycemia?

13. What information would you consider when formulating an explanation to a client about how oral hypoglycemic agents lower blood glucose?

TRAINING FOR TEST TAKING

14. Dietary breakfast trays generally arrive on the nursing unit at 08:00. The nurse plans to administer a dose of regular insulin to the client between which of the following times?
    1. 08:00-08:15
    2. 07:45-08:00
    3. 07:30-07:45
    4. 07:15-07:30

15. The nurse is conducting an admission interview on an adult client with a history of diabetes mellitus. The nurse concludes that this client is at risk for episodes of hypoglycemia when the client reports abuse of which of the following drugs?
    1. Cocaine
    2. Alcohol
    3. Marijuana
    4. Morphine

16. The nurse is teaching a diabetic client new to insulin therapy how to properly draw up the dose. The nurse would demonstrate which of the following during this teaching session?
    1. Shake both vials energetically before drawing up the insulins.
    2. Inspect the vial of NPH insulin to ensure that it is clear.
    3. Draw up the regular insulin before NPH insulin into the same syringe.
    4. Insert air first into the vial of regular insulin.

17. The nurse has an order for metformin (Glucophage) for a client with diabetes mellitus. The nurse would question the order if the client has a history of which of the following disorders?
    1. Renal insufficiency
    2. Hypertension
    3. Increased intraocular pressure
    4. Peptic ulcer disease

174

18. An adult client newly diagnosed with diabetes mellitus has been unable to control blood glucose using diet and will be starting drug therapy with glyburide (DiaBeta). The nurse explains that which of the following is the most frequent adverse effect of this class of drug?
    1. Photosensitivity
    2. Hypoglycemia
    3. Muscle cramps
    4. Increased fatigue

19. An adult client is taking rosiglitazone (Avandia) for control of type 2 diabetes mellitus. The nurse would place highest priority on reporting to the prescriber which of the following manifestations?
    1. Elevated liver function studies
    2. Fluid retention
    3. Anemia
    4. Muscle and back pain

20. The nurse determines that the family of a child with diabetes mellitus understands instructions on the use of glucagon after they state to do which of the following?
    1. Use a 3-mL syringe.
    2. Inject at a 90-degree angle.
    3. Use within 30 days of expiration date.
    4. Use this drug as the preferred treatment for hypoglycemia.

50 Overview of the Male and Female Reproductive Systems

1. Complete the following puzzle.

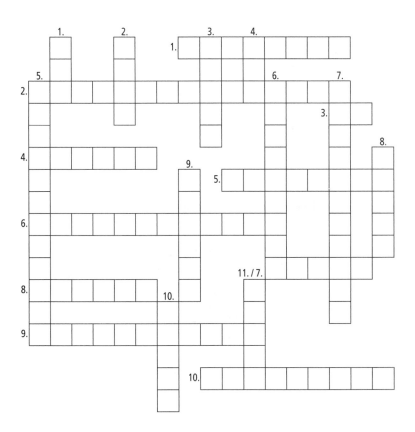

Across

1. Forms on ovary and releases ovum
2. Part of autonomic nervous system controlling orgasm
3. Abbreviation for luteinizing hormone
4. Gamete-producing gland
5. Common site for cancer in older men
6. Male hormone
7. Meaning "seed"
8. Pleasurable end to sexual act
9. Release of semen
10. Cutting of vas deferens

Down

1. Egg
2. Abbreviation of interstitial cell-stimulating hormone
3. Gland which releases ova
4. Abbreviation for luteotropic hormone
5. Female hormone increased in pregnancy
6. Female hormones
7. Male "menopause"
8. Fluid containing sperm
9. Womb
10. Folds of skin at opening of vagina
11. Erectile organ of the male

2. The reproductive system of the human female consists of the _____, _____ tubes, _____, and _____.

3. The male reproductive system consists of the _____, _____ vesicles, _____ gland, _____ glands, and _____.

4. In the female, _____ _____ hormone stimulates the development of the ovarian (graafian) follicles up to the point of ovulation and, in the male, the development of the seminiferous tubules.

5. _____ hormone acts in the female to promote growth of the interstitial cells in the follicle and the formation of the corpus luteum; in the male, it stimulates growth of interstitial cells in the testes and promotes formation of androgen (testosterone).

6. _____ occurs when the mature ovarian follicle ruptures and releases its ovum.

7. For both males and females, _____ stimulation and _____ stimulation are necessary for a satisfactory sexual experience.

8. Erectile tissue is located in the introitus (vaginal opening) and clitoris, and is under _____ nerve control.

9. _____ glands situated near the labia minora, produce mucus secretion inside the introitus, which helps to serve as a _____ during sexual intercourse.

10. _____, an androgen, aids in developing and maintaining the male secondary sex characteristics and male accessory organs.

11. Depending on sexual activity, sperm can be stored in the _____ _____ for more than 1 month without losing fertility.

12. In later life, women undergo _____, and men experience the _____ _____.

51 Drugs Affecting Women's Health and the Female Reproductive System

STAYING ON TOP OF TERMINOLOGY

1. Match the definition at the right with the term at the left.

_____ Anovulation
_____ Biphasic
_____ Estrogen
_____ Monophasic
_____ Oral contraception
_____ Progestogen
_____ Triphasic

a. A luteal hormone derived from the corpus luteum formed in the ovary from the ruptured follicle
b. Oral contraceptive formulations that offer two different concentrations of progestin (and sometime estrogen) through the cycle
c. The absence of ovulation
d. Oral contraceptive formulations with identical concentrations of estrogen/progestin for 21 days
e. Oral contraceptive formulations that offer three different concentrations of progestin (and sometime estrogen) through the cycle
f. A type of hormone secreted by the ovary produced by the cells of the developing graafian follicle
g. A medication taken by mouth to prevent pregnancy

FOCUSING ON THE FACTS

2. Gonadotropin releasing hormone (GnRH) stimulates the synthesis and release of _____ hormone (LH) and _____-_____ hormone from the _____ _____ gland.

3. Gonadorelin is a synthetic GnRH used as an adjunct to other tests to diagnose _____ in males and females.

4. Nafarelin is indicated for the treatment or management of _____ and _____ _____ _____.

5. Ganirelix (Antagon) is a GnRH antagonist that suppresses LH and gonadotropic secretion and prevents _____ _____.

6. The gonadotropin secreted by the placenta during pregnancy is called _____ _____.

Chapter **51** **Drugs Affecting Women's Health and the Female Reproductive System**

7. Chorionic gonadotropin is used for prepubertal _____ and hypogonadotropic _____ to stimulate androgen production in the testes.

8. In combination with chorionic gonadotropins, _____ are indicated for female infertility caused by ovulatory dysfunction.

9. The beneficial effects of supplemental estrogen include improving _____ symptoms of _____ .

10. Supplemental estrogen has significant risk, including increased _____ events, and increased risk for certain _____ .

CONNECTING WITH CLIENTS

11. You are working with a client who is taking oral contraceptives. For each potential symptom below, indicate whether it would be considered an adverse effect (**A**) or a contraindication (**C**) to taking birth control pills.

    _____ Coronary artery disease
    _____ Weight gain
    _____ Breast tenderness
    _____ Nausea
    _____ Tiredness
    _____ Depression
    _____ Pregnancy
    _____ Acne
    _____ Decreased menses
    _____ Abdominal bloating
    _____ Hot flashes
    _____ High blood pressure

12. What would you include in a teaching plan for a client who is beginning drug therapy with clomiphene citrate (Clomid) for female infertility?

13. What adverse effects would you include in a discussion with a female client with infertility who is taking urofollitropin (Bravelle)?

14. The nurse working with a client just beginning drug therapy with gonadorelin (Factrel) would teach the client to report immediately which adverse drug effect?
    1. Hives
    2. Pain at injection site
    3. Abdominal cramping
    4. Fever

15. The nurse is reinforcing an explanation about how to properly take the newly prescribed drug nafarelin (Synarel) to a female client with endometriosis. The nurse explains that this drug should be taken:
    1. subcutaneously, in the morning.
    2. orally three times per day.
    3. intranasally, in the morning and at night.
    4. as a vaginal cream at bedtime.

16. The nurse would formulate which of the following goals for a client receiving ganirelix (Antagon)?
    1. Client has relief of pain from endometriosis.
    2. Client has slowed rate of bone loss.
    3. Client will conceive.
    4. Client will develop secondary sexual characteristics.

17. A female client is considering hormone replacement therapy with estrogen. The nurse anticipates that this client will not be eligible for this type of drug therapy based on a history of which of the following?
    1. Chronic obstructive pulmonary disease
    2. Hepatitis
    3. Osteoporosis
    4. Coronary artery disease

18. A 42-year-old client would benefit from estrogen therapy. The nurse explains that the client's habitual use of which of the following increases the risk of adverse drug effects?
    1. Alcohol
    2. Cigarettes
    3. Coffee
    4. Herbal tea

19. A client will be using an estrogen transdermal patch. The client indicates an understanding of where to apply the patch by stating to place it:
    1. At the waistline.
    2. On the lower abdomen.
    3. On the breast.
    4. Behind the ear.

20. A client will be using progestin therapy (21-day cycle) for oral contraception. The nurse teaches the client to do which of the following to effectively manage drug therapy?
    1. Take the pill at the same time each day.
    2. Keep a 3-month supply of pills on hand.
    3. Use a back-up contraceptive method for the first 6 months.
    4. Take three tablets on the day following a missed dose.

181

Chapter **51** **Drugs Affecting Women's Health and the Female Reproductive System**

52 Drugs for Labor and Delivery

STAYING ON TOP OF TERMINOLOGY

1. Match the definition at the right with the term at the left.

_____ dinoprostone	a. One of two hormones secreted by the posterior pituitary gland, whose name means "rapid birth"
_____ Oxytocics	
_____ oxytocin	b. A drug indicated to prevent and treat uncomplicated premature labor in pregnancies of 20 or more weeks' gestation
_____ ritodrine	
_____ Tocolytics	c. Drugs that inhibit premature labor
	d. A drug indicated to promote cervical ripening prior to labor induction
	e. Agents that stimulate contraction of the smooth muscle of the uterus, resulting in contractions and spontaneous labor

FOCUSING ON THE FACTS

2. The _____ of drugs may be altered during labor and delivery.

3. The smooth muscle fibers of the _____ extend longitudinally, circularly, and obliquely.

4. Drugs that act on the uterus include _____ and _____.

5. In addition to other functions, oxytocin facilitates _____ _____ during lactation.

6. A suppository formulation of _____ has been used as part of protocols to terminate pregnancy.

7. _____ _____, which occurs before the 37th week of pregnancy, is defined as regular uterine contractions every 5 to 10 minutes or 6 to 10 in 1 hour, with progressive cervical effacement or dilatation.

8. The goal of tocolysis is to stop _____ and delay _____ for at least _____ to _____ hours in most women.

9. Clinical trials have shown that only one agent, _____, an NSAID, significantly prolongs gestation for more than 7 days.

10. Pretreatment considerations for tocolysis include _____-_____ status, _____ age, and the clinical resources.

CONNECTING WITH CLIENTS

11. What adverse effects would you assess for in a client who is receiving ergonovine (Ergotrate)?

12. A client will be taking terbutaline (Brethine) at home. What safety factors would be important to teach this client?

13. A client is receiving ritodrine (Yutopar) for premature labor. What nursing diagnoses might you formulate for this client?

TRAINING FOR TEST TAKING

14. The nurse would assess a client in labor receiving oxytocin (Pitocin) by the intravenous route for which of the following adverse effects?
    1. Fetal tachycardia
    2. Maternal bradycardia
    3. Nausea and vomiting
    4. Leg muscle cramping

15. The nurse determines that an oxytocin (Pitocin) infusion for a woman in labor most likely needs to be stopped after noting which of the following assessment data?
    1. Drop in fetal heart rate
    2. Increase in maternal pulse by 5 beats/min
    3. Discomfort with uterine contractions
    4. Respiratory rate of 24 with contractions

16. The nurse explains to a client who will be starting drug therapy with methylergonovine (Methergine) that which of the following is a common adverse effect of this drug?
    1. Constipation
    2. Sensation of flushing
    3. Nausea
    4. Fatigue

17. The nurse overhears the physician at the nurses' station stating that a client will be started on ritodrine (Yutopar). The nurse anticipates that the order is being written for the client with which of the following conditions?
    1. Preterm labor at 24 weeks' gestation
    2. Lack of cervical dilation
    3. Hypotonic uterine contractions
    4. Postpartum hemorrhage

18. A client is receiving magnesium sulfate during labor. The nurse plans to assess this client regularly for which of the following early signs of hypermagnesemia?
    1. Tachycardia
    2. Hypertension
    3. Sudden increase in urine output
    4. Slurred speech and weakness

19. A client in labor is being treated with dinoprostone (Prepidil). The nurse plans to monitor which data to determine effectiveness of the drug?
    1. Fetal heart rate
    2. Strength of uterine contractions
    3. Cervical dilation
    4. Whether amniotic sac has ruptured

20. A client is being treated with bromocriptine (Parlodel) after delivery of an infant. The nurse determines that the client understands the intended effect of the drug when the client states that it will:
    1. Reduce discomfort in breasts.
    2. Suppress production of breast milk.
    3. Reduce postpartum pain.
    4. Treat postpartum hemorrhage.

STAYING ON TOP OF TERMINOLOGY

1. Complete the following word search.

ANDROGENS
ANEMIA
ANTINEOPLASTIC
ASSESSMENT
BPH
CANCER
DEPRESSION
DIZZINESS
ERECTIONS
FINASTERIDE
GYNECOMASTIA

HYPOGONADISM
INDICATIONS
JAUNDICE
LIBIDO
NURSING
PROSTATE
PROTEIN
PUBERTY
REACTIONS
SAW
TESTOSTERONE

```
U T K P N I I B G E G C C O D I B I L
T B A V R R D P F N E I U Y V L S W Y
P S S R G G Z H C C I T F Q F B S W O
T Q J Z C R H M N A S S E S S M E N T
H A C F N O E K U P E A R N S L N A M
T Q H S L Y V C U I D L W U H Q I A D
V R A B P L Z B P N I P J Q N F Z I E
J C F D R M E A N D R O G E N S Z T P
L U C J O R L N A I E E E K H M I S R
E P D H T M L E Y C T N C Z R E D A E
M R O Y E X M M S A S I I N E R J M S
I O N N I Q X I P T A T D P A E Q O S
D S T I N D Q A C I N N N U C C X C I
W T Y H V J S U X O I A U R T T S E O
O A X S D B T T Z N F O A R I I X N N
Y T B L D D O X V S C U J N O O V Y K
T E S T O S T E R O N E I X N N A G O
F U J A I A M P Y R S D B G S S Q Y K
O V O U Z O O H Y P O G O N A D I S M
```

2. _____ are male sex hormones necessary for the normal development and maintenance of male sex characteristics.

3. When prescribed for conditions other than deficiency states, the most common undesirable effect of androgens is _____.

4. Finasteride (Proscar) is a drug used in the treatment of _____ _____ _____, which until recently had been almost exclusively surgical.

5. _____, a naturally occurring androgenic hormone produced primarily by the testes, regulates male development.

6. Androgens are potent _____ agents because they stimulate the formation and maintenance of muscular and skeletal protein.

7. Most androgens are classified as Schedule _____ drugs in the United States.

8. Androgens may enhance the _____ effects of warfarin and _____ effects of insulin and oral hypoglycemics.

9. Benign prostatic hyperplasia (BPH) obstructs the bladder _____ and compresses the _____, which results in urinary _____ and increases the risk of _____.

10. Symptoms of BPH include _____, _____, and _____.

CONNECTING WITH CLIENTS

11. The nurse recalls that which of the following are possible uses for testosterone, after hearing that a client will begin drug therapy with this androgen?

12. What nursing diagnoses would you consider for a client receiving testosterone therapy?

Chapter **53** **Drugs Affecting the Male Reproductive System**

13. What side/adverse effects would you assess for in a client receiving finasteride (Proscar)?

TRAINING FOR TEST TAKING

14. A client has begun therapy with oxandrolone (Oxandrin). The nurse expects which of the following changes in laboratory values based on known drug effects?
    1. Increased hemoglobin and hematocrit
    2. Decreased serum cholesterol
    3. Increased blood glucose
    4. Decreased liver enzymes

15. A client will be using a matrix type of testosterone (Testoderm) patch. The nurse explains to the client that it should be applied to which of the following areas?
    1. Abdomen
    2. Back
    3. Thighs
    4. Scrotum

16. A client taking testosterone therapy should be taught by the nurse that which of the following conditions would require temporary withdrawal of the drug because of excessive dosing?
    1. Urinary frequency
    2. Atrophy of the testicles
    3. Priapism
    4. Impotence

17. The nurse explains to an adolescent client taking prescribed testosterone therapy that ongoing monitoring will include assessment for which of the following musculoskeletal complications?
    1. Increased serum calcium levels
    2. Early epiphyseal closure
    3. Delayed linear bone growth
    4. Nocturnal muscle cramps

18. A 29-year-old female client is considering androgen therapy as adjunct treatment for breast carcinoma. The nurse ensures that the client understands that this classification of drugs carry which of the following pregnancy category ratings?
    1. B
    2. C
    3. D
    4. X

19. The nurse explains to a client beginning drug therapy with finasteride (Proscar) that full effects of the drug on urinary symptoms may not be seen for how long?
    1. 2 weeks
    2. 4 weeks
    3. 6 months
    4. 12 months

20. The nurse ensures that which of the following laboratory assessments is made as a baseline before beginning drug therapy with finasteride (Proscar)?
    1. Liver function studies
    2. Thyroid function studies
    3. Serum calcium
    4. Serum glucose

54 Drugs Affecting Sexual Behavior

1. Match the definition at the right to the term at the left.

_____ alprostadil
_____ Impotence
_____ Libido
_____ Premenstrual dysphoric disorder
_____ propranolol
_____ sildenafil

a. A ß-adrenergic blocker that has been associated with decreased libido and erectile dysfunction
b. A key oral drug indicated for the treatment of erectile dysfunction in men
c. The inability of the adult male to achieve or maintain a penile erection, along with decreased sexual function
d. A drug used in the treatment of erectile dysfunction in men by intracavernous injection
e. The sex drive
f. A female disorder characterized by anxiety, irritability, and depression

FOCUSING ON THE FACTS

2. _____ is an integral part of one's identity; it is a reflection of how one feels about oneself and how one interacts with others.

3. Sexual function refers to the _____ and _____ ability to perform in a sexually satisfying manner, with or without a partner.

4. Sexuality and sexual behavior have _____, _____, and _____ dimensions that reflect a complexity beyond drug-related effects.

5. Decreased _____ is common in both genders and may be secondary to depression, drug therapy or other factors.

6. Among the physical factors affecting sexual dysfunction are _____ _____, _____ _____, and _____.

7. Men with vascular complications of chronic diseases (particularly those with diabetes) report a higher incidence of _____ _____.

8. In the male, parasympathetic (cholinergic) stimulation controls _____ _____.

9. Many physiologic functions significant to sexual pleasure are controlled by the _____ and the _____ nervous system.

10. The embryo is characteristically _____ initially and does not differentiate until fetal androgens begin to _____ tissues (seventh to twelfth weeks of pregnancy).

CONNECTING WITH CLIENTS

11. A female client with a history of depression tells the nurse she has less interest in sexual activity than is typical of her. She states she began taking an antidepressant a few months ago. How can you explain the relationship between antidepressant therapy and reduced sexual interest?

12. A client reports decreased libido during a routine physical examination. In reviewing the client's medication list, what types of drugs could impair sexual behavior and how do they accomplish this effect?

13. When working with clients in regard to human sexuality, what would be your nursing goals?

TRAINING FOR TEST TAKING

14. A client with erectile dysfunction is considering the drug sildenafil (Viagra). The nurse concludes that the client is ineligible to take this drug after noting which of the following concurrent drugs listed on the medical history form?
    1. nitroglycerin (Nitrostat)
    2. theophylline (Theo-Dur)
    3. furosemide (Lasix)
    4. magnesium hydroxide (Milk of Magnesia)

15. A client is beginning drug therapy with tadalafil (Cialis). The nurse explains to the client to avoid which of the following breakfast juices while taking this medication?
    1. Orange
    2. Grapefruit
    3. Apple
    4. Tomato

16. A neonate has a medication order for alprostadil (Prostin VR Pediatric). The nurse concludes that the infant has which of the following congenital disorders?
    1. Spina bifida
    2. Club foot
    3. Patent ductus arteriosus
    4. Tetralogy of Fallot

17. A client who has been given a new prescription for vardenafil (Levitra) indicates an understanding of drug interactions by stating to avoid if possible taking which of the following antimicrobials concurrently?
    1. gentamicin
    2. cefazolin
    3. penicillin
    4. ketoconazole

18. A client will be dosed with alprostadil (Caverject) by insertion of urethral pellets. The nurse explains in advance that which of the following is the most common adverse effect of this drug?
    1. Headache
    2. Penile pain
    3. Urethral edema
    4. Hypotension

19. The client who is starting drug therapy with sildenafil (Viagra) reports using various substances in the past to enhance sexual performance. The nurse teaches the client that which of the following substances is absolutely contraindicated while taking sildenafil?
    1. vitamin E
    2. cantharis
    3. amyl nitrite
    4. levodopa

20. A male client with decreased libido tells the nurse that his friends have said that marijuana can be used as an aphrodisiac. Which of the following should the nurse include in a reply?
    1. Marijuana is, indeed, an aphrodisiac.
    2. Marijuana has no effect at all on sexual functioning.
    3. The type of plant and growing conditions affect its usefulness.
    4. The client's state of mind and expectations influence its usefulness.

STAYING ON TOP OF TERMINOLOGY

1. Match the definition at the right with the term at the left.

_____ Cancer
_____ Combination chemotherapy
_____ Gompertzian growth
_____ Ivasive growth
_____ Metastasis
_____ Persistent proliferation

a. The rapid growth of cancer in the early stages until it nearly outgrows its blood and nutrient supply, followed by decreased growth or plateau phase for the tumor
b. Unrestrained growth and division; probably the most distinguishing characteristic of cancer cells
c. Spreading of the cancer from the original site
d. A group of more than 300 diseases characterized by the uncontrolled growth and spread of abnormal cells
e. A hallmark of cancer cells, whereby they often penetrate into adjacent tissue
f. The use of two or more anticancer drugs at the same time

FOCUSING ON THE FACTS

2. Choices for treatment of cancer include _____ interventions, _____ , and _____ .

3. Pharmacologic interventions include _____ chemotherapy, _____ interventions, targeted therapies which block specific enzyme or receptor function, _____ agents, and the _____ _____ modifiers.

4. Cytotoxic chemotherapy targets _____ _____ cancer cells and may or may not be specific for a particular point in the dividing _____ _____ .

5. Cancer cells often display altered _____ as a result of genetic mutation, exposure to chemical carcinogens, irradiation, viruses, or other insults.

6. The Papanicolaou (Pap) smear is a cytologic test capable of detecting carcinoma of the _____ and _____ in the subclinical stages.

7. Antineoplastic agents that are active against both proliferating and resting cells are called _____ _____-_____ agents.

8. Hormonal and targeted therapies bind to specific_____, affect specific _____ function or inhibit angiogenesis.

9. The GI toxicities associated with cancer chemotherapy may manifest at oral ulcers or _____, _____, and/or _____ syndromes.

10. _____ to chemotherapy is common with repeated cycles of drug therapy, often because of mutations that occur in the tumor.

CONNECTING WITH CLIENTS

11. When explaining to a client how chemotherapy affects normal cells, what would you say about how chemotherapy affects the gastrointestinal tract, the bone marrow, the hair follicles, and the mouth?

12. Can you identify at least one nursing intervention to manage constipation, alopecia, and stomatitis as adverse effects of chemotherapy?

13. A client receiving chemotherapy as an outpatient experiences vomiting after each treatment. How should you instruct the client or caregiver to handle soiled bedpans or containers contaminated by vomitus?

TRAINING FOR TEST TAKING

14. A client receiving chemotherapy as treatment for cancer experiences drug-related nausea and vomiting. In addition to antiemetic therapy, the nurse should try which of the following approaches to control this problem?
    1. Increase intake of red meat and other proteins
    2. Plan the largest meal of the day at noon.
    3. Serve foods at room temperature or cooler.
    4. Rest for 15 to 20 minutes after eating.

15. The nurse would encourage the client who has cancer chemotherapy-related diarrhea to increase intake of which of the following foods?
    1. Bananas
    2. Beans
    3. Whole grain toast
    4. Fresh apples

196

16. A client receiving cancer chemotherapy has a platelet count of 75,000/mm³. The nurse should write which of the following interventions in the plan of care for this client?
    1. Use regular toothbrush for mouth care and floss daily.
    2. Avoid taking rectal temperatures.
    3. Use nail clippers carefully.
    4. Give medications by parenteral injection whenever possible.

17. A client who is on a chemotherapy regimen for cancer has a low neutrophil count. The nurse would avoid doing which of the following to appropriately care for this client?
    1. Carefully wash hands each time room is entered and exited.
    2. Provide canned fruits in place of fresh ones.
    3. Apply topical antibiotics to skin abrasions.
    4. Give acetaminophen (Tylenol) for low-grade fever.

18. The nurse determines that a client receiving chemotherapy who is at risk for impaired oral mucous membranes is using proper self-care measures when which of the following is noted?
    1. Avoids commercial mouthwash products.
    2. Wears dentures most of the day.
    3. Sips on hot soups and broth.
    4. Tries to eat a large breakfast.

19. The nurse is providing anticipatory guidance to a client who will be taking a chemotherapy regimen that can lead to alopecia. The nurse would include which point in discussions with the client?
    1. Hair will begin to grow back in approximately 6 to 9 months after the last treatment.
    2. Hair will have the same color after chemotherapy.
    3. It is important to buy a wig within 1 month of hair loss.
    4. It is important to avoid using curling irons for the equivalent of two haircut lengths.

20. The nurse would alert the oncologist after noting which of the following blood urea nitrogen (BUN) and creatinine levels in a client receiving chemotherapy that has nephrotoxicity as an adverse effect?
    1. BUN 22 mg/dL and creatinine 1.8 mg/dL
    2. BUN 12 mg/dL and creatinine 2.8 mg/dL
    3. BUN 16 mg/dL and creatinine 0.5 mg/dL
    4. BUN 28 mg/dL and creatinine 2.2 mg/dL

56 Antineoplastic Chemotherapy Agents

STAYING ON TOP OF TERMINOLOGY

1. Match the definition at the right with the term at the left.

_____ Alkylating agents	a. Drugs accepted by the cell as necessary for cell growth but are impostors that interfere with normal DNA production
_____ Antibiotic antitumor agents	
_____ Antimetabolites	b. A treatment that reduces the time that normal cells are exposed to toxic effects of high-dose methotrexate treatments
_____ Extravasation	
_____ Leucovorin rescue	c. Plant alkaloids that block cell division in metaphase
_____ Mitotic inhibitors	
_____ Nadir	d. Drugs that substitute an alkyl chemical structure for a hydrogen atom in DNA
	e. The lowest point of something being measured, such as a laboratory value
	f. Pain or redness at an injection site from infiltration that can result in tissue cellulitis, fibrosis and necrosis
	g. Drugs that interfere with DNA functioning by blocking the transcription of new DNA or RNA

FOCUSING ON THE FACTS

2. _____ agents do not directly kill tumor cells; they act by interfering with cell reproduction or replication at some point in the cell cycle.

3. _____ interferes with synthesis of DNA and RNA.

4. _____ prevents cell division and protein synthesis.

5. _____ binds DNA and inhibits RNA synthesis.

6. _____ and _____ inhibit mitosis during the M-phase of the cell cycle.

7. _____ inhibits virus replication, decreases cell proliferation, and enhances phagocyte activity.

8. _____ produces stable microtubule bundles and interferes with the late G-2 mitotic phase in cell.

9. A number of _____ _____ agents are available and include cyclophosphamide, chlorambucil, ifosfamide, melphalan, and methchloramine.

10. Monitoring for myelosuppression as in clients receiving chemotherapy involves reviewing laboratory test results for decreased _____, _____ count, and total and differential _____ count.

CONNECTING WITH CLIENTS

11. You are working on an oncology unit and you are assigned to four clients who are receiving chemotherapy as part of their treatment. If each client reported one of the side or adverse effects below, which drug would you associate it with? Write your answers below.

_____ Dark discoloration of skin and fingernails   a. cisplatin
_____ Tinnitus   b. 5-FU
_____ Chills   c. cyclophosphamide
_____ Paresthesias of hands and feet   d. vincristine

12. The intravenous line of a client receiving doxorubicin has infiltrated. How would you care for the site knowing that there could be some drug extravasation?

13. You are preparing chemotherapy for a client and accidentally spill some of the drug. What procedure would you use to clean the spill?

TRAINING FOR TEST TAKING

14. The nurse would assess for which of the following relatively unique adverse effects in a female client receiving cisplatin (Platinol) as part of a chemotherapy regimen for cancer?
1. Abdominal pain
2. Hypertension
3. Leg cramps
4. Numbness and tingling in the toes

15. A client with a history of myocardial infarction and heart failure will be starting chemotherapy for treatment of breast cancer. The nurse would be especially vigilant in performing ongoing cardiac assessments if the client will be receiving which drug?
1. bleomycin (Blenoxane)
2. methotrexate (Folex PFS)
3. fludarabine (Fludara)
4. doxorubicin (Adriamycin)

16. A client with lung cancer has an order for methotrex-ate (Folex PFS) as a chemotherapy agent. The nurse looks for an accompanying order for which of the following drugs?
    1. cyclophosphamide (Cytoxan)
    2. leucovorin (Wellcovorin)
    3. etoposide (Toposar)
    4. paclitaxel (Taxol)

17. The nurse would assess the client receiving vin-cristine (Oncovin) would assess the client for which of the following major adverse effects of this chemotherapy drug?
    1. Decreased white blood cell count
    2. Nausea and vomiting
    3. Numbness and tingling in the extremities
    4. Ringing in the ears and hearing loss

18. The nurse anticipates that a client with ovarian can-cer scheduled to receive paclitaxel (Taxol) will also receive which of the following as pretreatment for paclitaxel?
    1. Hydration with 2 liters of normal saline
    2. Leucovorin (Wellcovorin)
    3. Corticosteroid and histamine receptor blocker
    4. Antiemetics and furosemide (Lasix)

19. The medication administration record for a client lists tamoxifen (Nolvadex) as a scheduled medica-tion. The nurse realizes that this client either has or is at risk for which of the following types of cancer?
    1. Breast
    2. Prostate
    3. Lung
    4. Liver

20. A client has just received a scheduled dose of cyclophosphamide (Cytoxan). The nurse would do which of the following as an important part of care at this time?
    1. Watch for sudden diarrhea.
    2. Encourage increased fluid intake to 3 liters per day.
    3. Ask the client about dizziness or headaches.
    4. Keep the client on bedrest for at least 8 hours.

57 Overview of Infections, Inflammation, and Fever

STAYING ON TOP OF TERMINOLOGY

1. Fill in the blanks describing the body temperature control mechanism.

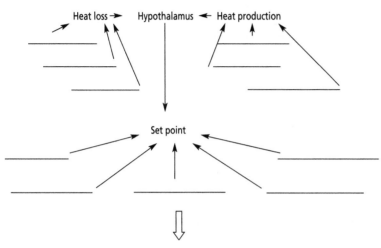

Heat loss → Hypothalamus ← Heat production

Set point

Normal body temperature

FOCUSING ON THE FACTS

2. _____ is the invasion and multiplication of pathogenic microorganisms in body tissues that cause disease by local cellular _____, secretion of a _____, or an _____-_____ reaction in the host.

3. _____ is a protective mechanism of body tissues in response to invasion or toxins produced by colonizing microorganisms.

4. Although _____ may lead to septicemia in the immunocompromised host, it is usually a short-lived, self-limited process (depending on the pathogen) in clients with normally functioning immune systems.

5. In immunocompetent hosts, _____ therapy is seldom required to treat the colonization of nonpathogenic organisms or transient bacteremia without tissue invasion.

6. _____, _____, and _____ (which arrive later) are the granulocytes that affect the injured area by acting as the cellular mediators of infection.

203

7. The chemical mediators of infection are part of the _____ system, which enhances chemotaxis, increases blood vessel _____, and eventually causes cell _____.

8. The _____ sets the point at which body temperature is maintained, but body temperature regulation depends on a balance between heat _____ and heat _____.

9. Drugs that inhibit the synthesis of _____ have antipyretic activity (e.g., acetaminophen, salicylates).

10. _____ reduce fever by causing the hypothalamic center to reestablish a normal set point.

CONNECTING WITH CLIENTS

11. A nursing assistant asks you after inter-shift report what "fever of unknown origin" means, which is a diagnosis of a client on the nursing unit. What information could you include in a response?

12. A client is seen in the ambulatory clinic for an infected foot wound after stepping on a shard of glass the previous week. The client states she used over the counter products to treat the wound but admits confusion over the labels on some of the products. How would you explain to her the differences among the terms antibacterial, bacteriostatic, and bactericidal?

13. What information would you include in a teaching plan being developed for a client receiving an antimicrobial agent?

TRAINING FOR TEST TAKING

14. A client is beginning antimicrobial therapy for pneumonia. The nurse would assess for which of the following as a sign of hypersensitivity after administration of the first dose?
   1. Rash and itching
   2. Increased cough
   3. Failure of fever to drop
   4. Diminished breath sounds

15. The client has developed a hypersensitivity reaction following administration of an antimicrobial. The nurse would ensure that which of the following drugs are available for immediate use as ordered?
   1. Acetaminophen and a corticosteroid
   2. Aspirin and an antihistamine
   3. Antihistamine and epinephrine
   4. Antipyretic and corticosteroid

204

16. A client taking antibiotic therapy is at risk for super-infection with *Clostridium difficile*. The nurse assesses this client for which symptom that is consistent with *C. difficile* infection?
    1. Vaginal itching
    2. Diarrhea
    3. White patches in the mouth
    4. Sore throat

17. The nurse evaluates that a client being treated with antimicrobial therapy for an infected right leg ulcer is experiencing the *best* outcome if which of the following is noted?
    1. Temperature of 99.4°F
    2. Drainage changed from purulent to cloudy yellow
    3. Right leg circumference half inch larger than left
    4. White blood cell count of 8,600/mm³

18. A client with a history of heart failure and diabetes is receiving an antimicrobial drug by intermittent IV infusion every 6 hours. The drug needs to be diluted in 100mL of normal saline to prevent vein irritation. The nurse should assess this client for which of the following based on history?
    1. Lung crackles
    2. Infiltration of the IV
    3. Hyperglycemia
    4. Decreasing pulse

19. The client has an order to begin IV antimicrobial therapy for infection of a surgical incision. Which of the following actions should the nurse take first?
    1. Look in the medication refrigerator to see if a dose is available.
    2. Ask the client about past need to take an antihistamine.
    3. Ensure that the ordered culture and sensitivity specimen has been obtained.
    4. Ask the client about current signs and symptoms of infection.

20. The client who will be receiving intravenous penicillin tells the nurse he has never had this drug before. The allergy record states no allergies. Which of the following actions by the nurse is most appropriate?
    1. Ask the client about allergies to antiviral agents.
    2. Remain with the client for the first 30 minutes of the dose.
    3. After hanging the dose, tell the client to call for any itching or rash.
    4. Ask about family history of allergy to penicillin.

205

58 Antibacterials

STAYING ON TOP OF TERMINOLOGY

1. Identify on the following figure the area indicating the therapeutic range, the area that represents the trough, and the area that represents the peak.

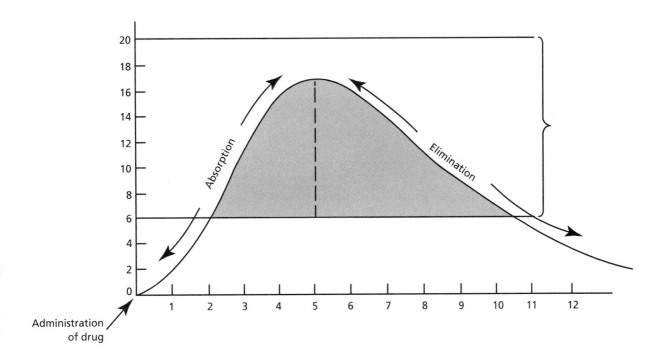

FOCUSING ON THE FACTS

2. _____ collection and _____ should be completed before initiating antibiotic therapy.

3. _____, particularly penicillins, have been associated with serious hypersensitivity and allergic reactions.

4. Reducing or eliminating normal flora by antibiotic therapy provides an environment conducive to the growth of undesirable _____, _____, or _____ in a condition known as _____.

5. Special attention must be given to the interactions of oral antibacterials with _____ or other _____ .

6. The times of antibacterial drug administration should be spaced as _____ as possible over a _____-_____ period to ensure stable and consistent serum levels.

7. As a general rule, antibacterials should be administered within _____ minutes of the scheduled time.

8. Penicillins are among a broad group of agents that share a _____-_____ _____ in their chemical structure.

9. All tetracyclines are contraindicated in children younger than the age of ___ years since the drug deposits in bone and teeth _____ and can result in permanent _____ of developing teeth.

10. Significant adverse effects of the _____ include nephrotoxicity and ototoxicity.

CONNECTING WITH CLIENTS

11. You are assigned to a client receiving an aminoglycoside antibiotic who has peak and trough drug levels ordered. What is the relationship and the importance of these to the client?

12. A client is due for a dose of intravenous vancomycin. What side or adverse effects would you monitor for?

13. You need to hang a scheduled dose of intravenous metronidazole (Flagyl) for a client with an indwelling IV that has 5% dextrose in 0.45% sodium chloride hanging. What is important to remember to give this dose correctly?

14. The culture and sensitivity report for a client with a wound infection indicates that the microorganism is sensitive to several cephalosporins. Before calling the physician with the test results, the nurse should check the client's record for history of allergy to which of the following antibiotics?
    1. Penicillin
    2. Sulfonamides
    3. Erythromycin
    4. Clindamycin

15. A client needs to take a course of cefotetan (Cefotan) for an infection. The nurse should teach the client to avoid which item during the course of therapy?
    1. Milk products
    2. Alcohol
    3. Excess sodium
    4. Grapefruit juice

16. The nurse assesses a client receiving intravenous vancomycin for which of the following adverse effects that would be related to excessive speed of infusion?
    1. Taste alterations
    2. Hearing loss
    3. Nausea and vomiting
    4. Reddened face and neck

17. The client is beginning a course of antibiotic therapy with erythromycin (E-mycin). The nurse explains to the client to self-assess for which most frequent adverse effect?
    1. Muscle aches
    2. Hearing loss
    3. GI upset
    4. Red discoloration of urine

18. A client has been prescribed clindamycin (Cleocin) for a joint infection. The nurse teaches the client which of the following information about how to take the oral tablet?
    1. On an empty stomach
    2. With meals
    3. With a full glass of water
    4. Without milk

19. A client who is beginning a course of drug therapy with ciprofloxacin (Cipro) indicates an understanding of proper use of the drug by stating to take it:
    1. with a full glass of water.
    2. with milk.
    3. with meals.
    4. on an empty stomach.

20. The nurse would attribute which of the following client's abnormal laboratory values to an adverse effect of tobramycin (Nebcin)?
    1. Sodium 153 mEq/L
    2. Albumin 3.4 g/dL
    3. Serum creatinine 2.2 mg/dL
    4. White blood cell count of 13,000/mm^3

59 Antifungal and Antiviral Drugs

STAYING ON TOP OF TERMINOLOGY

1. Match the definition on the right to the term at the left.

_____ acyclovir	a. The most widely used of the azole anti-fungals
_____ amphotericin B	b. A common drug used to treat the herpes-related viruses
_____ Candidiasis	c. A protease inhibitor that is used in combination with the nucleoside analogues to treat advanced HIV infection in selected individuals
_____ Chemoprophylactic	
_____ enfuvirtide	
_____ fluconazole	
_____ Mycoses	d. Infections with fungi that can range from mild and superficial to severe and life threatening
_____ nevirapine	
_____ saquinavir	e. The first available and prototype agent in the treatment of HIV
_____ zidovudine	f. Treats HIV-1 infection when combined with other antiretrovirals but not recommended for women with CD4 counts above 250 because of risk for serious hepatotoxicity

g. An infection that is also called thrush

h. The first available fusion inhibitor that as of yet has a limited role in the management of HIV disease

i. Using a drug as a preventive agent before disease appears or early in the disease process

j. An antifungal that can be fungistatic or fungicidal and binds to sterols in the fungus cell membrane

FOCUSING ON THE FACTS

2. Human infections with _____ can be caused by any of approximately 50 species of plantlike, parasitic microorganisms.

3. Oral _____ is common in newborn infants and immunocompromised clients, whereas vaginal _____ is common in women who are pregnant, have diabetes mellitus, or take oral contraceptives.

4. Among the most common risk factors for systemic fungal infection is an _____ state, which can occur in clients who are neutropenic for various reasons.

5. _____ play a clear role in a number of inflammatory states, including hepatitis, encephalitis and meningitis.

6. Viruses are true parasites; they replicate within the _____ cell and use the _____ systems of the host cells.

7. Drugs used in the treatment of HIV disease include _____ and those used to prevent or treat opportunistic infections associated with advanced AIDS.

8. Frequently, infectious disease specialists test the HIV strain to establish _____ before using an initial regimen with a client.

9. HIV is transmitted sexually via _____ and _____ _____ or from a mother with AIDS to her child during birth.

10. The _____ _____ _____ inhibitors are diverse chemicals that act by binding directly to, or very near, the active site of the enzyme and rendering it inactive.

CONNECTING WITH CLIENTS

11. What would you include in a teaching plan for a client receiving amphotericin B?

12. What side or adverse effects would you assess for in a client receiving zidovudine?

13. What nursing interventions would you implement when administering didanosine tablets to a client?

TRAINING FOR TEST TAKING

14. To assess for a key adverse effect of amphotericin B therapy, the nurse would vigilantly monitor which of the following laboratory test results?
    1. Liver enzymes
    2. Hemoglobin and hematocrit
    3. Blood urea nitrogen and creatinine
    4. Uric acid and bilirubin levels

15. The nurse would question a newly written order for itraconazole (Sporanox) to be administered to a client with which of the following health problems?
    1. Heart failure
    2. Kidney stones
    3. Irritable bowel syndrome
    4. Glaucoma

16. After noting an order for valacyclovir (Valtrex), the nurse anticipates that a review of the client's medical record will reveal which health problem?
    1. Herpes simplex (cold sores)
    2. Herpes genitalis
    3. Disseminated zoster
    4. Acquired immunodeficiency syndrome

17. The pediatric nurse hears during inter-shift report that an infant diagnosed with respiratory syncytial virus (RSV) is receiving ribavirin (Virazole). The nurse plans to administer the scheduled dose by which of the following standard routes?
    1. Intravenous
    2. Inhalation
    3. Intramuscular
    4. Intranasal

18. A client who has no history of Parkinson's disease or medications that cause extrapyramidal reactions is beginning drug therapy with amantadine (Symmetrel). The nurse questions the client about its use to prevent which of the following disorders?
    1. Guillain Barré syndrome
    2. Hepatitis C
    3. Pneumococcal pneumonia
    4. Influenza A

19. A client with acquired immunodeficiency syndrome (AIDS) is taking antiviral therapy to manage the disease. The nurse concludes that the client understands how to manage this medication regimen after the client states to:
    1. Space medications as evenly as possible while awake but try to sleep 10 hours nightly.
    2. Adjust dosages upward temporarily when symptoms get worse.
    3. Do not take any over-the-counter (OTC) medications without consulting prescriber.
    4. Take medications at variable times to minimize the incidence of adverse effects.

20. A client with acquired immunodeficiency syndrome (AIDS) is adding indinavir (Crixivan) to the medication regimen. The nurse should teach this client about which most serious acute onset adverse effect?
    1. Nephrolithiasis
    2. Nausea and vomiting
    3. Flu-like symptoms
    4. Elevated blood glucose levels

60 Other Antimicrobial Drugs and Antiparasitic Drugs

1. Complete the following word search.

AMEBIASIS
AMINOSALICYLATE
CBC
CHILDREN
CHLOROQUINE
COMMUNITY
DISEASE
EDUCATION
ERYTHROCYTIC
GRANULOMATOUS
HANSEN
HELMINTHS

MALARIA
PARASITE
PATHOGENESIS
PINWORMS
PREGNANCY
PYRAZINAMIDE
RIFAMPIN
SAFETY
TOXOPLASMOSIS
TRICHOMONIASIS
TUBERCULOSIS

```
D J G R U H D S I S O L U C R E B U T Y
L W N X D D G I P A T H O G E N E S I S
I M I H R Y P F Z R M P I T G I R S G X
Y K S W V D Y X M A L A R I A P V I T Z
O Y R V J V T L W T I R C A F M E S O X
L T U E T I S A R A P N E P U A D A X L
A E N I U Q O R O L H C O Y R F I I O F
M F O E R Y T H R O C Y T I C I M N P O
E A T R C O M M U N I T Y O N R A O L W
B S F N P H Y D D G E C E R S S N M A O
I M L B V N I H A B B F C H P E I O S U
A M I N O S A L I C Y L A T E Y Z H M X
S I L Y E N D P D U H Q E S Q J A C O T
I F Y A S K U L Z R C T L G D P R I S B
S U S E E Z C Q P R E G N A N C Y R I T
G E N E D U C A T I O N K A U R P T S K
J A S U O T A M O L U N A R G S M F A K
H E L M I N T H S M R O W N I P L N D V
D L D W L T S K S G V Q S A T E D B B Q
Q O G F V L J Y K J F O B L J G Z K G B
```

2. Malaria is the most important of the _____ diseases in humans, with more than 41% of the world's population at risk of acquiring it each year.

3. Malaria may be transmitted to humans by the _____ of an infected female *Anopheles* mosquito, by _____ _____, congenitally, or by contaminated _____ commonly used by substance abusers.

4. _____, the first drug used to treat malaria, is derived from natural sources of the South American _____ tree.

5. Drug therapy to suppress malaria is initiated ____ week before exposure, continued while traveling in a malarious area, and for ____ weeks after leaving the region.

6. _____ is a chronic granulomatous infection caused by the _____-_____ bacillus *Mycobacterium tuberculosis*.

7. The bacteria that causes TB most commonly affects the _____, but other body areas can also be infected, and this is referred to as _____ TB.

8. Tubercle bacilli droplets are transmitted when an infected person _____ or _____.

9. The smear test can detect mycobacterial organisms, but culture and sensitivity testing takes much longer—from _____ weeks to detect growth and _____ weeks to be certain.

10. Leprosy, or _____ disease, is a chronic infectious disease that is caused by *Mycobacterium leprae* in humans.

CONNECTING WITH CLIENTS

11. You are assigned to the care of a client who has pulmonary tuberculosis. How is the tubercle bacillus of this infection transmitted?

12. What important learning needs should you plan to meet for a client who is beginning drug therapy with isoniazid (INH)?

216

13. What adverse effects of dapsone (Avlosulfon) would you assess for in a client who began therapy with this drug recently?

TRAINING FOR TEST TAKING

14. The nurse working in a traveler's clinic explains to a client that which of the following drugs will most likely be ordered before traveling to a country where risk of contracting malaria is high?
    1. chloroquine (Aralen)
    2. pyrazinamide (PZA)
    3. ethambutol (Myambutol)
    4. quinine sulfate (generic)

15. The nurse in the traveler's clinic sees an order for a client to begin taking mefloquine (Lariam) before leaving the country. The nurse questions the order after noting that the client takes which of the following cardiovascular medications?
    1. metoprolol (Lopressor)
    2. quinidine (Quinidex)
    3. enalapril (Vasotec)
    4. nifedipine (Adalat)

16. The nurse explains to a client with tuberculosis being treated with isoniazid (INH) that the adverse effect of peripheral neuritis can be decreased by increasing intake of which of the following B vitamins?
    1. thiamine (B_1)
    2. niacin (B_3)
    3. pyridoxine (B_6)
    4. cyanocobalamin (B_{12})

17. The nurse would include which of the following statements when teaching a client about the expected adverse effects of rifampin (Rifadin), which is being prescribed as part of treatment for tuberculosis?
    1. Muscle twitching is common in the early weeks of treatment.
    2. The urine may change to a red-orange color and is not of concern.
    3. Report ringing in the ears to the prescriber.
    4. Optic neuritis is the greatest risk of therapy with this drug.

18. A client diagnosed with tuberculosis is taking ethambutol (Myambutol) as part of the drug therapy regimen. The nurse verifies that the client is keeping regular appointments with which health professional to detect the most serious adverse drug effect?
    1. Endocrinologist
    2. Cardiologist
    3. Dentist
    4. Ophthalmologist

19. The nurse notes that a client with tuberculosis is receiving therapy with a second-line drug after seeing an order for which of the following on the medical record?
    1. pyrazinamide (PZA)
    2. ethambutol (Myambutol)
    3. rifampin (Rifadin)
    4. capreomycin (Capastat)

20. A client will be beginning drug therapy with dapsone (Avlosulfon) along with rifampin (Rifadin) for treatment of leprosy. Before administering the dose of dapsone, the nurse checks the client's allergy list to ensure that the client does not have an allergy to which type of drug?
    1. Sulfonamides
    2. Penicillins
    3. "Azole" antifungals
    4. Aminoglycosides

61 Overview of the Immunologic System

STAYING ON TOP OF TERMINOLOGY

1. Match the cells/tissues of the immune system to their major function. There may be more than one choice.

_____ IgG		a. Organs of immunity
_____ Thymus		b. Cell-mediated immunity
_____ IgM		c. Humoral immunity
_____ T-helper		d. Antibodies
_____ Spleen		
_____ T-cytotoxic		
_____ IgE		
_____ Tonsils		
_____ IgD		
_____ T-memory		

FOCUSING ON THE FACTS

2. Mononuclear _____ cells and _____ cells and the _____ _____ are involved in the immune response.

3. In humans, stem cells from the bone marrow are transformed to T cells (T lymphocytes) in the _____ gland and B cells (B lymphocytes) elsewhere in the _____.

4. Three major groups of T cells include (1)_____, (2)_____, and (3) _____.

5. Helper T cells may also secrete _____, a cytokine that is capable of stimulating the action of other T cells, such as cytotoxic T cells and some suppressor T cells.

6. The _____ response to an antigen may be slow, weak, and of short duration. The _____ response is much more rapid and far more potent and prolonged.

7. _____ are gamma globulins (a type of protein) called immunoglobulins.

8. _____ is the major immunoglobulin in the blood and is capable of entering tissue spaces, coating microorganisms, and activating the _____ system, thus accelerating phagocytosis.

9. _____ binds to histamine-containing _____ cells and _____ . It can mediate histamine release in the immune response to parasites (helminths) and in some allergic conditions.

10. The second part of _____ immunity is activation of the complement system, a series of approximately 20 proteins that circulate in the blood in an inactive form.

11. Artificially acquired _____ immunity is often chosen for susceptible individuals following a known exposure.

12. A number of products used in artificial passive immunization cause adverse effects because of individual hypersensitivities to _____ products, to the _____ used in a medication, or to an _____ .

62 Serums, Vaccines, and Other Immunizing Agents

STAYING ON TOP OF TERMINOLOGY

1. Identify each vaccine as either active (**A**) or passive (**P**) immunity.

_____ Varicella-zoster
_____ Botulism antitoxin
_____ Cholera
_____ Influenza
_____ Hepatitis B immune globulin
_____ Rabies
_____ Measles immune globulin
_____ Haemophilus influenza
_____ Diphtheria antitoxin
_____ Typhoid
_____ Rho (D) immune globulin
_____ Polio

FOCUSING ON THE FACTS

2. The body's first defense against invasion by potentially lethal microorganisms is intact _____ and _____ _____.

3. _____ _____ exists when the body produces specific antibodies to combat infections caused by specific antigens or microbes.

4. _____ _____ occurs when antibodies are transferred from a human or animal to a susceptible person.

5. Increasing the vaccination rates in the general population serves to reduce risk for clients who are not vaccinated, and this concept is referred to as _____ _____.

6. Vaccines contain whole _____ that are not pathogenic but can induce the formation of _____.

7. _____ contain detoxified microbe by-products that are antigenic and also induce antibody production.

8. _____ and _____, which contain exogenous antibodies or immunoglobulins, are used to provide artificially acquired passive immunity.

9. Minor expected reactions to vaccines can be treated with _____ and _____. Severe fevers (greater than 103°F) can be treated with _____ and _____ _____ to reduce body temperature.

10. Rare but serious _____ reactions are characterized by urticaria, dyspnea, cyanosis, shock, or unconsciousness that occurs within minutes of injection; any recipient of a vaccine should be observed for up to _____ minutes after therapy.

CONNECTING WITH CLIENTS

11. What are the potential learning needs of parents of a child receiving immunizations?

12. What special considerations should you keep in mind when administering vaccines to an infant or child?

13. A client is scheduled for a vaccination. What assessments should you make to determine whether the client has any contraindications to receiving a vaccine at this time?

TRAINING FOR TEST TAKING

14. The pediatric nurse teaches the parent of a child receiving a DTaP vaccine that which of the following is among the most frequently reported adverse effect to watch for?
    1. Swelling and redness at the site of injection
    2. High fever
    3. Intolerance of milk products
    4. Irritability for 30 minutes after the injection

15. The nurse considers that which of the following clients requiring influenza virus vaccines in the ambulatory care center is the best candidate for the nasal formulation (FluMist)?
    1. A 54-year-old client who had a kidney transplant.
    2. A 29-year-old administrative assistant.
    3. A client receiving chemotherapy for cancer.
    4. A client working as an RN in the local hospital.

16. Which of the following clients can safely receive the measles-mumps-rubella (MMR) vaccine?
    1. A child with cancer receiving chemotherapy.
    2. A child with an organ transplant.
    3. A child with allergy to egg protein.
    4. A child with cystic fibrosis.

17. The nurse determines that a client with an allergy to which of the following substances is not eligible to receive the inactivated poliovirus vaccine (IPV)?
    1. Aspirin
    2. Neomycin
    3. Penicillin
    4. Ragweed

18. A client seeks treatment in the emergency department following a jagged laceration of the hand with a rusty nail while doing a home remodeling project. The nurse assesses that this client would need a tetanus boost injection if the client's last dose was longer than how many years?
    1. 2
    2. 5
    3. 10
    4. 15

19. A pediatric client in the well-child clinic is due for routine 2-month immunizations. The nurse explains to the mother the need to keep the infant in the examination room for up to how long after the immunizations are given?
    1. 10 minutes
    2. 20 minutes
    3. 30 minutes
    4. 60 minutes

20. The nurse working in an immunization clinic is storing a new batch of vaccines that just arrived. The nurse plans to put these doses in which of the following locations?
    1. Middle shelf of refrigerator
    2. Refrigerator door
    3. Cool, dark closet
    4. In a cabinet near a sharps disposal container

63 Immunosuppressants and Immunomodulators

STAYING ON TOP OF TERMINOLOGY

1. Match the definition on the right to the term at the left.

_____ Cyclosporine
_____ Immune globulin
_____ Immunocompromised state
_____ Immunosuppressant agents

a. Specific ones are used as postexposure treatment for a particular infectious condition, including hepatitis B, rabies and tetanus
b. May result from inhibition of granulocyte formation, impairment of synthesis and antibody production, loss of mucocutaneous barriers, and impairment of cellular immunity
c. A potent immunosuppressant used to prevent of organ transplant rejection (renal, hepatic, or cardiac allografts)
d. Drugs that decrease or prevent an immune response

FOCUSING ON THE FACTS

2. _____ immunodeficiency may be induced by a variety of drugs, such as chemotherapeutic and immunosuppressant agents or radiation therapy, or through viral infections such as AIDS.

3. Although _____ contributes to morbidity in many conditions, it can be helpful in cases in which an overactive immune response is problematic.

4. The body activates an immune response by releasing _____ to phagocytize and process foreign substances; additionally, a number of _____ are involved in the immune response.

5. The care of a client with secondary immunodeficiency focuses on _____ and on treatment of the underlying _____ .

6. Before administering an immunosuppressant drug, determine that a client does not have, has not recently had, or has not been exposed to either_____ _____ , _____ _____ , or other infection.

7. In clients receiving immunosuppressive drugs, assess for symptoms of _____ infections, such as night sweats, fever, fatigue, involuntary weight loss, persistent diarrhea, headache, persistent cough, thrush and green or yellow sputum.

8. Careful _____ asepsis is a priority with an immunosuppressed client.

9. Do not give _____ _____ vaccines to a client receiving immunosuppressive therapy.

10. For clients taking immunosuppressants to prevent transplant rejection, emphasize that the duration of drug therapy is _____ .

CONNECTING WITH CLIENTS

11. What would you consider when trying to explain to a client how HIV causes immunodeficiency?

12. What criteria should you include in an education plan for an immunocompromised client?

13. What most frequently reported adverse effects of cyclosporine would you teach to a client requiring immunosuppressive therapy?

TRAINING FOR TEST TAKING

14. A client will be using an oral solution of cyclosporine (Sandimmune) following organ transplant. The nurse teaches the client to do which of the following to administer this drug appropriately?
    1. Mix the dose in water.
    2. Mix the dose in orange juice.
    3. Use a disposable paper cup for the dose.
    4. Wash the measuring device well after use.

15. The nurse instructs the client who will be taking cyclosporine (Sandimmune) to avoid which of the following fruit juices because of drug-food interaction?
    1. Tomato
    2. Apple
    3. Grapefruit
    4. Pineapple

16. The nurse explains to a client beginning drug therapy with azathioprine (Imuran) that which of the following laboratory tests needs to be drawn on a weekly basis initially?
    1. Serum electrolytes
    2. Liver function studies
    3. Uric acid level
    4. Complete blood count

17. A client has an order for muromonab-CD3 (Orthoclone). The nurse explains to the client that this drug frequently causes which of the following first dose effects?
    1. Fever and chills
    2. Ringing in the ears
    3. Flank pain
    4. Numbness and tingling in the digits

18. A client who had a renal transplant is due for a first dose of mycophenolate (CellCept) today. The breakfast meal trays on the nursing unit arrive at 08:00. The nurse should schedule the dose for which of the following times?
    1. 07:00
    2. 08:00
    3. 08:30
    4. 09:00

19. The nurse notes that a client who underwent organ transplant has an order for parenteral tacrolimus (Prograf). The nurse would question the order if the client had hypersensitivity to which of the following oils?
    1. Corn
    2. Sunflower
    3. Castor
    4. Mineral

20. A client is receiving an injection of immune globulin. The nurse would be most concerned about the development of which reaction after administration?
    1. Aching at the injection site
    2. Swelling at the injection site
    3. Temperature 99.4° F oral
    4. Confusion

64 Overview of the Integumentary System

STAYING ON TOP OF TERMINOLOGY

1. Identify the anatomic structures of the skin on the diagram below.

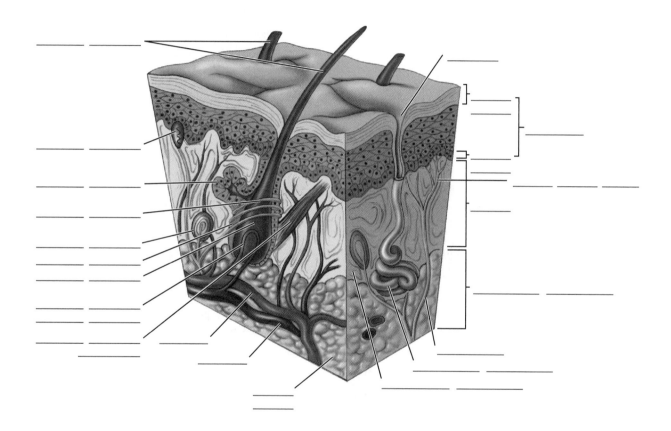

Copyright © 2006, 2001 Mosby, Inc. All rights reserved.

Chapter **64** Overview of the Integumentary System

2. The _____, or _____, has been described as the largest organ in the body.

3. The _____, or outer skin layer, consists of four strata or layers: *stratum corneum, lucidum, granulosum,* and *germinativum.*

4. The more _____ that is present, the deeper the brown skin color; it is also a protective agent, blocking ultraviolet rays to prevent injury to the underlying tissues.

5. The _____ has no direct blood supply of its own; it is nourished only by _____.

6. The _____ lies between the epidermis and subcutaneous fat and provides skin support from its blood vessels, nerves, lymphatic tissue, and elastic and connective tissues.

7. _____ glands produce sebum, the oil or film layer that covers the epidermis; they are especially abundant in the scalp, face, anus, and external ear.

8. The _____ glands, or _____ glands, help to regulate body temperature by promoting cooling through evaporation of their secretion; they also help to prevent excessive skin dryness.

9. The _____ glands, which are located mainly in the axillae, genital organs, and breast areas, are odoriferous and are believed to represent scent or sex glands.

10. The skin maintains body temperature homeostasis by regulating heat _____ or heat _____.

11. Skin excretes _____ and _____, stores _____, synthesizes _____, and provides a site for drug _____.

12. A disfiguring skin condition can lead to _____ problems, and a chronic skin condition may also lead to _____.

65 Dermatologic Drugs

1. Match the description or example to the type of lesion.

_____ Raised, 1 to 2 cm diameter	a. Macule
_____ Herpes	b. Nodule
_____ Melanoma	c. Papule
_____ Lipomas	d. Plaques
_____ Flat, vary in color	e. Vesicle
_____ Psoriasis	f. Wheals
_____ Raised, irregular shape	
_____ Acne	
_____ Freckles	
_____ Raised, less than 1 cm diameter	
_____ Deep in dermis	
_____ Urticaria	
_____ Raised, fluid-filled	
_____ Burns	
_____ Raised, hard, rough	
_____ Scabies	
_____ Atopic dermatitis	

FOCUSING ON THE FACTS

2. Dermatologic diagnosis includes _____ assessment; _____, _____, and _____ history; and _____ tests, _____, and cytodiagnosis.

3. A _____ _____ carcinoma is most common on the face, but occasionally it occurs on the _____.

4. _____ attacks only those areas of the face that flush.

5. Clients with an acute inflammation that is _____ or _____ often need a drying and soothing lotion, such as a saline, aluminum acetate, or calamine lotion.

6. A lichenified, oozing skin problem (eczema) may need a _____ and _____ agent, such as coal tar paste, Lassar's paste, or zinc compound paste.

7. If the skin problem is _____, _____, and located on an _____ or _____, a dusting powder such as talcum or starch may be appropriate to reduce friction and help to dry the area.

8. To render baths soothing in irritative conditions, _____, _____, or _____ may be added—usually 1 to 2 ounces per gallon of water.

9. _____ are fatty or oily substances that soften or soothe irritated skin and mucous membranes.

10. Skin _____ are used to coat minor skin irritations or to protect the person's skin from chemical irritants such as urine or stool.

CONNECTING WITH CLIENTS

11. What are the various forms of skin preparations that are available to clients who wish to use them?

12. What nursing diagnoses might you formulate for a client receiving dermatologic agent therapy?

13. A client seeks care in the ambulatory clinic for recent onset of an unsightly skin condition. What could be the possible etiologies of skin conditions such as these?

TRAINING FOR TEST TAKING

14. The nurse has conducted preventive health teaching on the use of sunscreens to the mother of two small children. The nurse evaluates that the mother needs additional information after stating to:
    1. Apply the sunscreen at least 15 minutes before going into the sunshine.
    2. Use whenever the weather is sunny rather than cloudy.
    3. Reapply every 2 hours or as needed after swimming.
    4. Avoid use of sunscreens that have SPF ratings of less than 12.

15. A female client has been prescribed acyclovir (Zovirax Ointment 5%) for treatment of herpes genitalis lesions. The nurse advises the client to do which of the following?
    1. Begin use of the ointment within 24 hours of symptom appearance.
    2. Have a partner use condoms during sexual activity while lesions are present.
    3. Use a finger cot or rubber glove to apply the ointment.
    4. Have a Pap smear done at least every other year.

16. The nurse working in a dermatology practice anticipates that a client being seen for which of the following conditions will mostly likely benefit from a
topical corticosteroid product?
    1. Fungal infection
    2. Atopic dermatitis
    3. Molluscum contagiosum
    4. Acne vulgaris

17. A client who will be using isotretinoin (Accutane)
for treatment of cystic acne should be taught by the
nurse to avoid intake of which of the following
dietary supplements?
    1. Calcium
    2. Vitamin A
    3. Thiamine
    4. St. John's wort

18. The respiratory rate of a client receiving mafenide
(Sulfamylon) as topical therapy for a burn wound
increases to 26 breaths/min. The nurse anticipates
that this finding will require which of the following
actions?
    1. Reduction in dressing changes to once every other
    day.
    2. Assessing the urine for sulfa crystals.
    3. Washing the mafenide from the burn wound with
    sterile saline.
    4. Increasing fluid intake to 3 liters daily.

19. A 10-month-old infant who has been receiving care
at a licensed day care facility has been diagnosed
with head lice and an over-the-counter (OTC) product has not been effective. Which of the following
products does the nurse expect to be prescribed?
    1. permethrin (Nix)
    2. lindane (Kwell)
    3. crotamiton (Eurax)
    4. malathion (Ovide)

20. A client has been prescribed efalizumab (Raptiva)
for treatment of psoriasis. The nurse would be most
concerned about risk of adverse drug effects after
noting which of the following trends in laboratory
test results?
    1. Decreasing white blood cell count.
    2. Decreasing hemoglobin.
    3. Decreasing erythrocyte sedimentation rate.
    4. Decreasing platelet count.

Chapter **65** **Dermatologic Drugs**

66 Debriding Agents

1. Match the definition on the right to the term at the left.

_____ Debridement	a. Used for chemical debridement because they digest or liquefy necrotic tissue
_____ Eschar	
_____ Granulation tissue	b. Healthy pink, soft new tissue
_____ Pressure ulcer	c. A process used to remove dirt, foreign objects, damaged tissue, and cellular debris from a wound or burn to prevent infection and promote healing
_____ Proteolytic enzyme	
	d. Another term for a crust on the skin
	e. A break in the skin and underlying subcutaneous and muscle tissue

FOCUSING ON THE FACTS

2. _____, _____, and _____ of the wounds are necessary when pressure ulcers do occur.

3. Wound _____ is the process of using fluid to remove inflammatory contaminants from the wound surface.

4. Exposure to _____ weakens the outer layers of skin and nutritional depletion contributes to the risk of _____ _____.

5. Pressure ulcers most commonly affect _____, _____, _____, or _____ clients.

6. _____ -_____ _____ devices are nondrug therapies used to treat wounds or to prepare them for surgery.

7. The prevention and treatment of pressure ulcers are focused on treating the underlying _____, providing well-balanced _____, and minimizing or eliminating the _____or _____ that is causing the tissue damage.

8. The treatment of pressure ulcers depends on the _____ of the ulcer and condition of the _____ _____.

9. Clients with _____ resulting from a pressure ulcer may present with bone pain, drainage, and/or systemic manifestations of infection including fever, chills, leukocytosis, and bacteremia.

10. Most enzymes contain the suffix "_____" in their name plus the name of the substrate on which they act.

CONNECTING WITH CLIENTS

11. What adverse effects would you assess for in a client being treated with proteolytic enzyme preparations?

12. What are the stages of pressure ulcers that a client could develop and how would you treat each stage?

13. What nursing interventions would you use to prevent the development of a pressure ulcer in an assigned client?

TRAINING FOR TEST TAKING

14. Which of the following solutions is the first choice of the nurse when irrigating a pressure ulcer?
    1. Half-strength povidone iodine
    2. Half-strength hydrogen peroxide
    3. Saline solution
    4. Dakin's solution

15. A client with a pressure ulcer on the hip is receiving topical treatment with collagenase (Santyl). The nurse determines that the topical agent should be discontinued when which of the following is noted during assessment?
    1. White blood cell count decreased to 12,000/mm^3
    2. Eschar less than one-eighth-inch thick
    3. Presence of pale yellow drainage
    4. Bleeding during gentle cleansing

16. During cleansing of a pressure ulcer being treated with collagenase (Santyl), the nurse notes that the skin around the ulcer is erythematous. The nurse should apply which of the following substances to the skin to protect it from the collagenase in the ulcer bed?
    1. Mineral oil
    2. Petrolatum jelly
    3. Nitrofurazone
    4. Zinc oxide paste

17. The nurse has an order to do an irrigation on a pressure ulcer with application of a topical debriding agent and a topical antibacterial agent. After removing the dressing, the nurse should take which of the following actions?
    1. Irrigate the wound, then apply the antibacterial followed by the debriding agent.
    2. Irrigate the wound, then apply the debriding agent followed by the antibacterial.
    3. Mix the debriding agent and antibacterial together and apply them after the irrigation.
    4. Apply the debriding agent, then irrigate the area, then apply the antibacterial.

18. The family member of a client with a pressure ulcer being treated with collagenase (Santyl) asks how long the treatment will be necessary. The nurse explains that in many cases, the length of treatment before granulation occurs is approximately:
    1. 4 days
    2. 7 days
    3. 11 days
    4. 21 days

19. A client with an infected wound is going to be treated with topical fibrinolysin and desoxyribonuclease (Elase) ointment. Before using this agent for the first time, the nurse checks the medical record to be sure that the client does not have an allergy to which of the following?
    1. Pork
    2. Sulfa
    3. Thimerosal
    4. Thiazides

20. The nurse determines that which of the following assigned clients with wounds would best benefit from the use of a flexible hydroactive dressing (DuoDERM)?
    1. A client with active vasculitis.
    2. A client with arterial insufficiency.
    3. A client with an infected ulcer.
    4. A client with an ulcer that has muscle exposed.

237

67 Vitamins and Minerals

STAYING ON TOP OF TERMINOLOGY

1. Although vitamins have been given a letter of the alphabet to identify them, they all have one or more scientific names, depending on the number of chemicals making up that vitamin category. Fill in the following chart with the proper names of the vitamins.

Vitamin | Other names or chemical names

A

B_1

B_2

B_3

B_6

B_9

B_{12}

C

D

E

FOCUSING ON THE FACTS

2. The nutritional needs of the individual are best met by adequate oral ingestion of _____ and _____, _____ meals.

3. Subtle deficiencies in several vitamins (at levels below that which cause classic vitamin deficiency syndromes) put the individual at risk for chronic degenerative diseases such as _____, _____, and _____.

4. _____ are organic compounds that help to maintain normal metabolic functions, growth, and tissue repair.

5. A commonly prescribed IV solution of dextrose 5% in water delivers only _____ calories/L, and it is delivered purely in the form of a _____.

6. Most vitamins must either be ingested in _____ or taken as _____ _____.

7. Vitamin D deficiency is common in older adults; supplements of vitamin D with calcium have been shown to reduce _____ and increase _____.

8. _____, a major risk factor for cardiovascular disease, can be lowered by one RDA of folic acid daily.

9. Vitamin and mineral requirements may change with _____ and _____ status.

10. Vitamins _____ and _____ possess antioxidant properties, although health benefits related to their antioxidant activity has been questioned.

CONNECTING WITH CLIENTS

11. How would you explain the term "RDA" found on a food label to a client?

12. What would you include in an educational plan for a client receiving iron?

13. What nursing diagnosis/diagnoses would be appropriate to use for a client who is diagnosed with a vitamin deficiency?

TRAINING FOR TEST TAKING

14. A client reports having difficulty with seeing properly while driving at night. The nurse recommends which of the following vitamins that would help if the condition is because of a deficiency state?
   1. Vitamin K
   2. Vitamin E
   3. Vitamin D
   4. Vitamin A

15. A client who eats a poorly balanced diet reports that her skin bruises very easily. The nurse concludes that a deficiency of which of the following vitamins might be responsible for this symptom?
   1. Vitamin K
   2. Vitamin E
   3. Vitamin D
   4. Vitamin A

16. The nurse who is preparing to administer medications notes that a client has an order for a vitamin D supplement. The nurse would question the order if the client has which of the following documented health problems?
    1. Hyponatremia
    2. Hypercalcemia
    3. Hypochloremia
    4. Hyperkalemia

17. A client with a long-standing history of alcohol abuse is admitted to the hospital and requires fluid volume expansion and nutritional support. The nurse anticipates an order for which of the following vitamins that is a priority need for this client?
    1. Cyanocobalamin
    2. Riboflavin
    3. Thiamine
    4. Niacin

18. The nurse anticipates that an assigned client with which of the following health problems will have an order to receive parenteral cyanocobalamin (vitamin B_{12})?
    1. Esophageal varices
    2. Duodenal ulcer
    3. Polyps of the colon
    4. Malabsorption syndrome

19. A client with kidney stones is trying to acidify the urine. The nurse recommends increased intake of which of the following vitamins?
    1. Vitamin B_6
    2. Vitamin C
    3. Vitamin E
    4. Vitamin A

20. A client has an order for an injections of iron dextran (INFeD). The nurse would do which of the following to properly administer this medication?
    1. Use a 25- to 27-gauge needle.
    2. Use the deltoid muscle as the injection site.
    3. Change the needle after withdrawing the drug from the vial.
    4. Ensure that the needle length is between 1/2 inch and 1 inch.

68 Fluids and Electrolytes

STAYING ON TOP OF TERMINOLOGY

1. Match the symptoms at the left to the electrolyte imbalance (there may be more than one correct answer).

_____ Lethargy	a. Hypocalcemia
_____ Weakness	b. Hypermagnesemia
_____ Peaked T waves	c. Hyponatremia
_____ Tetany	d. Hyperkalemia
_____ Flushing	e. Hypercalcemia
_____ Athetoid movements	f. Hypokalemia
_____ Amnesia	g. Hypomagnesemia
_____ Paralysis	h. Hypernatremia
_____ Seizures	
_____ Oliguria	

FOCUSING ON THE FACTS

2. The intracellular electrolytes are _____ and _____.

3. The extracellular electrolytes are _____, _____, and _____.

4. A few reasons for administering intravenous solutions are to replace _____ and _____, and correct _____ _____ imbalances.

5. Depending on the amount of adipose tissue present, water accounts for _____ % to _____ % of the total body weight in humans.

6. If the water gained exceeds the water lost during a period of time, _____ fluid volume or _____ and edema occur.

7. Although _____ is complex and not well understood, it is induced by a _____ in saliva and _____ of the mouth and throat.

8. The principal way that fluid is lost from the body is via the _____ in the form of _____.

9. Water travels from less concentrated areas to areas with higher concentrations of solutes or dissolved substances by _____.

10. _____ refers to the total solute concentration usually expressed per liter of serum.

CONNECTING WITH CLIENTS

11. You are assigned to three clients, each of which needs one of the intravenous solutions outlined in the categories below. For each category, give an example of an appropriate solution and why each client might require its use.

Category	Solution	Use
Hydrating solution		
Isotonic solution		
Maintenance solution		

12. You are assigned to a group of debilitated clients who are at risk for dehydration. Which type of dehydration would you suspect if the client exhibited each of the items on the left? Write in the corresponding letter next to the symptom.

_____ Thirst   a. Isotonic
_____ Increased intracellular fluid   b. Hypotonic
_____ Shock   c. Hypertonic
_____ Confusion
_____ Dry, furrowed tongue
_____ Low sodium
_____ Irritability
_____ Regular pulse

13. How can you as a nurse protect your clients from the hazard of overdosing with electronic infusion devices (EIDs)?

TRAINING FOR TEST TAKING

14. A client is scheduled to receive a unit of packed red blood cells. The nurse obtains which of the following solutions from the supply storage area to use when priming the blood transfusion line?
1. 5% dextrose in 0.45% sodium chloride
2. 5% dextrose in 0.9% sodium chloride
3. 0.9% sodium chloride
4. 0.45% sodium chloride

15. The client who has an order for NPO status requires hydration. The nurse anticipates that which of the following solutions will most likely be ordered?
1. 5% dextrose in water
2. 5% dextrose in 0.225% sodium chloride
3. 5% dextrose in 0.45% sodium chloride
4. 5% dextrose in 0.9% sodium chloride

16. An adult client who is hypokalemic has an order for IV infusion of 5% dextrose in 0.45% sodium chloride with 60 mEq potassium chloride to infuse at 125 mL/hr. The nurse ensures that which of the following items is in use during the infusion?
    1. Infusion set with a drop factor of 60 drops/mL
    2. In-line IV filter
    3. Pulse oximeter
    4. Cardiac monitor

17. A client is scheduled for a dose of liquid potassium for supplementation of deficiency. To disguise the taste, the nurse should mix it into which of the following items?
    1. Pudding
    2. Gelatin
    3. Orange juice
    4. Milk

18. A client needs to take calcium carbonate tablets for calcium replacement. The nurse suggests that the client take the tablets at which of the following times to enhance absorption?
    1. 1 hour before meals
    2. With meals
    3. 2 hours after meals
    4. Bedtime

19. An older adult client is receiving intravenous infusion therapy. On routine assessment, the nurse notes that the client is tachycardic, tachypneic, and auscultation of the lungs reveals dependent crackles. Which of the following actions should the nurse take first?
    1. Measure the blood pressure.
    2. Notify the physician.
    3. Slow the IV infusion rate to KVO.
    4. Discontinue the IV.

20. A client with hypertonic dehydration has undergone fluid replacement therapy. The nurse determines that this problem has been resolved after noting that which symptom unique to hypertonic dehydration is absent?
    1. Dry, furrowed tongue
    2. Increased pulse rate
    3. Vomiting
    4. Abdominal cramps

69 Enteral and Parenteral Nutrition

STAYING ON TOP OF TERMINOLOGY

1. Match the definition on the right to the term at the left.

_____ Amino acid
_____ Enteral nutrition
_____ Essential amino acids
_____ Negative nitrogen balance
_____ Nonessential amino acids
_____ Protein-sparing nutrition
_____ Semiessential amino acids
_____ Total parenteral nutrition

a. A condition in which more nitrogen is excreted than is taken in, indicating the wasting of tissue
b. Usually reserved for clients who have minimal protein deficiencies and sufficient fat stores
c. The IV approach to complete nutrition, may also be referred to as hyperalimentation
d. Substances that can be synthesized from a nitrogen source
e. Histidine and arginine, which are not synthesized in adequate amounts during growth periods
f. The provision of liquid formula diets into the GI tract
g. Necessary substances to promote the production of proteins (anabolism), to reduce protein breakdown (catabolism), and to help promote wound healing
h. Substances that the body cannot synthesize

FOCUSING ON THE FACTS

2. To achieve and maintain good health requires a regular intake of sufficient amounts of _____, _____, _____, _____ and _____.

3. Malnutrition is reflected in laboratory values such as reduced total _____ count, serum _____, and _____ levels (or iron-binding capacity).

4. _____ or _____ tubes are ideal for clients who require short-term (less than 2 weeks) enteral nutrition.

5. _____ syndrome is the result of a sudden influx of feeding and the creation of a high _____ gradient within the small intestine, leading to fluid shifts from the vascular compartment to the intestinal lumen.

6. Numerous different enteral formulations are available, and they can be broadly divided into _____, _____, _____, _____, and _____ - _____ formulations.

7. For intermittent enteral feeding administration, measure the _____ _____ halfway between feedings.

8. Concentrations of dextrose solutions above _____% are hyperosmolar and are too irritating to be given continuously peripherally; thus they should be administered through _____ _____ catheters.

9. _____ usually occurs when dextrose is administered without lipids as the primary source of calories.

10. Although some commercial parenteral nutrition solutions contain _____ _____ or _____, clients who are placed on long-term administration should be evaluated for deficiencies in these.

CONNECTING WITH CLIENTS

11. What data would you consider it important to assess in a client receiving total parenteral nutrition?

12. What education needs would you be prepared to meet for a client being discharged to home while receiving tube (enteral) feedings?

13. What complications of parenteral nutrition could arise in an assigned client from infection and sepsis?

TRAINING FOR TEST TAKING

14. An adult client will be started on full strength continuous enteral feedings that provide 1 cal/mL. The nurse anticipates that the flow rate at the beginning of the infusion will be how many mL/hour?
    1. 25
    2. 50
    3. 75
    4. 100

15. A client with inflammatory bowel disease requires enteral feedings. Which of the following types of products will most likely be ordered for this client?
    1. Modular
    2. Monomeric
    3. Oligomeric
    4. Polymeric

248

16. The nurse is providing care to a client receiving enteral nutrition. Which of the following actions by the nurse upholds the standard of care for this client?
    1. Elevate the head of the bed at least 30 to 45 degrees during feeding.
    2. Warm the refrigerated feeding for 5 minutes prior to use.
    3. Chart the volume infused in the intake column used for oral fluids.
    4. Label the feeding bag with the name and volume of fluid in the feeding bag.

17. Which of the following clients assigned to the nurse would be the best candidate for peripheral parenteral nutrition?
    1. A client who has gastric surgery and cannot have oral intake for 5 days.
    2. A client with an enterocutaneous fistula.
    3. A client who was critically injured in a motor vehicle accident.
    4. A client who sustained burns to 50% of the body surface area.

18. A client who began total parenteral nutrition (TPN) at 10:00 should have a blood glucose level checked by the nurse no later than which of the following times on the same day?
    1. 14:00
    2. 18:00
    3. 20:00
    4. 22:00

19. The nurse is monitoring the status of a client with a history of heart failure who is receiving total parenteral nutrition (TPN). The nurse would alert the physician for which of the following data?
    1. Intake greater than output of 300 mL.
    2. Temperature of 99° F oral.
    3. Crackles in bases of lungs.
    4. Weight gain of 1 pound in 4 days.

20. Which of the following laboratory values for a client receiving total parenteral nutrition (TPN) should be reported by the nurse to the physician?
    1. Serum sodium 145 mEq/L
    2. Blood glucose 158 mEq/L
    3. Serum potassium 3.1 mEq/L
    4. Blood urea nitrogen 21 mg/dL

70 Antiseptics, Disinfectants, and Sterilants

STAYING ON TOP OF TERMINOLOGY

1. Match the definition on the right to the term at the left.

_____ Antiseptics
_____ Bactericidal
_____ Bacteriostatic
_____ Disinfectants
_____ Medical asepsis
_____ Nosocomial infection
_____ Sterilization
_____ Surgical asepsis

a. A practice that results in the absence of pathogenic organisms

b. Substances that are typically applied only to living tissue; they must be less potent or made more dilute to prevent cell damage.

c. A process that destroys all forms of life on an instrument or utensil, in a liquid, or within a substance

d. Acquired in the hospital and most commonly result from gram-negative infections including *Pseudomonas, Proteus, Serratia, Providencia,* and others

e. Substances that are used only on nonliving objects because they are toxic to living tissue

f. A description for products that actually kill bacteria, but perhaps not all types, and often not fungi, viruses, or spores

g. A practice that results in the absence of all organisms

h. A description for products that slow the growth and replication of bacteria but do not kill off the entire bacteria population

FOCUSING ON THE FACTS

2. Urinary tract infections and postoperative wound infections account for the majority of the _____ infections detected in a _____ setting.

3. The focus in _____ _____ is to keep all organisms out of a designated area (e.g., fresh wound), whereas in _____ _____ the goal is to remove or destroy the pathogens in the area and contain the remaining nonpathogens by conscious efforts.

4. Several acceptable and practicable sterilization methods now exist, although _____ or _____ is preferred as the most effective method.

251

5. The current criteria for an effective disinfectant include the ability to destroy within _____ minutes all vegetative bacteria (not _____) and fungi, tubercle bacilli, animal parasites, and viruses (except _____ viruses).

6. Thorough _____ still predominates as the most effective measure for controlling the spread of infection.

7. The relative usefulness of various antiseptics can be compared based on their _____ index, the relationship between the specific antiseptic concentration effective against microorganisms without irritating _____ or interfering with _____.

8. _____ is an all-encompassing term for agents that work against many types of "germs"—bacteria, fungi, viruses, and spores.

9. The ideal all-around antiseptic/disinfectant would need to destroy all forms of _____ without being toxic to human cells, and have a low incidence of _____.

10. _____ is an antiseptic found in a number of consumer products including soaps, dishwashing liquids, detergents, toothpastes, lotions, creams, cosmetics, and plastics.

CONNECTING WITH CLIENTS

11. How do the various antiseptics and disinfectants that you use in a hospital or other health care setting work?

12. What nursing interventions would you employ if you were using iodine compounds?

13. What nursing considerations would you keep in mind when using oxidating agents?

14. A client has been given hexachlorophene to use as a scrub before surgery. The nurse assesses the client for which of the following symptoms as an adverse effect if absorption through the skin occurs?
    1. Palpitations
    2. Hearing loss
    3. Confusion
    4. Muscle aches

15. A newborn infant has been treated with silver nitrate 1% solution. The nurse determines that the infant has the expected outcome of treatment after noting which of the following?
    1. The umbilical cord is drier.
    2. Conjunctiva are pink and moist.
    3. Lanugo has decreased.
    4. Ear canals are patent and clean.

16. A client is being admitted to the preoperative holding area for surgery. The client showered at home the previous night with povidone iodine (Betadine) scrub. The nurse would assess the client for which of the following to see if an adverse effect occurred?
    1. Skin rash
    2. Blister formation
    3. Skin tenderness
    4. Reddish discoloration of skin

17. A daughter of a client with a pressure ulcer asks the nurse why hydrogen peroxide is not being used to clean the wound, because that is what was used for an aunt about 5 years ago. The nurse replies that hydrogen peroxide is not being used because it has which of the following adverse effects?
    1. Increases eschar formation.
    2. Increases bleeding in the ulcer base.
    3. Harms normal tissue forming in the ulcer.
    4. Is no longer effective against many microorganisms.

18. The nurse is orienting a nursing assistant to the nursing unit. When explaining the procedure on hand hygiene using chlorhexidine (Hibiclens), the nurse states to apply the product, add water, and use friction for how long?
    1. 5 seconds
    2. 15 seconds
    3. 30 seconds
    4. 60 seconds

19. The nurse would question an order to use which of the following substances as an antiseptic?
    1. povidone-iodine (Betadine)
    2. isopropanol (isopropyl alcohol)
    3. chlorhexidine (Hibiclens)
    4. benzalkonium chloride

20. The home health nurse would recommend which of the following common substances to a client for use as an antiseptic?
    1. Acetic acid
    2. Benzoic acid
    3. Lactic acid
    4. Boric acid

71 Diagnostic Agents

STAYING ON TOP OF TERMINOLOGY

1. Complete the following word search.

ANERGY
ANTIHISTAMINES
CHOLANGIOGRAPHY
CONTRAST
DETECTION
DIAGNOSTICS
EPINEPHRINE
FLUSHING
FUNCTIONING
IMMUNOSUPPRESSED
INDICATIONS
MRI
NURSING

ORGANS
RADIOACTIVE
RADIONUCLIDES
RADIOPAQUE
RADIOPHARMACEUTICAL
ROENTGEN
SCREENING
TOMOGRAPHY
TREATMENT
TUMORS
ULTRASONOGRAPHY
VISUALIZATION

```
S  N  O  I  T  A  C  I  D  N  I  G  L  R  B  E  G  G  N  G  H
D  E  S  S  E  R  P  P  U  S  O  N  U  M  M  I  C  N  N  I  U
L  R  U  M  B  F  N  E  G  T  N  E  O  R  T  F  Q  I  D  U  U
S  G  P  S  X  Y  V  T  D  C  M  Y  I  C  H  A  X  N  Q  Y  L
M  X  O  C  F  Y  Z  A  A  O  T  H  Z  W  G  F  J  O  B  D  T
I  M  K  R  Q  Z  B  W  N  N  R  P  Z  N  K  R  R  I  E  D  R
R  L  N  E  C  R  V  X  T  T  E  A  Y  N  J  G  V  T  M  I  A
P  A  Y  E  B  N  Q  V  I  R  A  R  R  B  A  B  E  C  B  A  S
R  T  D  N  X  X  T  D  H  A  T  G  G  N  U  C  P  N  F  G  O
A  O  S  I  W  U  M  W  I  S  M  O  S  Y  T  E  I  U  L  N  N
D  M  R  N  O  Z  M  D  S  T  E  I  R  I  I  A  N  F  U  O  O
I  O  T  G  U  A  M  R  T  C  N  G  O  L  K  D  E  H  S  S  G
O  G  C  W  T  R  C  V  A  N  T  N  M  D  A  F  P  I  H  T  R
N  R  N  B  V  Y  S  T  M  D  V  A  U  J  K  F  H  T  I  I  A
U  A  S  U  S  A  G  I  I  T  I  L  T  C  S  S  R  W  N  C  P
C  P  I  B  X  Q  G  W  N  V  L  O  N  G  H  X  I  U  G  S  H
L  H  N  X  S  D  R  R  E  G  E  H  P  Y  J  X  N  Q  E  A  Y
I  Y  G  F  S  R  F  K  S  O  F  C  C  A  Z  A  E  R  P  J  H
D  A  Q  E  X  Z  F  F  W  G  K  L  E  F  Q  M  J  U  M  B  G
E  U  R  A  D  I  O  P  H  A  R  M  A  C  E  U  T  I  C  A  L
S  X  V  V  I  S  U  A  L  I  Z  A  T  I  O  N  E  B  H  E  H
```

FOCUSING ON THE FACTS

2. _____ _____ are chemical substances used to diagnose or monitor a client's condition or disease.

3. Ordinary _____ _____ are useful only for studies of dense materials such as bone; however, when injected or instilled, _____ agents make the body cavity, compartment, or blood vessels appear more dense or opaque than neighboring anatomic structures.

4. Many diagnostic agents contain molecular _____ in the radiopaque contrast medium to provide the opacity necessary to outline internal organ cavities, lumens, or ducts.

5. Barium contrast media consist of _____ _____ powder and a vehicle such as _____ _____, which are mixed with a prescribed volume of water to provide a suspension for oral or rectal administration.

6. Because they are not absorbed internally, barium sulfate preparations are only potentially hazardous when administered to persons with _____ _____ or _____.

7. The most common clinical use of iodinated contrast media is _____.

8. A _____ is a photographic recording that shows the distribution and intensity of radioactivity in various tissues and organs following administration of a radiopharmaceutical.

9. _____ are used as tracers to evaluate the physiologic and biochemical functioning of organ systems.

10. The time it takes for the original radioactivity to decay to one half its original value is known as the physical or radioactive _____ _____ of the particular radionuclide.

CONNECTING WITH CLIENTS

11. What are some common tests that are used to screen for health conditions?

Chapter **71**   **Diagnostic Agents**

12. What would be the secondary effects of nonradioactive agents that you would be assessing for in an assigned client?

13. What nursing interventions would you employ for a client receiving a radiopaque agent?

TRAINING FOR TEST TAKING

14. A client will receive contrast material iohexol (Omnipaque-140) during an upcoming diagnostic angiography. The nurse assesses the client for which of the following allergies before the procedure?
    1. Shellfish
    2. Cod
    3. Haddock
    4. Scallops

15. A client is scheduled for an upper GI series with barium as a contrast agent. The nurse should request from the physician an order for which of the following types of medications following the procedure?
    1. Analgesic
    2. Antiemetic
    3. Laxative
    4. Histamine receptor antagonist

16. The client will undergo diagnostic testing using injectable iodinated contrast medium. The nurse explains to the client that which of the following common adverse effects may be noted during injection?
    1. Nausea and flushing
    2. A drop in pulse rate
    3. Transient electrocardiogram changes
    4. Petechiae on the skin

17. A client is undergoing testing of gastric function using histamine as the diagnostic aid. Which of the following secondary effects of histamine should the nurse be prepared to manage?
    1. Dyspnea
    2. Fever
    3. One-sided weakness
    4. Blurred vision

18. A client is undergoing intradermal allergy testing. The nurse would determine that the client has had a positive result to one of the allergens injected after noting which of the following findings at the injection site?
    1. Ecchymoses
    2. Pain and pallor
    3. Redness and induration
    4. Induration and cool temperature

19. An older adult client who is homeless was admitted for pneumonia and malnutrition. On intradermal testing with candida, the client had no response. Which conclusion by the nurse would be best initially?
    1. The client is not at risk for candida infection.
    2. The client does not have candida infection.
    3. The client needs retesting in 6 months.
    4. The client's condition may be causing anergy.

20. The nurse needs to administer an intradermal tuberculin test with purified protein derivative (PPD). Which of the following actions by the nurse is correct?
    1. Use a 20- to 22-gauge needle.
    2. Draw up a 0.6-mL test dose.
    3. Insert at an angle as flat against the skin as possible.
    4. Insert the needle bevel down until it disappears.

72 Poisons and Antidotes

STAYING ON TOP OF TERMINOLOGY

1. Match the sign to the toxin.

_____ Seizures or muscle twitching	a.	Iron
_____ Abdominal colic	b.	Phenytoin
_____ Bitter almond breath odor	c.	Aspirin
_____ Ataxia	d.	Botulism
_____ Salivation	e.	Cyanide
_____ Coma and drowsiness	f.	Mercury

FOCUSING ON THE FACTS

2. Toxicology is the study of _____, their _____ and _____, methods of _____, and the _____ and _____ of poisoning.

3. Poison is any substance that in _____ amounts can cause _____ or_____.

4. Toxidromes are _____.

5. Ipecac syrup is the most commonly used _____; it tastes _____.

6. Apomorphine is a/an _____ that causes _____.

7. Gastric lavage is _____.

8. Activated charcoal is instilled or swallowed following _____ or _____ to act as _____.

9. SLUDGE refers to the symptoms of _____, which are _____, _____, _____, _____, _____, and_____.

10. Complications associated with emesis are problematic for agents that suppress _____ _____ _____ function, produce local _____ (e.g., acids, bases, and other caustic agents), or agents that are more likely to be _____ (e.g., gasoline, petroleum based products).

CONNECTING WITH CLIENTS

11. How would you describe your role as a nurse in the emergency care of a client with a drug poisoning/overdose?

12. A client who was transported to the emergency department following an overdose is being considered for treatment with activated charcoal. Under what circumstances would this type of therapy be contraindicated?

13. A client who experienced an overdose may be treated with an antidote. What do you recall about the various ways in which antidotes can work?

TRAINING FOR TEST TAKING

14. A client who took a drug overdose is comatose with stable vital signs. When the nurse conducts neurologic assessment, the client has no pain response and depressed deep tendon reflexes, and pupils are reactive by slightly dilated. The nurse documents on the client care flow-sheet that the client is in which category of coma?
    1. Grade I
    2. Grade II
    3. Grade III
    4. Grade IV

15. The home health nurse is making a routine visit to an older adult man who lives with his daughter's family. On arrival, the daughter is distraught because her 5-year-old just drank some household cleaner that looked like apple juice. The nurse should take which of the following correct actions?
    1. Wait for 10 minutes to see if symptoms appear.
    2. Call the poison control center before taking any specific action.
    3. Immediately induce vomiting.
    4. Read the container and follow antidote instructions immediately.

16. The nurse working in an emergency department concludes that inducing emesis may be appropriate following overdose in which of the following situations?
    1. Client exhibits seizure activity.
    2. Client is comatose.
    3. Client ingested an alkali .
    4. Client is an awake 8-year-old.

17. A client who took an overdose of a substance is brought to the emergency department. The client is comatose and has pinpoint pupils. The nurse suspects which of the following substances is involved?
    1. Opioids
    2. Salicylates
    3. Antihistamines
    4. Cocaine

18. A client is brought to the emergency department with an overdose of cyanide. The nurse hearing the ambulance radio transmission while in transit would prepare which of the following antidotes for use on arrival of the client?
    1. Glucagon
    2. Flumazenil
    3. Methylene blue
    4. Deferoxamine (Desferal)

19. A client requires treatment for iron toxicity. Which of the following substances would the nurse prepare as ordered for an antidote?
    1. trientine (Syprine)
    2. edetate calcium disodium (Versenate)
    3. D-penicillamine (Cuprimine)
    4. succimer (Chemet)

20. The nurse would assess a client with suspected salicylate overdose for which of the following odors on the breath?
    1. Acetone
    2. Alcohol
    3. Bitter almonds
    4. Garlic

Answer Key

CHAPTER 1

Orientation to Pharmacology

1.

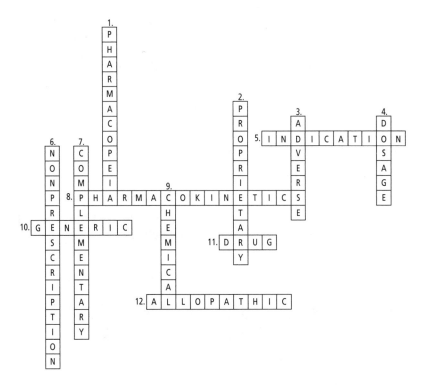

2. Pharmacology
3. Hippocrates
4. pharmacopeia
5. drug
6. generic, nonproprietary
7. prescription, legend
8. key, prototype
9. indications
10. assessment

11. **Suggested Answer:** You should look up information about the drug, including usual dosage, route of administration, indication(s), significant adverse effects, major drug interactions, contraindications, and the appropriate nursing assessment, planning, implementation, and evaluation techniques necessary to administer the drug safely.

12. **Suggested Answer:** Drugs have two commonly used names. The generic name identifies a drug based on pharmacologic and/or chemical relation-ships. This name is the same regardless of who the manufacturer is. However, when drug companies market a particular drug product, they often select and copyright a trade, brand, or proprietary name for their drug, which is the name associated with the drug produced only by that pharmaceutical company.

13. **Suggested Answer:** When implementing the plan of care for a drug regimen, you should incorporate the nursing activities of monitoring, intervention, and education. These activities need to be planned to administer specific drugs safely and accurately.

14. **Answer:** 4

Rationale: A nursing drug handbook gives brief overviews of drugs in outline format. It is helpful as a quick refresher on the unit to remind the nurse of important points related to a drug. It is also helpful because information is formatted according to the nursing process and gives nursing considerations.

Cognitive Level: Application

263

Nursing Process Step: Implementation
NCLEX: Physiological Integrity: Pharmacological and Parenteral Therapies

15. **Answer:** 2
Rationale: It is important to select Internet sites carefully when seeking drug information, because erroneous information may be posted. There is no screening tool for Internet information, and thus the best approach is to use sites where the provider is reputable. For example, use drug information from drug information centers; pharmacy, medical, or nursing school posted information; professional journals; and the American Cancer Society, the Food and Drug Administration (FDA), the National Institutes of Health, and numerous other organizations.
Cognitive Level: Application
Nursing Process Step: Implementation
NCLEX: Physiological Integrity: Pharmacological and Parenteral Therapies

16. **Answer:** 3
Rationale: Nurses seeking to protect clients from harm during medication therapy will chart drug effects clearly and accurately, question an order that is clear or could harm the client, and refer to authoritative sources, such as drug literature or pharmacists or the prescriber, for questions about an ordered drug.
Cognitive Level: Application
Nursing Process Step: Implementation
NCLEX: Physiological Integrity: Pharmacological and Parenteral Therapies

17. **Answer:** 1
Rationale: Manufacturers often place an identification code consisting of letters or numbers on their solid oral dosage forms. Although these markings may not be meaningful to the practicing nurse or client, pharmacists and local drug information centers can use them to assist in identifying generic and trade products.
Cognitive Level: Application
Nursing Process Step: Implementation
NCLEX: Physiological Integrity: Pharmacological and Parenteral Therapies

18. **Answer:** 3
Rationale: During the planning step of the nursing process, the nurse writes goals that directly relate to the client's nursing diagnoses and specific outcome criteria for medication therapy.
Cognitive Level: Comprehension
Nursing Process Step: Planning
NCLEX: Physiological Integrity: Pharmacological and Parenteral Therapies

CHAPTER 2

Legal and Ethical Aspects of Medication Administration

1.

2. Controlled Substances Act
3. abuse
4. animals
5. therapeutic index
6. X
7. drug reactions or adverse effects
8. informed consent
9. valid
10. beneficence
11. **Suggested Answer:** Although the detection of chemical defects is usually outside the nurse's province, the detection of observable physical

defects is not. You should learn to be keenly aware of the physical characteristics of drugs you administer and make comparisons before administering them. For example, unusual discolorations, precipitates, other inconsistencies, or foreign bodies in parenteral fluids should be considered suspect. Such observations warrant withholding the drug and contacting the pharmacy department or other authoritative source. Recall of defective drugs is necessary to prevent client harm.

12. **Suggested Answer:** The drug is in the stage of extended clinical evaluation. The drug is now ready for testing in various centers in the United States in larger numbers of individuals. Standards (protocols) have been developed and are to be followed at all investigative sites. The three objectives for this phase are to: (1) determine clinical effectiveness, (2) determine drug safety, and (3) establish tolerated dosage or dosage range.

13. **Suggested Answer:** Drugs in Pregnancy Category C fall under the following criteria. Animal reproduction studies have reported an adverse effect on the fetus, but there are no adequate and well-controlled studies in humans; the benefits of the drugs in pregnant women may be acceptable despite its potential risks.

14. **Answer:** 1
Rationale: The Kefauver-Harris Amendment required proof of both the safety and efficacy of a new drug before it could be approved for use. It tightened controls over drug safety and statements about adverse effects and contraindications, drug testing methods, and drug effectiveness criteria. The Orphan Drug Act allowed drug companies to take tax deductions for about three-quarters of the cost of clinical studies for drugs that may offer little or no profit, but may benefit people with rare diseases. The Durham-Humphrey Amendment of 1952 distinguished more clearly between drugs that can be sold with or without a prescription and those that cannot be refilled. The Controlled Substances Act of 1970 categorized controlled substances on the basis of their relative potential for abuse.
Cognitive Level: Knowledge
Nursing Process Step: General
NCLEX: General

15. **Answer:** 2
Rationale: Schedule II drugs often include opioids with a high risk for dependence. By federal law, no refills are allowed. Schedule I drugs are not safe for use, and drugs in Schedules III and IV may be allowed limited refills according to which group they are in.
Cognitive Level: Application
Nursing Process Step: Analysis

NCLEX: Physiological Integrity: Pharmacological and Parenteral Therapies

16. **Answer:** 4
Rationale: The nurse would follow agency protocol for counting controlled substances, which then keeps the organization in compliance with federal law. Controlled substances are counted at the beginning and end of the work shift with an off-going and on-coming nurse, respectively.
Cognitive Level: Application
Nursing Process Step: Implementation
NCLEX: Physiological Integrity: Pharmacological and Parenteral Therapies

17. **Answer:** 3
Rationale: The nurse should replace the IV solution with a new bag and then call the pharmacy. The bag would be handled according to agency policy, which often consists of returning it to pharmacy, who will not discard it. An incident report would be written after immediate client concerns are attended to.
Cognitive Level: Analysis
Nursing Process Step: Implementation
NCLEX: Physiological Integrity: Pharmacological and Parenteral Therapies

18. **Answer:** 1
Rationale: A drug that is pregnancy category A is one in which adequate and well-controlled studies indicate no risk to the fetus in the first trimester of pregnancy, and there is no evidence of risk in later trimesters. For this reason, the nurse should administer the dose.
Cognitive Level: Application
Nursing Process Step: Implementation
NCLEX: Physiological Integrity: Pharmacological and Parenteral Therapies

19. **Answer:** 3
Rationale: The responsibility of obtaining informed consent belongs to the researcher, who gives a full explanation and answers pertinent questions.
Cognitive Level: Comprehension
Nursing Process Step: Analysis
NCLEX: Physiological Integrity: Pharmacological and Parenteral Therapies

20. **Answer:** 2
Rationale: The nurse should contact the prescriber to clarify the order. The other options either do not protect the client or involve a significant delay in seeking appropriate treatment for the client.
Cognitive Level: Application
Nursing Process Step: Implementation
NCLEX: Physiological Integrity: Pharmacological and Parenteral Therapies

CHAPTER 3

Principles of Drug Action

1.

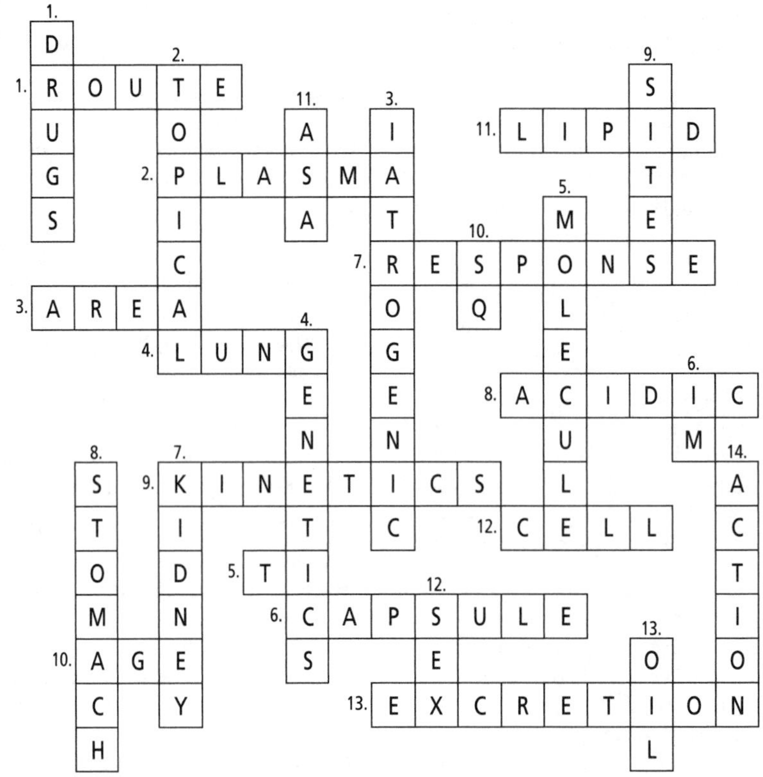
1. ROUTE
2. PLASMA
3. AREA
4. LUNG
5. TI
6. CAPSULE
7. RESPONSE
8. ACIDIC
9. KINETICS
10. AGE
11. LIPID
12. CELL
13. EXCRETION
1. DRUGS
2. TOPICAL
3. IATROGENIC
4. GENETICS
5. MOLECULAR
6. IM
7. KIDNEY
8. STOMACH
9. SITES
10. SQ
11. ASA
12. SE
13. OIL
14. ACTION

2. functions
3. Pharmacokinetics
4. passive
5. loading
6. enteric or film
7. intradermal
8. first pass
9. water
10. kidney, liver
11. **Suggested Answer:** Drugs can affect different tissues in the body that have cells with similar receptors. Depending on the function of that receptor in that tissue, a drug that has a helpful effect in one location may be harmful in another. In this case, the β blocking effect that lowers blood pressure then limits bronchodilation in the lungs, and can worsen respiratory symptoms.
12. **Suggested Answer:** Gastroparesis or delayed gastric emptying time is often observed in individuals with diabetes and delayed onset of drugs given orally to these individuals is often observed. To counteract this effect, administer drugs on an empty stomach with sufficient water (8 ounces) to ensure dissolution, rapid passage into the small intestine, and drug absorption in the larger surface area. After administering pills or tablets (solid drug forms), have the client sit upright for at least 30 minutes to hasten gastric emptying time (time required for the drug to reach the small intestine) and to reduce the potential for tablets or capsules to lodge in the esophageal area.
13. **Suggested Answer:** By pressing on the side of the eye near the nose, known as the inner canthus, there will be less absorption of the medication into the bloodstream. Ophthalmic medications are intended to produce a local effect on the conjunctiva or anterior chamber of the eye.
14. **Answer:** 4

Rationale: An antagonist is an agent that has an affinity for the receptor (or an area near the receptor) and counteracts the action of other drugs or substances at the receptor. Antagonists may be either competitive (e.g., compete with agonists to bind to the receptor) or noncompetitive (e.g., bind to a site near the receptor and change the three-dimensional structure of the receptor in a way that renders the receptor inactive). The remaining terms refer to other principles of drug binding.

Cognitive Level: Comprehension
Nursing Process Step: Analysis
NCLEX: Physiological Integrity: Pharmacological and Parenteral Therapies

15. **Answer:** 3
Rationale: Blood circulation at the site of administration is a significant factor in drug absorption. A client in shock may not respond to drugs administered intramuscularly or subcutaneously because of poor peripheral circulation. Intravenous administration is desirable when speedy drug effects are necessary, such as in shock states. Not all drugs are absorbed appropriately by the intratracheal route.

Cognitive Level: Application
Nursing Process Step: Planning
NCLEX: Physiological Integrity: Pharmacological and Parenteral Therapies

16. **Answer:** 1
Rationale: Drugs such as warfarin (Coumadin) that are highly protein bound may quickly rise to toxic levels in the presence of hypoalbuminemia. For this reason, the nurse should be aware of the client's albumin level, if ordered, whenever administering a drug that has greater than 90% protein binding.

Cognitive Level: Analysis
Nursing Process Step: Assessment
NCLEX: Physiological Integrity: Pharmacological and Parenteral Therapies

17. **Answer:** 4
Rationale: The serum level of a drug is usually drawn just before the first dose of the day. In this case, the level would be drawn just prior to the 8 AM dose.

Cognitive Level: Application
Nursing Process Step: Planning
NCLEX: Physiological Integrity: Pharmacological and Parenteral Therapies

18. **Answer:** 2
Rationale: Adverse reactions are unintended, undesirable, and often unpredictable drug effects that can range from mild (e.g., rashes, phototoxic or photosensitivity reactions to light) to potentially fatal (anaphylaxis). Side effects are usually predictable and often unavoidable secondary effects produced by a drug at the usual therapeutic drug doses. The most commonly reported side effects are anorexia, nausea, vomiting, dizziness, drowsiness, dry mouth, abdominal gas or distress, constipation, and diarrhea.

Cognitive Level: Application
Nursing Process Step: Implementation
NCLEX: Physiological Integrity: Pharmacological and Parenteral Therapies

19. **Answer:** 3
Rationale: Antihistamines, epinephrine, and bronchodilators are indispensable in the treatment of ana-

phylactic shock. Ranitidine is a histamine-1 antagonist and is used to reduce gastric acid. Digoxin is a cardiac glycoside used to treat heart failure. Acetylcysteine is a mucolytic drug (not a bronchodilator), which is also useful in treating acetaminophen (Tylenol) overdose.

Cognitive Level: Application
Nursing Process Step: Planning
NCLEX: Physiological Integrity: Pharmacological and Parenteral Therapies

20. **Answer:** 1
Rationale: Drugs that are known to irritate the gastrointestinal tract should be administered with meals. The other times listed are those when the stomach is more likely to be empty.

Cognitive Level: Application
Nursing Process Step: Planning
NCLEX: Physiological Integrity: Pharmacological and Parenteral Therapies

CHAPTER 4

Medication Errors

1. c, d, b, a
2. prescribing
3. dispensing
4. errors
5. name, date of birth
6. three
7. given or administered
8. five
9. client safety or incident
10. blame

11. **Suggested Answer:** You should compare the list of medications written on the physician order sheet against the admission orders, to ensure that all client medications that are necessary have been ordered. You would also check all previously written medication orders that were written, to be sure that they were completed (if one time or stat doses) or to determine when they were last given (such as pain medication or antibiotics).

12. **Suggested Answer:** Have another nurse check the dose to ensure it is correct. Check the client's identify before administration and give it in the right site at the right time, and document the dose correctly in the medical record.

13. **Suggested Answer:** You should stop, refrain from administering the medication, and recheck the medication against the original order.

14. **Answer:** 4
Rationale: The Lasix order is free of unapproved abbreviations. The Digoxin order has a trailing zero; it should read 0.25 mg. The lisinopril order should read "daily" instead of QD. The insulin order should have

267

the word "units" spelled out, rather than using the abbreviation "U."
Cognitive Level: Analysis
Nursing Process Step: Implementation
NCLEX: Physiological Integrity: Pharmacological and Parenteral Therapies

15. **Answer:** 2
Rationale: The advantage or benefit to the client of computerized physician order entry systems is the reduced risk for drug interactions, which is flagged by the computer program. Reduced need to clarify orders, take telephone orders, and the reduced risk for transcription errors are benefits to the nurse.
Cognitive Level: Comprehension
Nursing Process Step: Analysis
NCLEX: Physiological Integrity: Pharmacological and Parenteral Therapies

16. **Answer:** 3
Rationale: The medications are different and giving the drug sent by the pharmacy would constitute a medication error. The nurse should contact the pharmacy to have the dose replaced. Later the nurse may write an incident report according to hospital policy. Each of the other options indicates an action consistent with administering the wrong medication, and does therefore not represent safe practice.
Cognitive Level: Application
Nursing Process Step: Implementation
NCLEX: Physiological Integrity: Pharmacological and Parenteral Therapies

17. **Answer:** 1
Rationale: In some instances, clients have a prescriber's order allowing them to keep certain medications (e.g., nitroglycerin and antacids) at the bedside and take them as necessary. These are examples of medications that are ordered to treat a specific symptom, and would not be used on a regular schedule. Digoxin (a cardiac glycoside), famotidine (a histamine receptor antagonist), and furosemide (a diuretic) would be ordered on a regular schedule and would not be left at the bedside of the client.
Cognitive Level: Application
Nursing Process Step: Analysis
NCLEX: Physiological Integrity: Pharmacological and Parenteral Therapies

18. **Answer:** 2
Rationale: The next step that the nurse should take is to label the syringe as part of safe practice. One other nurse (not two) may be asked to check the dose. The vial should not be discarded before the medication is labeled. The medication should not be charted until after it is administered.
Cognitive Level: Analysis
Nursing Process Step: Implementation
NCLEX: Physiological Integrity: Pharmacological and Parenteral Therapies

19. **Answer:** 3
Rationale: The nurse administering the medications is responsible for assuring that the client takes them. The nurse should not leave the client unattended to swallow the medications, nor should the nurse delegate this to a nursing assistant. It is better client-centered care to remain with the client until all medications are swallowed than to leave and return with them after the phone call.
Cognitive Level: Application
Nursing Process Step: Implementation
NCLEX: Physiological Integrity: Pharmacological and Parenteral Therapies

20. **Answer:** 4
Rationale: Within an institutional setting, the nurse should return any unused medication to the pharmacy. Institutional policy and, in some states, the law requires the unused portion to be credited to the client's account. The other options do not allow for this responsibility to be met.
Cognitive Level: Application
Nursing Process Step: Planning
NCLEX: Physiological Integrity: Pharmacological and Parenteral Therapies

CHAPTER 5

The Nursing Process and Pharmacology

1. A Chief complaint of the client
   I Checking an identification bracelet before drug administration
   D Nausea related to chemotherapy
   E Recording secondary effects
   D Noncompliance with prescribed steroid therapy
   E Monitoring therapeutic response to a drug
   A History of allergy
   P Behavioral objectives for the client
   I Instillation of eye drops
   I Calculating flow rate for oxygen therapy
   A Vital signs
   E Observing a client demonstrate proper self-medication with insulin
2. contraindication
3. stat
4. lower
5. sublingual
6. 26 to 27
7. 2
8. infiltration
9. filter
10. blood pressure

11. **Suggested Answer:** More than half of the 100 most commonly prescribed drugs contain at least one ingredient known to interact adversely with imbibed alcohol. An interaction is probable if the drug is

known to affect the central nervous system (CNS) or is metabolized by the liver. The effects are dose related, and also depend on whether quantities of alcohol are used habitually, chronically, or only occasionally. Patterns of alcohol consumption are also likely to affect the client's compliance with drug treatment and follow through. Alcohol use should be avoided if a client is taking opioids, tranquilizers, sedatives, and other CNS depressant–type drugs, which may cause additive or synergistic respiratory and CNS depression.

12. **Suggested Answer:** As a nurse you could encourage increased mobility (such as ambulation in the hall) provided the client has an order to be out of bed. You could also encourage increased intake in the diet of fluids and high-fiber foods.

13. **Suggested Answer:** Antibiotics should be evenly spaced around the clock to maintain steady therapeutic serum levels. You would also want to try to avoid interrupting the client's sleep pattern to whatever extent possible. For example, an antibiotic ordered every 6 hours would be better scheduled at hours 12-6-12-6 than at 9-3-9-3.

14. **Answer:** 4
Rationale: A drug known to cause blood dyscrasias warrants assessment of the client's baseline complete blood count, which identifies the number of red blood cells, white blood cells, and platelets. If blood dyscrasias do occur, a change would occur in one or more of these blood elements. Serum electrolytes provide a general client baseline that is not specific to blood dyscrasias, whereas liver enzymes and serum creatinine evaluate liver and renal function, respectively.
Cognitive Level: Application
Nursing Process Step: Assessment
NCLEX: Physiological Integrity: Pharmacological and Parenteral Therapies

15. **Answer:** 1
Rationale: Cholestyramine (Questran) and colestipol (Colestid), drugs indicated for hypercholesteremia, adsorb other medications, and the fat-soluble vitamins A, D, E, and K; these substances are then excreted from rather than absorbed into the body. The other problems listed would not occur because of the process of binding or chelation.
Cognitive Level: Application
Nursing Process Step: Assessment
NCLEX: Physiological Integrity: Pharmacological and Parenteral Therapies

16. **Answer:** 4
Rationale: Ineffective therapeutic regimen management is a pattern in which the individual experiences or is at high risk to experience difficulty integrating into daily living a program for the treatment of illness and its

sequelae. Factors that contribute to ineffective management may be a lack of trust in health care providers or insufficient confidence, knowledge, or resources. In this question, the barrier is a financial resource. The other nursing diagnoses do not address resource issues.
Cognitive Level: Application
Nursing Process Step: Analysis
NCLEX: Physiological Integrity: Pharmacological and Parenteral Therapies

17. **Answer:** 2
Rationale: Central nervous system (CNS) stimulants cause nausea, nervousness, tremors, tachycardia, extra systoles, increased blood pressure, diuresis, and visual disturbances. CNS depressants can cause dizziness, drowsiness, hypotension, and confusion and progress to respiratory depression, coma, and death.
Cognitive Level: Application
Nursing Process Step: Evaluation
NCLEX: Physiological Integrity: Pharmacological and Parenteral Therapies

18. **Answer:** 3
Rationale: A troche is a medication that dissolves in the mouth. A sublingual medication is placed under the tongue. A few medications, such as antacid tablets, may be chewed. Pills, tablets, and capsules are drug forms that should be swallowed with 8 ounces of water.
Cognitive Level: Application
Nursing Process Step: Implementation
NCLEX: Physiological Integrity: Pharmacological and Parenteral Therapies

19. **Answer:** 1
Rationale: Blood samples may be obtained at the drug's peak level (the highest concentration) and/or at the trough/residual level (the lowest concentration) after a steady state of the drug has been reached in the client. For this client, the lowest concentration would be just prior to the next dose, making 9:30 the only appropriate choice.
Cognitive Level: Application
Nursing Process Step: Planning
NCLEX: Physiological Integrity: Pharmacological and Parenteral Therapies

20. **Answer:** 1
Rationale: Daily doses of diuretics should be given in the morning to reduce the risk that the client's sleep will be disturbed by drug action during the late evening and nighttime. With this in mind, the 08:00 timeframe is the only time that occurs before midday.
Cognitive Level: Application
Nursing Process Step: Planning
NCLEX: Physiological Integrity: Pharmacological and Parenteral Therapies

Biocultural Aspects of Drug Therapy

1.

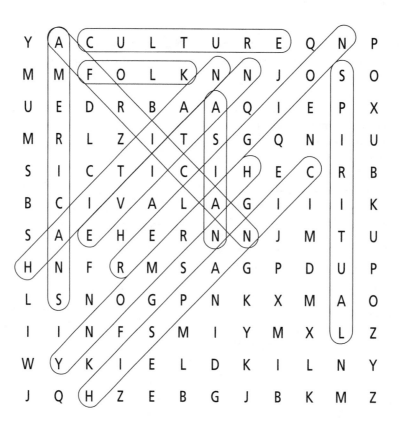

2. health beliefs
3. disparities
4. Curandero
5. outcomes
6. Western
7. Tuskegee
8. luck, behavior
9. yin, yang
10. nature

11. **Suggested Answer:** Muslims maintain a highly structured lifestyle based on religious beliefs. They believe in self-help and the need for self-discipline, and they highly value life and good health. This belief system fosters the effective management of a therapeutic regimen. Dietary restrictions are similar to a kosher diet—abstinence from pork or pork products, and from beans (e.g., black-eyed, kidney, and lima beans), which are considered to be for animal consumption. Alcohol ingestion is not permitted because it is believed to cause illness.

12. **Suggested Answer:** "Could you tell me about yourself and your family?" "How do you keep well?" "What made you become ill?"

13. **Suggested Answer:** Mexican Americans tend to believe that imbalance in the body relates to the four aspects of the body: blood, which is hot and wet; yellow bile, which is hot and dry; phlegm, which is cold and wet; and black bile, which is cold and dry. According to the "imbalance" theory, equilibrium can be regained if cold remedies or foods are taken for "hot" illnesses and vice versa. However, perceptions of what foods or medications are hot or cold may vary from client to client because these terms do not refer to temperature but are qualities assigned to particular substances. Cold illnesses are treated with hot medications (e.g., penicillin), or hot foods (e.g., chicken soup, hot tea), but they are not treated with orange juice, fruit, or other cold remedies that are commonly recommended by American health care providers.

14. **Answer:** 2
Rationale: People of the Jewish faith do not ingest pork or pork products. For this reason, they should not receive pork insulin. There is no contraindication to any of the other types listed.
Cognitive Level: Application

Nursing Process Step: Planning
NCLEX: Physiological Integrity: Pharmacological and Parenteral Therapies

15. **Answer:** 3
Rationale: Thiazide diuretics and long-acting calcium channel blockers (CCBs) seem to have greater blood pressure–lowering effects than other classes of antihypertensive agents in African American clients. The other drug groups listed as less effective, according to the results of current research.
Cognitive Level: Application
Nursing Process Step: Analysis
NCLEX: Physiological Integrity: Pharmacological and Parenteral Therapies

16. **Answer:** 3
Rationale: Mal ojo (evil eye), an example of an illness caused by magic, has symptoms of malaise, lethargy, and headaches and is thought to be the result of being excessively admired by another. Empacho is an example of a dislocation of a part of the body being a cause of illness. Symptoms of abdominal discomfort, pain, and cramping (option 1), are thought to be caused by a ball of food clinging to the wall of the stomach and are treated by massaging the spine while prayers are spoken. "Susto" is a state of depression caused by a strong emotional state of fright (option 2). Option 4 is not specific to any culturally influenced illness.
Cognitive Level: Application
Nursing Process Step: Assessment
NCLEX: Physiological Integrity: Pharmacological and Parenteral Therapies

17. **Answer:** 2
Rationale: Acupuncture, a practice that has been mainstreamed into allopathic medicine, is a method of producing analgesia or altering the function of a body system by inserting fine, wire-thin needles into the skin at specific sites on the body along a series of lines called meridians. In moxibustion, pulverized wormwood is heated and placed on the skin over specific meridian points. Herbal therapies may be prescribed to treat problems of either yin or yang.
Cognitive Level: Application
Nursing Process Step: Analysis
NCLEX: Physiological Integrity: Pharmacological and Parenteral Therapies

18. **Answer:** 1
Rationale: Some clients of Asian origin may nod during instructions as a sign of respect. This does not necessarily mean that the client is agreeing with or understands what is being said. The nurse should verify what the client knows by asking the client to repeat the instructions. Asking the client if he understand the instructions may or may not be effective (option 2). Documenting that the client understood (option 3) is a false assumption, and option 4 (following up 1 day later) does not meet the client's need for current and accurate information.

Cognitive Level: Application
Nursing Process Step: Implementation
NCLEX: Physiological Integrity: Pharmacological and Parenteral Therapies

19. **Answer:** 1
Rationale: Because Native Americans have maintained their rich history through an oral tradition, note taking is not viewed favorably; the nurse should rely on memory rather than on notes when in the client's presence. Documentation should be done later at the end of the interview. In most Western cultures maintaining direct eye contact during communication is seen as demonstrating interest in the client; however, this practice may be considered inappropriate by many Native Americans. Keeping questions limited exclusively to those on the form (option 4) may lead to insufficient data and is not good nursing practice; occasional follow-up questions may be needed.
Cognitive Level: Application
Nursing Process Step: Assessment
NCLEX: Psychosocial Integrity

20. **Answer:** 4
Rationale: Areas in which genetic variations in response to medication therapy have been discovered include oncology (in which tumor response to drug is in part genetically determined), and epilepsy (in which approximately one-third of individuals with seizures do not respond adequately to pharmacotherapy). Genetic variations may also affect a client's response to β-adrenergic pulmonary drugs, angiotensin-converting enzyme (ACE) inhibitors used to treat hypertension and heart failure (HF), antipsychotic drugs that affect dopaminergic receptors, some drugs that affect clotting and bleeding, and drugs affecting serotonin receptors (some antidepressants and drugs for nausea and vomiting).
Cognitive Level: Analysis
Nursing Process Step: Analysis
NCLEX: Physiological Integrity: Pharmacological and Parenteral Therapies

CHAPTER 7

Maternal and Child Drug Therapy

1. a, e, b, d, c, a ,c
2. teratogenicity
3. umbilical cord
4. carcinogenic
5. pregnancy
6. conception
7. fat
8. weight, body surface area
9. sitting
10. 20, 30

11. **Suggested Answer:** Medication administration will result in planned absorption and distribution in the

271

maternal circulation. Most drugs readily cross into breast milk. If human milk contains small, fixed amounts of drugs absorbed by the mother, it is usually recommended that breastfeeding be temporarily interrupted (usually for 24 to 72 hours) and the breasts pumped to remove drug-containing milk.

12. **Suggested Answer:**

Adult dose	Clark	BSA
Atropine sulfate grain 1/150	Grain 1/5	Grain 1/5
Aminophylline 0.5 g	0.126 g	0.2 g
Gentamicin 80 mg	15 mg	27 mg

13. **Suggested Answer:** Health care professionals often divide suppository doses by cutting them. This is dangerous practice because all of the medication might be contained in one area of the suppository. If divided doses must be administered, the pharmacist should be contacted for alternate product advice and guidance.

14. **Answer:** 4

Rationale: The period of greatest danger for drug-induced developmental defects is the first trimester of pregnancy—a time when many women may not realize they are pregnant.

Cognitive Level: Analysis

Nursing Process Step: Analysis

NCLEX: Physiological Integrity: Pharmacological and Parenteral Therapies

15. **Answer:** 4

Rationale: Pregnancy does not seem to have much effect on drug absorption from the gastrointestinal (GI) tract, but protein binding is decreased for some substances, which increases the amount of drug available for placental transfer. Biotransformation of drugs in the liver is probably delayed in pregnancy, but renal excretion may be more rapid because renal blood flow dramatically increases glomerular filtration rate.

Cognitive Level: Application

Nursing Process Step: Implementation

NCLEX: Physiological Integrity: Pharmacological and Parenteral Therapies

16. **Answer:** 1

Rationale: The nurse would not need to be concerned about the risk of withdrawal in the infant whose mother took acetaminophen (Tylenol) during pregnancy. Each of the other drugs listed can lead to fetal withdrawal, as outlined in Table 7-1 of the textbook.

Cognitive Level: Analysis

Nursing Process Step: Assessment

NCLEX: Physiological Integrity: Pharmacological and Parenteral Therapies

17. **Answer:** 3

Rationale: The FDA has issued recommendations that all infant formulations contain at least 0.3 to 0.5 mg/L of iron (the lowest iron level found in human milk) and that the iron be in a bioavailable form. Infants at risk for iron deficiency should be given supplements containing 1 to 2 mg/100 kcal of iron, or approximately 6 to 12 mg/L. Most iron-supplemented infant formulas today contain 12 or 13 mg/L.

Cognitive Level: Application

Nursing Process Step: Planning

NCLEX: Physiological Integrity: Pharmacological and Parenteral Therapies

18. **Answer:** 2

Rationale: Children 4 years old or over may choose to hold their own medicine cup or drink unassisted and to take pills from the container without any assistance from the nurse. Children of this age are motivated by social reinforcers, such as being praised for their cooperation or being told that "your job is to stay very still," which enhance their self-esteem and feelings of competence.

Cognitive Level: Application

Nursing Process Step: Planning

NCLEX: Physiological Integrity: Pharmacological and Parenteral Therapies

19. **Answer:** 2

Rationale: It is best to avoid putting medications in essential foods such as milk, cereal, or orange juice, because the child may refuse to accept that food in the future. With this in mind, the best choice is to place the medication in a nonessential food such as pudding.

Cognitive Level: Application

Nursing Process Step: Implementation

NCLEX: Physiological Integrity: Pharmacological and Parenteral Therapies

20. **Answer:** 2

Rationale: Mild pressure for 30 seconds over the inner canthus next to the nose prevents premature drainage of the medication away from the eye and may also retard systemic absorption. The other measures stated are not likely to serve a useful purpose.

Cognitive Level: Application

Nursing Process Step: Implementation

NCLEX: Physiological Integrity: Pharmacological and Parenteral Therapies

CHAPTER 8

Drug Therapy for Older Adults

1.

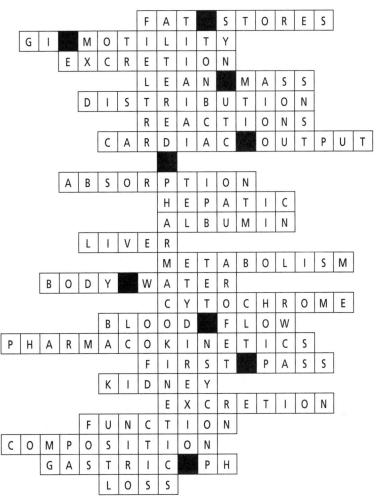

ANSWER: ALTERED PHARMACOKINETICS

2. polypharmacy
3. Beers
4. albumin
5. biotransformation
6. central nervous
7. misuse
8. low, slow
9. medications
10. index

11. **Suggested Answer:** Factors could include the following:
    - Absorption: changes in gastric pH and intestinal blood flow
    - Distribution: changes in lean body mass, adipose stores, total body water, and serum albumin
    - Biotransformation or metabolism: changes in liver size, blood flow, and functions
    - Excretion: changes in kidney function

12. **Suggested Answer:** Older adults are living longer, have one or more chronic diseases, receive prescriptions from two or more prescribers, undergo physiologic changes, have limited income, and on average use prescription and over-the-counter (OTC) drugs in greater amounts than the general public, and are therefore more at risk for polypharmacy.

13. **Suggested Answer:** This can be accomplished by a thorough assessment of the client's health status, current medication regimen, environmental factors, and implementation of appropriate interventions, client education, and counseling.

14. **Suggested Answer:** Review all medications with the client and/or caregiver; have the client/caregiver repeat the name, use, and dosing instructions for each; perform a functional assessment to determine if the client needs a compliance aid, and discuss with

the prescriber possible changes to simplify the medication regimen if it is complicated.

15. **Answer:** 2

Rationale: Age-related changes in physiology that affect medication distribution include decrease in lean body mass, increase in adipose stores, decrease in total body water, decrease in serum albumin, and decrease in blood flow and cardiac output. The other options refer to absorption, biotransformation, and excretion respectively.

Cognitive Level: Application

Nursing Process Step: Implementation

NCLEX: Physiological Integrity: Pharmacological and Parenteral Therapies

16. **Answer:** 4

Rationale: It is important to identify all prescribers for an older adult client at risk for polypharmacy. This information should be verified by checking prescription labels when the client is confused, because the client may not be a reliable source of this information. Because a relative or the primary care provider may or may not be aware of all prescribers, reading the name of the prescribing physician on each prescription label is likely to yield the most accurate data.

Cognitive Level: Application

Nursing Process Step: Assessment

NCLEX: Physiological Integrity: Pharmacological and Parenteral Therapies

17. **Answer:** 2

Rationale: Diphenhydramine (Benadryl) is an anticholinergic type of antihistamine that may cause confusion and excessive sedation in the older adult client. Therefore it should not be used as a hypnotic and another medication should be substituted. The other options do not reflect this specific concern.

Cognitive Level: Application

Nursing Process Step: Implementation

NCLEX: Physiological Integrity: Pharmacological and Parenteral Therapies

18. **Answer:** 3

Rationale: The older adult client is most at risk for gastrointestinal bleeding when taking the nonsteroidal antiinflammatory drug Naprosyn. Acetaminophen is not associated with this risk, and the other medications listed (Naprosyn and oxybutynin) are associated with excessive sedation in the older adult client.

Cognitive Level: Application

Nursing Process Step: Assessment

NCLEX: Physiological Integrity: Pharmacological and Parenteral Therapies

19. **Answer:** 1

Rationale: The nurse should ask the client for permission to discard the expired medications as a priority, and after that is done, should assess why duplicate medications are in the home. The nurse would not support use of expired medications in any way.

Cognitive Level: Application

Nursing Process Step: Planning

NCLEX: Physiological Integrity: Pharmacological and Parenteral Therapies

20. **Answer:** 3

Rationale: The client should be positioned upright to enhance swallowing. Tilting the head back could lead to aspiration; the chin should remain in the normal position or be tucked down. Sufficient water should be given before and after medication to aid in swallowing. Medications may need to be given one at a time to aid in swallowing.

Cognitive Level: Application

Nursing Process Step: Implementation

NCLEX: Physiological Integrity: Pharmacological and Parenteral Therapies

Substance Misuse and Abuse

1.

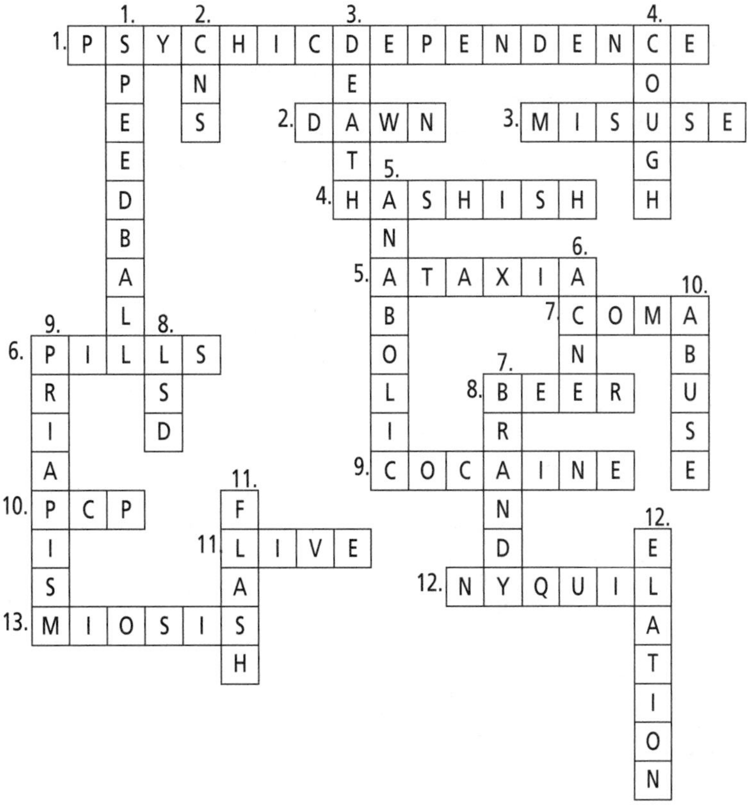

The crossword grid:

Across:
1. PSYCHIC DEPENDENCE
2. DAWN
3. MISUSE
4. HASHISH
5. ATAXIA
7. COMA
8. BEER
9. COCAINE
6. PILLS
10. PCP
11. LIVE
12. NYQUIL
13. MIOSIS

Down words visible in grid:
1. (P)SYCHIC → column: P, P, E, E, D, B, A, L
- SPEEDBALL
- CNS (C,N,S...)
- DETHANOL / DEPENDENCE
- COUGHSYRUP
- ANSTABOLISM
- STANABOL...
- CONANDRONE
- PRIASP...
- FLASH
- ABUSE
- ELATION
- MOMABUSE

2. Physical
3. Psychologic
4. mandatory reporting
5. Chain of custody
6. xanthines, caffeine
7. predatory drugs
8. amphetamines
9. nausea, vomiting
10. benzodiazepine

11. **Suggested Answer:** Collectors ensure the specimen is collected from the correct individual, obtain samples, determine if certain forms of adulteration have occurred, and establish a chain of custody for the specimen. Identification (ID) is done using a photo ID or by having the donor sign a certification statement on the specimen's custody and control form. The collector ensures that the room where the specimen is obtained is "clean." The donor is usually allowed to urinate in private, but direct observation may be necessary if the donor appears intoxicated, is suspected of specimen adulteration, or has abused drugs. The temperature of the specimen must be between 90°F and 100°F, measured within 4 minutes of donation. The specimen is sealed with tamper-resistant tape and initialed on the bottle label and dated by the collector and initialed by the donor. Each bottle has a unique ID number. The specimen may be split into two specimens, one for testing now and one for testing at a later date. Both bottles are labeled as above, and specimen "A" and specimen "B" are designated. Chain of custody forms are maintained for both portions.

12. **Suggested Answer:** The four characteristics of substance abuse are:
1. Altered state of consciousness
2. Development of tolerance
3. Rapid onset of action of desired effects
4. Possible abstinence syndrome if drug is discontinued abruptly after extended period of use

13. **Suggested Answer:** Acute alcohol withdrawal typically presents 48 to 72 hours into ethanol withdrawal. Clients often experience intense anxiety, confusion, nightmares, sweating, depression, hallucinations, and possibly panic type attacks. The client may have a sensation of room spinning or floor movement, and is

at high risk for falls or injury. Delirium may be mild, moderate or severe, and is often accompanied by tachycardia and elevated temperatures. Alcohol withdrawal seizures are not uncommon and usually manifest as generalized tonic-clonic seizure activity.

14. **Answer:** 2

Rationale: This reaction begins with flushing of the face and develops into intense vasodilation of the face, neck, and upper body. Hyperventilation and increased pulse rate may occur. Nausea occurs in 30 to 60 minutes along with facial pallor, hypotension, and copious vomiting. There is usually an intense feeling of discomfort, a pulsating headache, palpitations, dyspnea, syncope, and a constrictive feeling in the neck.

Cognitive Level: Application
Nursing Process Step: Implementation
NCLEX: Physiological Integrity: Pharmacological and Parenteral Therapies

15. **Answer:** 3

Rationale: The most important adverse effects of cocaine abuse are cardiovascular with a high risk for myocardial infarction, dysrhythmias, thrombosis, hypertension, tachycardia, and sudden death. For clients with chest pain associated with cocaine risk, this is particularly true, and risk for myocardial infarction or another serious adverse effect is highest for the following 12 hours. Other body systems are affected, including respiratory (pulmonary abscesses, lung infections, pulmonary edema and hemorrhage, and pneumonitis); renal (rhabdomyolysis—the release of skeletal muscle contents into the plasma, which results in generalized muscle aches and pains and, in one third of the reports, acute renal failure); and neurologic (seizures, stroke, and intracranial hemorrhage). Psychiatric conditions and other miscellaneous conditions may also occur.

Cognitive Level: Analysis
Nursing Process Step: Assessment
NCLEX: Physiological Integrity: Pharmacological and Parenteral Therapies

16. **Answer:** 1

Rationale: A "talk-down" approach in a quiet, relaxed environment is often used to reassure the client that he or she is safe and that the drug effects will dissipate in a few hours. If talking down cannot help the panic, then drug therapy with an oral benzodiazepine might be considered, but this is only used as an adjunct to crisis intervention psychotherapy. The use of phenothiazines, especially chlorpromazine (Thorazine) is avoided because such agents can potentiate the panic reaction, induce postural hypotension, and perhaps induce anticholinergic toxicity. The practice of administering massive doses of tranquilizers, applying restraints, and isolating such individuals should be avoided because they may be more traumatic rather than therapeutic.

Cognitive Level: Application
Nursing Process Step: Planning
NCLEX: Physiological Integrity: Pharmacological and Parenteral Therapies

17. **Answer:** 2

Rationale: The CAGE questions include the following:

1. Have you ever felt the need to **C**ut down your drinking (use of drugs)?

2. Have you ever felt **A**nnoyed by criticism of your drinking (drug use)?

3. Have you ever had **G**uilt feelings about drinking (drug use)?

4. Have you ever taken a morning **E**ye opener (required a drink or drug fix to get on with your day's activities)?"

Cognitive Level: Application
Nursing Process Step: Assessment
NCLEX: Physiological Integrity: Pharmacological and Parenteral Therapies

18. **Answer:** 4

Rationale: Typical alterations in laboratory values in the client who abuses anabolic steroids include increased hemoglobin concentration, increase in liver enzymes, hyperglycemia (hyperinsulinemia), and decreased high-density lipoproteins (HDLs).

Cognitive Level: Application
Nursing Process Step: Assessment
NCLEX: Physiological Integrity: Pharmacological and Parenteral Therapies

19. **Answer:** 1

Rationale: Naloxone, a pure opioid antagonist, reverses opioids toxicity. The usual adult dose is 0.4 to 2 mg IV, which may be repeated a 2- to 3-minute intervals if necessary. Larger doses may be required to treat acute overdoses of butorphanol (Stadol), nalbuphine (Nubain), propoxyphene (Darvon and Darvocet products), and pentazocine (Talwin). Norepinephrine raises blood pressure and Naprosyn is a nonsteroidal antiinflammatory drug.

Cognitive Level: Application
Nursing Process Step: Planning
NCLEX: Physiological Integrity: Pharmacological and Parenteral Therapies

20. **Answer:** 3

Rationale: Amphetamines are central nervous system (CNS) stimulants, whereas alcohol, morphine (an opioid), and barbiturates are CNS depressants.

Cognitive Level: Application
Nursing Process Step: Assessment
NCLEX: Physiological Integrity: Pharmacological and Parenteral Therapies

CHAPTER 10

Client Education for Self-Administration of Medication

1.

```
T  G  J  O  U  P  L  A  N  N  I  N  G  A
H  H  N  X  T  X  U  X  Y  K  R  K  N  L
L  N  O  I  T  P  E  C  R  E  P  K  I  K
M  V  N  U  R  S  I  N  G  S  J  R  H  O
R  P  F  O  G  O  D  R  T  O  B  X  C  Z
R  A  T  P  O  H  T  D  D  W  Q  R  A  A
L  N  N  O  K  W  T  I  F  W  Z  E  E  P
A  S  S  E  S  S  M  E  N  T  C  D  T  V
N  B  A  R  R  I  E  R  S  O  G  H  R  J
O  H  C  W  M  P  L  Q  M  L  M  T  E  D
I  D  E  V  E  L  O  P  M  E  N  T  A  L
T  B  F  A  B  B  L  B  R  A  H  P  D  A
A  Y  M  V  R  I  S  I  C  R  S  N  I  N
U  J  J  E  A  I  K  V  N  N  O  Z  N  G
L  G  X  N  M  S  N  U  X  I  P  B  E  U
A  R  C  U  O  O  Q  G  S  N  E  B  S  A
V  E  Q  N  A  L  R  I  U  G  Y  S  S  G
E  D  E  U  N  Q  V  Y  M  O  M  W  U  E
I  M  P  L  E  M  E  N  T  A  T  I  O  N
```

2. medications, diet, and follow-up care
3. behaviors
4. assessment
5. medication regimen
6. family, visitors
7. cultural
8. vision, hearing
9. therapeutic seeding
10. Documentation

11. **Suggested Answer:** Clients have difficulty with having most medication teaching done by a community pharmacist because of the lack of privacy and the busy environment of the pharmacy setting. Some health care providers, including nurses, are concerned because the pharmacist does not have access to the client's medical history.

12. **Suggested Answer:** If the client has a cognitive impairment that could interfere with retention of medication information, the nurse should identify a caregiver who might be able to participate in the learning-teaching process.

13. **Suggested Answer:** Three of the most common nursing diagnoses in relation to clients and the self-administration of medications are deficient knowledge, noncompliance, and ineffective therapeutic regimen management. Deficient knowledge is the state in which the individual has a deficiency in cognitive knowledge or psychomotor skills regarding

the condition or treatment plan; this is somewhat different from noncompliance. Noncompliance is the state in which an individual or group desires to comply but is prevented from doing so by factors that deter adherence to health-related advice given by health care professionals. Ineffective therapeutic regimen management is a pattern of regulating and integrating into daily living a program for treating illness and the sequelae of illness that is unsatisfactory for meeting specific health goals.

14. **Answer:** 3

Rationale: Medications should be scheduled whenever possible to coincide with the client's schedule to increase compliance with taking prescribed medications. Option 1 will help to prevent polypharmacy. Options 2 and 4 are helpful for the nurse to assess as part of routine care for any client receiving medication therapy.

Cognitive Level: Analysis

Nursing Process Step: Implementation

NCLEX: Physiological Integrity: Pharmacological and Parenteral Therapies

15. **Answer:** 2

Rationale: Because antibiotics tend to assist a client to feel better within 2 to 3 days of beginning therapy, this client may be at risk for noncompliance with a medication regime that is to last 10 days. Although the other options are possible, option 2 has the highest priority because of the nature of the medication and its effects on the client.

Cognitive Level: Analysis

Nursing Process Step: Assessment

NCLEX: Physiological Integrity: Pharmacological and Parenteral Therapies

16. **Answer:** 1

Rationale: The client who will be going home within the next few hours has the greatest need for timely medication instructions. The client in option 2 should have greater pain relief before teaching begins. The clients in options 3 and 4 may require more time and therefore should not be placed first when planning teaching time.

Cognitive Level: Analysis

Nursing Process Step: Planning

NCLEX: Physiological Integrity: Pharmacological and Parenteral Therapies

17. **Answer:** 4

Rationale: Clients who are hearing impaired often benefit from written instructions, because they are hard of hearing and may not fully comprehend oral instructions, or those in videotaped materials. A pill box would be useful if the client forgets to take scheduled medication doses, and a magnifying glass may help a client who is visually impaired.

Cognitive Level: Application

Nursing Process Step: Implementation

NCLEX: Physiological Integrity: Pharmacological and Parenteral Therapies

18. **Answer:** 1

Rationale: Initially, the nurse should teach the client to associate taking medication with another daily routine, such as brushing the teeth or watching television news. If this does not work, the client can then be taught to use additional aids to remember medication doses, but these are not the initial steps.

Cognitive Level: Application

Nursing Process Step: Implementation

NCLEX: Physiological Integrity: Pharmacological and Parenteral Therapies

19. **Answer:** 2

Rationale: Goals need to be measurable to determine whether they have been met. The only goal with a measurable verb is the verb "states" in option 2.

Cognitive Level: Application

Nursing Process Step: Planning

NCLEX: Physiological Integrity: Pharmacological and Parenteral Therapies

20. **Answer:** 3

Rationale: The client is having a second visit so the medication information should not be new to the client. The process of therapeutic seeding as a teaching approach involves mentioning an idea to a client, allowing time to pass so the client has a chance to think about the idea, then reintroducing the idea. On the second opportunity the client may more easily identify the concept and see it as a learning need. Option 3 is the one that utilizes this technique, rather than general questions or statements.

Cognitive Level: Application

Nursing Process Step: Implementation

NCLEX: Physiological Integrity: Pharmacological and Parenteral Therapies

CHAPTER 11

Over-the-Counter Medications

1. c, d, e, a, b, a, b, b, c, b
2. Drug Facts
3. Food and Drug Administration (FDA)
4. safe, effective
5. 8
6. magnesium, aluminum, calcium
7. histamine-2 (H_2)
8. dextromethorphan
9. guaifenesin (Robitussin)
10. spermicides

11. **Suggested Answer:** If stomach distress occurs with aspirin use, it should be taken with meals or food. Do not use if it has a strong, vinegar-like odor. Never use aspirin products directly on tooth or gum surfaces. Stop taking aspirin 5 to 7 days before a surgical procedure as directed by the health care provider. Do not

share or give aspirin to anyone under age 17 without health care provider approval.

12. **Suggested Answer:** The nurse should counsel the client that adverse effects of decongestants include central nervous system (CNS) stimulation such as insomnia and restlessness, dizziness, headaches, and increased irritability.

13. **Suggested Answer:** Adsorbent antidiarrheal agents act by coating the walls of the gastrointestinal (GI) tract, adsorbing bacteria or toxins causing the diarrhea and expelling them with the stools.

14. **Answer:** 1
Rationale: The nurse should placed highest priority on teaching the pregnant client about cautions related to OTC drug use. Clients who are pregnant should not use any OTC products without first consulting the prescriber because of the risk of harm to the fetus. Each of the other clients should avoid products containing a particular ingredient. The client with diabetes should avoid products with sugar; the client on a low-sodium diet should avoid products with added sodium, and the client with alcoholism should avoid products containing alcohol.
Cognitive Level: Analysis
Nursing Process Step: Planning
NCLEX: Physiological Integrity: Pharmacological and Parenteral Therapies

15. **Answer:** 4
Rationale: Clients are most at risk for hepatotoxicity when daily intake of acetaminophen is greater than 4 grams or 4000 mg daily. The client in option 4 takes in 5 grams (5000 mg). The client in option 1 takes in 2000 mg, whereas the clients in options 2 and 3 are using a total of 2600 mg each day.
Cognitive Level: Analysis
Nursing Process Step: Analysis
NCLEX: Physiological Integrity: Pharmacological and Parenteral Therapies

16. **Answer:** 2
Rationale: Magnesium-based antacids are more likely to cause diarrhea than the other symptoms listed. Aluminum-based antacids are more likely to cause constipation, whereas oral candidiasis and abdominal pain are not expected.
Cognitive Level: Application
Nursing Process Step: Implementation
NCLEX: Physiological Integrity: Pharmacological and Parenteral Therapies

17. **Answer:** 3
Rationale: For infants younger than 2 months of age, malt soup extract is an acceptable alternative to medication use. Young infants should not be given bran (option 1). The nurse should not advise the use of electrolyte solutions such as Pedialyte because the problem is constipation, not diarrhea. The nurse would also not recommend a change in the infant's progression of diet (adding fruits or vegetables) without the advice of a pediatric health care provider.

Cognitive Level: Application
Nursing Process Step: Implementation
NCLEX: Physiological Integrity: Pharmacological and Parenteral Therapies

18. **Answer:** 3
Rationale: The health care provider should be aware of all drugs being taken, both prescription and OTC. The client should take an OTC medicine that will treat only the current symptoms. The medication should be taken EXACTLY as stated on the label. The client shouldn't use OTC medicines after the expiration date has passed.
Cognitive Level: Application
Nursing Process Step: Implementation
NCLEX: Physiological Integrity: Pharmacological and Parenteral Therapies

19. **Answer:** 4
Rationale: The client should avoid taking nonsteroidal antiinflammatory products for more than 10 days for pain, 3 days for fever, if painful area is inflamed, if pregnant or breastfeeding, if new symptoms occur or current symptoms worsen, or if abdominal pain occurs.
Cognitive Level: Analysis
Nursing Process Step: Planning
NCLEX: Physiological Integrity: Pharmacological and Parenteral Therapies

20. **Answer:** 2
Rationale: The primary ingredients products for PMS are acetaminophen for pain, a mild diuretic such as pamabrom or caffeine for fluid accumulation and pyrilamine, an antihistamine, antipruritic agent. Because large doses of caffeine can cause gastrointestinal irritation, nervousness, irritability, tachycardia, anxiety and insomnia, individuals with a history of peptic ulcer disease, insomnia or persons taking other caffeine containing food, beverages or medications (xanthines, theophylline, etc.) should avoid products containing caffeine.
Cognitive Level: Application
Nursing Process Step: Implementation
NCLEX: Physiological Integrity: Pharmacological and Parenteral Therapies

CHAPTER 12

Complementary and Alternative Pharmacology

1. i, e, b, k, a, d, j, f, c, h
2. Complementary, alternative
3. dietary supplements
4. Homeopathy
5. Ginger
6. Saw palmetto
7. ephedra
8. echinacea
9. garlic
10. serotonin syndrome

11. **Suggested Answer:** There is some controversy about the use of ginger in pregnancy because of its abortifacient effects, but this effect has not been documented in humans. A recent review of the literature found no reason for contraindicating ginger during pregnancy when it is taken at the usual therapeutic dose.

12. **Suggested Answer:** Glucosamine is a building block used in the biosynthesis of glycosaminoglycans and proteoglycans, important constituents of articular cartilage. It is often combined with chondroitin for the treatment of osteoarthritis, particularly osteoarthritis of the knee.

13. **Suggested Answer:** Valerian is known to produce headache and morning grogginess. Whether valerian can cause dependence similar to other sedative-hypnotics remains unclear. Like many other complementary and alternative preparations, valerian is not recommended for women who are pregnant or lactating because of potential safety concerns.

14. **Answer:** 1
Rationale: Clinical data based on double-blind clinical trials using matched client groups with peripheral arterial insufficiency (showing signs of intermittent claudication) have demonstrated the clinical efficacy of a standardized extract of *G. biloba*. Significant improvements in pain-free walking time and maximum walking distance were achieved. It is not as helpful in improving memory, and has no use reducing joint inflammation or improving vision.
Cognitive Level: Application
Nursing Process Step: Implementation
NCLEX: Physiological Integrity: Pharmacological and Parenteral Therapies

15. **Answer:** 2
Rationale: Feverfew in the treatment of migraine headaches poses no safety risks but has no clearly documented benefit. The other options contain incorrect statements.
Cognitive Level: Comprehension
Nursing Process Step: Implementation
NCLEX: Physiological Integrity: Pharmacological and Parenteral Therapies

16. **Answer:** 3
Rationale: St. John's wort has most recently been identified as an effective treatment for mild to moderate depression. Valerian may be used to aid in sleep, whereas red yeast rice may lower blood cholesterol levels. Ginseng has been used to improve psychological function, immune function, and conditions associated with diabetes although strong evidence is lacking.
Cognitive Level: Application
Nursing Process Step: Assessment
NCLEX: Physiological Integrity: Pharmacological and Parenteral Therapies

17. **Answer:** 3
Rationale: Lobelia produces behavioral stimulation and depression, cardiac acceleration, peripheral vasoconstriction, and elevated blood pressure. It is contraindicated for use in individuals with unstable cardiovascular conditions such as angina, dysrhythmias, post–myocardial infarction, and hypertension.
Cognitive Level: Application
Nursing Process Step: Implementation
NCLEX: Physiological Integrity: Pharmacological and Parenteral Therapies

18. **Answer:** 1
Rationale: Evidence exists that milk thistle may be hepatoprotective through a number of mechanisms: antioxidant activity, toxin blockade at the membrane level, enhanced protein synthesis, and possible antiinflammatory or immunomodulating effects. The other supplements listed do not have a protective effect on the liver.
Cognitive Level: Application
Nursing Process Step: Assessment
NCLEX: Physiological Integrity: Pharmacological and Parenteral Therapies

19. **Answer:** 4
Rationale: Green tea, high in vitamin K, is known to interfere with the effects of the anticoagulant warfarin (Coumadin). The other drugs listed do not have this effect.
Cognitive Level: Application
Nursing Process Step: Assessment
NCLEX: Physiological Integrity: Pharmacological and Parenteral Therapies

20. **Answer:** 3
Rationale: The American Society of Anesthesiologists (ASA) recommends that all herbal medications be discontinued 2 to 3 weeks before an elective surgical procedure.
Cognitive Level: Application
Nursing Process Step: Implementation
NCLEX: Physiological Integrity: Pharmacological and Parenteral Therapies

CHAPTER 13

Overview of the Central Nervous System

1. See Figure 13-4 in the textbook.
2. nerve cells, astrocytes, brain's capillary walls
3. somatic motor pathway located in the CNS; skeletal muscles, coordination of muscle group movements, posture
4. consciousness and arousal effect; alerting mechanism; filter process that allows for concentration
5. acetylcholine
6. pain
7. cerebral stimulation
8. cerebrum

9. thalamus
10. mind; body
11. brainstem
12. glial cells, neurons
13. dopamine, norepinephrine, and epinephrine

CHAPTER 14

Analgesics

1. See Figure 14-9 in the textbook.
2. pain
3. Acute
4. Neuropathic
5. muscles, ligaments or joints
6. physical, emotional, cultural
7. undertreatment
8. sympathetic nervous system
9. naloxone (Narcan)
10. normeperidine

11. **Suggested Answer:** Some serious adverse effects include seizures, tinnitus, jaundice (from hepatic toxicity), pruritus, skin rash or facial edema (allergic reaction), respiratory difficulty or depression, excitability (paradoxical reaction seen mainly in children), confusion, and tachycardia.

12. **Suggested Answer:** To treat aspirin overdose, the aspirin needs to be removed from the body using some means, such as gastric lavage or emesis, exchange transfusion, hemodialysis, peritoneal dialysis, or (in severe cases) hemoperfusion.

13. **Suggested Answer:** Mild pain is rated 1 to 3 by clients on a scale of 1 to 10. Mild pain is generally effectively treated with nonopioid and nonpharmacologic adjuvants. For moderate pain that is rated 4 to 6, the previous interventions can be used and a weak opioid combination can be added to the regime. For severe pain that is rated 7 to 10, the client would benefit from strong opioids along with nonpharmacologic adjuvants.

14. **Answer:** 1
Rationale: Opioids should also be used with extreme caution in conditions such as acute bronchial asthma or any respiratory impairment or chronic disease, increased intracranial pressure (may increase), or severe inflammatory bowel disease (risk of toxic megacolon). Migraine headaches and urinary frequency are not reasons to use opioids cautiously, and the client's back pain could possibly be alleviated to some extent by opioid use.
Cognitive Level: Analysis
Nursing Process Step: Planning
NCLEX: Physiological Integrity: Pharmacological and Parenteral Therapies

15. **Answer:** 2
Rationale: Codeine produces similar adverse effects as observed with other opioid agonists with a higher risk for constipation, particularly in older adults. For this reason, each of the other options is incorrect.
Cognitive Level: Application
Nursing Process Step: Assessment
NCLEX: Physiological Integrity: Pharmacological and Parenteral Therapies

16. **Answer:** 3
Rationale: The patch should be held in place for 10 to 20 seconds to ensure good attachment to the skin. The site should be cleansed beforehand with water only and it should be applied to the upper torso. After removal, the patch should be folded in half and flushed down the toilet or placed in a sharps container.
Cognitive Level: Application
Nursing Process Step: Implementation
NCLEX: Physiological Integrity: Pharmacological and Parenteral Therapies

17. **Answer:** 3
Rationale: A prescriber orders the analgesic dose and a set lockout interval of 5 to 20 minutes, not 2. The client should be encouraged to use the pump before the pain becomes intense. The lockout mechanism prevents an inadvertent overdose or excessive analgesic administration. This pump also records the number of times the button is pushed and the total cumulative dose delivered.
Cognitive Level: Analysis
Nursing Process Step: Evaluation
NCLEX: Physiological Integrity: Pharmacological and Parenteral Therapies

18. **Answer:** 4
Rationale: Naloxone, naltrexone, and nalmefene are opioid antagonists that competitively displace the opioid analgesics from their receptor sites, thus reversing their effects. Naltrexone is indicated for adjuvant treatment in detoxified, opioid-dependent clients and to manage ethanol dependence. Nalmefene and naloxone are administered parenterally, whereas naltrexone is available as an oral drug. Naprosyn is a nonsteroidal antiinflammatory drug.
Cognitive Level: Application
Nursing Process Step: Analysis
NCLEX: Physiological Integrity: Pharmacological and Parenteral Therapies

19. **Answer:** 1
Rationale: Like other nonselective COX inhibitors, ibuprofen poses a risk for gastrointestinal bleeding. It may also result in renal failure in clients with preexisting moderate renal impairment. Other adverse effects include edema, hypertension (usually modest), and gastrointestinal discomfort. It does not cause dizziness, increased intraocular pressure, or skeletal muscle weakness.

Cognitive Level: Application
Nursing Process Step: Implementation
NCLEX: Physiological Integrity: Pharmacological and Parenteral Therapies

20. **Answer:** 2
Rationale: Specific analgesics that are considered inappropriate for use in older adults include propoxyphene (Darvon products), pentazocine (Talwin), and meperidine (Demerol). These agents are more toxic in older adults and much safer analgesics are available.
Cognitive Level: Application
Nursing Process Step: Planning
NCLEX: Physiological Integrity: Pharmacological and Parenteral Therapies

CHAPTER 15

Anesthetics

1. a, a, b, c, b, b, c, d
2. regional or local
3. a lower reported incidence of postoperative nausea, vomiting, and pain
4. inhaled, fat-soluble
5. analgesia, amnesia, muscular relaxation
6. Nitrous oxide
7. Halothane
8. benzodiazepines
9. Ketamine
10. neuromuscular blockers

11. **Suggested Answer:** A combination of drugs is necessary to produce all of the desired effects sought with anesthesia. Analgesia, muscle relaxation, unconsciousness, and amnesic effects are not produced safely by a single anesthetic. Balanced anesthesia involves the induction of anesthesia with a combination of drugs, each for its own specific effect, rather than with a single drug that has multiple effects.

12. **Suggested Answer:** Nitrous oxide administration may result in postoperative nausea, vomiting, or delirium. At the termination of anesthesia, the rapid movement of large amounts of nitrous oxide from the circulation into the lungs may dilute the oxygen in the lungs. This dilution may result in a phenomenon known as diffusion hypoxia. To prevent this, the anesthetist usually administers 100% oxygen to clear nitrous oxide from the lungs. During recovery the nurse administers humidified oxygen by mask and encourages the client to breathe deeply to promote ventilation.

13. **Suggested Answer:** Benzodiazepines are most often used for conscious sedation in which full anesthesia is not required such as during endoscopy, or as a premedication or adjunct in balanced anesthesia.

14. **Answer:** 3
Rationale: Halothane is the only volatile anesthetic agent that sensitizes the myocardium to the effects of catecholamines (epinephrine, norepinephrine, or dopamine) or sympathomimetic agents (e.g., ephedrine, metaraminol), leading to risk of serious cardiac dysrhythmias in the presence of halothane. Levodopa, which increases the quantity of dopamine in the CNS, should be discontinued at least 6 to 8 hours before halothane is administered.
Cognitive Level: Comprehension
Nursing Process Step: Analysis
NCLEX: Physiological Integrity: Pharmacological and Parenteral Therapies

15. **Answer:** 1
Rationale: The most common adverse effects during the recovery period are shivering and trembling. Nausea, vomiting, prolonged somnolence, and headache are less commonly reported. Serious adverse effects include emergence delirium (increased excitability, confusion, and hallucinations), cardiac dysrhythmias (tachycardia, bradycardia, or myocardial depression), allergic response (bronchospasm, rash, hives, hypotension, and edema of eyelids, lips, or face), respiratory depression, and thrombophlebitis.
Cognitive Level: Application
Nursing Process Step: Assessment
NCLEX: Physiological Integrity: Pharmacological and Parenteral Therapies

16. **Answer:** 2
Rationale: Benzodiazepines such as midazolam (Versed) induce amnesia at higher doses. This is an advantage for clients who are undergoing painful or uncomfortable procedures because it diminishes recall of traumatic events while under the influence of the agent. The other statements are not true.
Cognitive Level: Application
Nursing Process Step: Implementation
NCLEX: Physiological Integrity: Pharmacological and Parenteral Therapies

17. **Answer:** 4
Rationale: Propofol is a respiratory depressant and may produce apnea and cardiac depression depending on the dose, rate of administration, and concurrent drugs administered. Bradycardia and hypotension may also occur frequently. Nausea, vomiting, and involuntary muscle movement are commonly reported.
Cognitive Level: Analysis
Nursing Process Step: Analysis
NCLEX: Physiological Integrity: Pharmacological and Parenteral Therapies

18. **Answer:** 1
Rationale: With muscle relaxation caused by vecuronium, the ventilated client may appear comfortable and relaxed, but unless he or she is receiving other medications (e.g., opioid analgesics, benzodiazepines, or other anesthetics), the client is likely to be very anxious and uncomfortable. As such, it is critical to

administer analgesics for pain and benzodiazepines or other anesthetics that affect level of consciousness and memory prior to and during treatment with neuromuscular blockers.

Cognitive Level: Application
Nursing Process Step: Planning
NCLEX: Physiological Integrity: Pharmacological and Parenteral Therapies

19. **Answer:** 3
Rationale: Malignant hyperthermia is a life-threatening condition with a mortality rate of 30% to 40%. The operating room team, within which the nurse has a key role, should have a preplanned course of action, including the availability of dantrolene sodium, a complete change of anesthesia circuit, hyperventilation with 100% oxygen, methods to lower body temperature rapidly, and other symptomatic treatment.

Cognitive Level: Analysis
Nursing Process Step: Planning
NCLEX: Physiological Integrity: Pharmacological and Parenteral Therapies

20. **Answer:** 2
Rationale: Vasoconstrictors such as epinephrine and norepinephrine are used with the local anesthetic to decrease systemic absorption and prolong the duration of action of the anesthetic. They are not used for nerve blocks in areas with end arteries (fingers, toes, ears, nose, and penis) because ischemia may develop, resulting in gangrene. Lidocaine is considered the prototype local anesthetic.

Cognitive Level: Application
Nursing Process Step: Planning
NCLEX: Physiological Integrity: Pharmacological and Parenteral Therapies

CHAPTER 16

Antianxiety, Sedative, and Hypnotic Drugs

1.

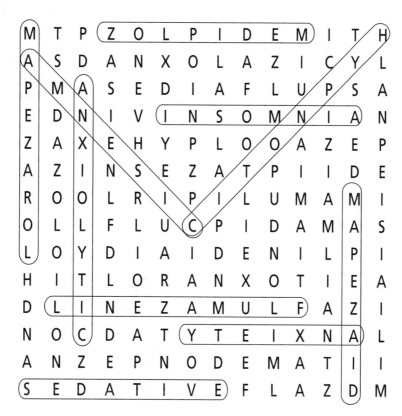

2. reduce feelings of anxiety
3. CNS-depressant; CNS depression
4. paradoxical; dreaming
5. older adults
6. benzodiazepines
7. GI tract, liver
8. Flumazenil (Romazicon)
9. insomnia
10. Buspirone (BuSpar)

11. **Suggested Answer:** It is important to find out what a client's sleep habits are and how he or she ensures good sleep at home. A thorough sleep history is required including environmental control, physical self-care/relaxation, eating habits, and quiet recreation.

12. **Suggested Answer:** In addition to standard aspects of the nursing care plan for antianxiety drugs, the pediatric considerations should include references to

the higher susceptibility of children to the CNS-depressant effects of benzodiazepines; danger of impaired functions with chronic use of clonazepam; the contraindications in children for buspirone, methyprylon, and, for hyperactive or psychotic children, diazepam; the importance of following manufacturer's dosage instructions; avoiding, when possible, concurrent use of other CNS depressants; monitoring excessive sedation, lethargy, or lack of coordination; monitoring for paradoxical reactions with use of barbiturates.

13. **Suggested Answer:** Nonpharmacologic supportive measures to induce sleep could include relaxation therapy, reduction of environmental stimuli, developing regular bedtime routines, and/or taking a warm decaffeinated drink.

14. **Answer:** 1
Rationale: The long-acting benzodiazepines (BZs) and their active metabolites are more apt to accumulate, especially in older adults, resulting in an increased risk for falls and hip fractures. BZs that do not undergo metabolism via conjugation and cytochrome P450 metabolism tend to have inactive metabolites and shorter durations of action (lorazepam [Ativan] and oxazepam [Serax]). These agents are often preferred in older adults and those with liver disease.
Cognitive Level: Application
Nursing Process Step: Analysis
NCLEX: Physiological Integrity: Pharmacological and Parenteral Therapies

15. **Answer:** 3
Rationale: Paradoxical neurologic reactions with benzodiazepines are rare but include insomnia, increased excitability, hallucinations, and apprehension. The most common adverse effects of benzodiazepines include drowsiness, hiccups (especially with midazolam [Versed]), lassitude, and loss of dexterity. Less common adverse effects include dry mouth, nausea, vomiting, headaches, constipation, abdominal cramping, unsteadiness, dizziness, and blurred vision.
Cognitive Level: Analysis
Nursing Process Step: Analysis
NCLEX: Physiological Integrity: Pharmacological and Parenteral Therapies

16. **Answer:** 2
Rationale: The most common indications for benzodiazepines include anxiety disorders, alcohol withdrawal, preoperative medication, insomnia, seizure disorders, and neuromuscular disease. They are also used to induce amnesia during cardioversion and endoscopic procedures.
Cognitive Level: Application

Nursing Process Step: Analysis
NCLEX: Physiological Integrity: Pharmacological and Parenteral Therapies

17. **Answer:** 4
Rationale: Individuals with a history of substance abuse often have concurrent anxiety, often in the context of other psychiatric conditions. For generalized anxiety disorder, many clinicians would consider the use of buspirone on a long-term basis, and a nonbenzodiazepine such as hydroxyzine for short-term management.
Cognitive Level: Application
Nursing Process Step: Assessment
NCLEX: Physiological Integrity: Pharmacological and Parenteral Therapies

18. **Answer:** 3
Rationale: Adverse effects include sedation, which usually disappears after a few days of therapy or when the dosage is reduced; and anticholinergic adverse effects such as dry mouth, blurred vision, and constipation.
Cognitive Level: Application
Nursing Process Step: Assessment
NCLEX: Physiological Integrity: Pharmacological and Parenteral Therapies

19. **Answer:** 2
Rationale: Chloral hydrate is indicated as a sedative and as a hypnotic. Chloral hydrate is unique among the sedatives in that it has minimal impact on electroencephalogram (EEG) readings, making it an ideal sedative for conscious sedation before EEG evaluations for seizure potential.
Cognitive Level: Application
Nursing Process Step: Planning
NCLEX: Physiological Integrity: Pharmacological and Parenteral Therapies

20. **Answer:** 3
Rationale: When possible, prescribers often suggest that older adults limit their intake of hypnotics to three or four times per week, which allows clients to select the nights on which they need to take their medication. This schedule usually results in enhanced effectiveness, less daytime drowsiness or sedation, and a decreased potential for inducing tolerance to the medication.
Cognitive Level: Application
Nursing Process Step: Implementation
NCLEX: Physiological Integrity: Pharmacological and Parenteral Therapies

Antiepileptic Drugs

1.

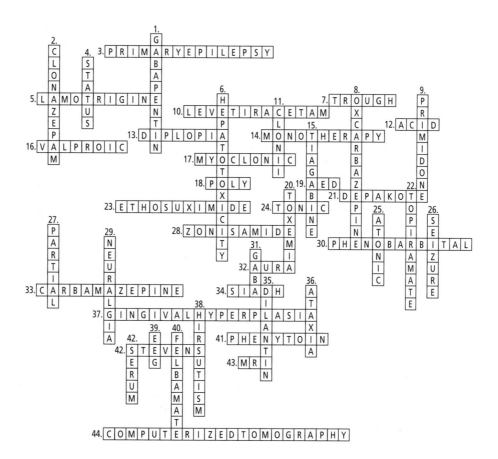

2. primary or idiopathic
3. apnea, respiratory depression, bronchospasms
4. absence
5. False
6. False
7. ethosuximide
8. phenobarbital
9. Diazepam
10. phenytoin

11. **Suggested Answer:** Epilepsy is a brain disorder in which clusters of nerve cells in the brain sometimes signal abnormally. This can lead to strange sensations, emotions, behavior changes, and possible seizures. Epilepsy is diagnosed after two or more seizures occur. Antiepileptic drugs will help by inhibiting how abnormal electrical impulses are conducted through the nervous system.

12. **Suggested Answer:** The following nursing interventions should be considered for this client:
    - Administer drugs safely and accurately
    - Assess the client for drug-specific adverse effects
    - Instruct the client about symptoms to be reported
    - Caution against activities requiring coordination and alertness until responses to drugs are known
    - Discourage self-altering of medication regimen
    - Explain the importance of carrying a Medic Alert identification

13. **Suggested Answer:** The client is at greater risk of developing toxicity with antiepileptic drugs (AEDs) for three reasons:
    - The client is an older adult and so drug metabolism is slower.
    - The history of liver disease may lead to slower drug metabolism.
    - The older adult may have lower serum albumin levels, which would decrease protein binding of bound drugs (such as phenytoin and valproic acid).
    All three of these circumstances indicate the need for lower drug doses to reduce the risk of developing toxicity or adverse effects.

14. **Answer:** 1
    Rationale: When an antiepileptic is ordered more than once a day, the serum drug level is often drawn before the first dose of the day. In this case, the first dose is

at 0800, so the nurse should plan on having the blood drawn at approximately 0730. If the drug were ordered on a once-daily dosing schedule, the nurse would schedule the lab work for a time greater than 8 hours since the daily dose.

Cognitive Level: Analysis
Nursing Process Step: Planning
NCLEX: Safe Effective Care Environment: Management of Care

15. **Answer:** 1

Rationale: A modest decline in leukocyte (white blood cell) count is an adverse effect of carbamazepine. Because the client is exhibiting signs of infection, the nurse should ask the client to come in for an evaluation visit. Options 2 and 4 delay treatment and could be harmful to the client. Option 3 is dangerous because the client should not double dose antiepileptic medications.

Cognitive Level: Analysis
Nursing Process Step: Implementation
NCLEX: Physiological Integrity: Pharmacological and Parenteral Therapies

16. **Answer:** 3

Rationale: When given intravenously, phenobarbital should be administered slowly to avoid respiratory depression; a rate of 60 mg/min should not be exceeded.

Cognitive Level: Application
Nursing Process Step: Implementation
NCLEX: Physiological Integrity: Pharmacological and Parenteral Therapies

17. **Answer:** 1

Rationale: Felbamate is indicated for treatment of Lennox-Gastaut syndrome in children, a condition of a variety of generalized seizures that appears in the first 5 years of life. It is an oral agent that increases seizure threshold and reduces the spread or progression of a seizure.

Cognitive Level: Application
Nursing Process Step: Analysis
NCLEX: Physiological Integrity: Pharmacological and Parenteral Therapies

18. **Answer:** 2

Rationale: Gabapentin is used more commonly for the treatment of neurogenic pain than other antiepileptic medications.

Cognitive Level: Application
Nursing Process Step: Analysis
NCLEX: Physiological Integrity: Pharmacological and Parenteral Therapies

19. **Answer:** 3

Rationale: Magnesium sulfate is used to control seizures in toxemia of pregnancy. Because magnesium can cause central nervous system depression, the nurse checks the patellar reflex or knee jerk in a client receiving magnesium sulfate. Assessment of deep tendon reflexes is not done during administration of the other antiepileptic medications listed.

Cognitive Level: Application
Nursing Process Step: Assessment
NCLEX: Physiological Integrity: Pharmacological and Parenteral Therapies

20. **Answer:** 4

Rationale: Blood levels of oxcarbazepine are not routinely monitored. It does not induce its own metabolism, and may cause drowsiness as other antiepileptic drugs do. It may also cause serum sodium levels to fall, so serum sodium levels need to be monitored periodically.

Cognitive Level: Application
Nursing Process Step: Implementation
NCLEX: Physiological Integrity: Pharmacological and Parenteral Therapies

Central Nervous System Stimulants
1.

```
N   O   R   A   D   E   F   A   N   I   T
A   M   P   H   E   T   A   M   I   N   E
N   A   R   I   F   O   N   T   R   O   N
R   S   I   S   I   R   A   N   O   R   I
O   N   C   R   C   L   L   O   C   S   T
N   T   N   A   I   X   E   R   O   N   A
A   R   C   O   T   A   P   H   E   T   O
T   A   T   T   E   N   T   I   O   N   L
S   C   A   F   F   E   I   N   E   T   A
Y   S   P   E   L   O   C   R   A   N   S
```

2. cerebral cortex
3. distractibility; short attention span; impulsive behavior; hyperactivity
4. daytime drowsiness; excessive sleep patterns
5. muscle weakness; narcolepsy
6. vivid auditory or visual dreams occurring at the onset of sleep
7. alertness, motor reaction
8. genetic
9. restlessness, anxiety
10. hypothalamus, limbic

11. **Suggested Answer:** Teach the client not to self-regulate the dose and stress the habit-forming potential of this type of drug. If effect seems to decrease, consult prescriber. Swallow sustained release tablet without breaking, chewing or crushing. Inform client of CNS and cardiovascular adverse effects; amphetamines may impair functioning in tasks requiring mental alertness and coordination. Caution client to store drug securely to avoid unintended use by another person.

12. **Suggested Answer:** Some of the more frequent adverse effects are anorexia, increased nervousness, insomnia (usually more frequent in children). Less frequent adverse effects are headache, nausea, abdominal pain, drowsiness, and dizziness.

13. **Suggested Answer:** Because this type of drug can increase heart rate and cardiac output, it is important to monitor the pulse and blood pressure. Overstimulation, especially in a client with preexisting heart disease, could lead to cardiac irregularities, which could be detected by onset of irregularities in the pulse or a change in cardiac rhythm as detected on a cardiac monitor or electrocardiogram.

14. **Answer:** 1
Rationale: Methylphenidate shares an adverse effect profile with other stimulants. Among the more common effects are nervousness and insomnia. Other potentially concerning effects include tachycardias, dysrhythmias, urticaria or rash, and hypersensitivity reactions.
Cognitive Level: Application
Nursing Process Step: Implementation
NCLEX: Physiological Integrity: Pharmacological and Parenteral Therapies

15. **Answer:** 2
Rationale: A recent warning was issued by the FDA about the risk for serious hepatotoxicity with atomoxetine. The potential for liver failure requiring transplant or leading to death is a concern with the use of this agent. Early warning signs include pruritus, jaundice, dark urine, abdominal tenderness, or unexplained "flu-like"

287

Answer Key

symptoms. These should be reported to the health care provider.

Cognitive Level: Application
Nursing Process Step: Implementation
NCLEX: Physiological Integrity: Pharmacological and Parenteral Therapies

16. **Answer:** 4
Rationale: Sibutramine (Meridia) is a norepinephrine and dopamine reuptake inhibitor in the CNS. It is indicated for the management of obesity when the Body Mass Index (BMI) is greater than 30 kg/m^2 or greater than 27 kg/m^2 if other risk factors (e.g., hypertension, diabetes) are present. Like other agents used for obesity management, it should be used in conjunction with a reduced calorie diet and other lifestyle modifications. Constipation is an adverse effect and the other statements are false.

Cognitive Level: Application
Nursing Process Step: Planning
NCLEX: Physiological Integrity: Pharmacological and Parenteral Therapies

17. **Answer:** 3
Rationale: Children in particular should be assessed on a regular basis for physical growth, because normal weight gain may be suppressed. The other items listed are routine and of lesser importance in relation to drug therapy, although a pulse rate would be needed to determine cardiovascular effects.

Cognitive Level: Analysis
Nursing Process Step: Assessment
NCLEX: Physiological Integrity: Pharmacological and Parenteral Therapies

18. **Answer:** 1
Rationale: The amphetamines, methylphenidate and modafinil (Provigil) have been used for narcolepsy. Pemoline (Cylert) has also been used for this purpose, although it does not possess an FDA-labeled indication for narcolepsy.

Cognitive Level: Application
Nursing Process Step: Analysis
NCLEX: Physiological Integrity: Pharmacological and Parenteral Therapies

19. **Answer:** 2
Rationale: A realistic goal for weight loss is 1 to 2 pounds per week, but some clients with obesity will tend to have a greater weight loss than this, at least initially. For planning purposes, this safe target range should be used.

Cognitive Level: Application
Nursing Process Step: Planning
NCLEX: Physiological Integrity: Pharmacological and Parenteral Therapies

20. **Answer:** 4
Rationale: Use of doxapram is typically limited to postanesthesia care and management of drug overdose in which respiratory depressants are involved and antagonists are not available (e.g., barbiturate overdose).

Occasionally, it is also used for very short periods of time (e.g., 1 to 2 hours) for clients with chronic obstructive pulmonary disease and elevated carbon dioxide levels.

Cognitive Level: Application
Nursing Process Step: Analysis
NCLEX: Physiological Integrity: Pharmacological and Parenteral Therapies

CHAPTER 19

Psychotherapeutic Drugs

1. c, a, d, b, b, a
2. behavioral, affective
3. dopamine
4. Tourette
5. Antipsychotic, neuroleptic
6. Abnormal Involuntary Movement
7. tapered
8. Reye
9. tricyclic
10. suicidality

11. **Suggested Answer:** The client should completely avoid aged cheeses, erring, broad beans, Chianti and sherry wines, and yeast. There are several other foods that must be restricted in the diet, which include beer, sardines, snails, anchovies, processed meats, fermented foods, liver, canned figs, raisins, coffee, sauerkraut, licorice, ripe avocado, and soy sauce. Up to 2 oz. per day of the following foods is acceptable: sour cream, yogurt, cottage cheese, American cheese, mild Swiss cheese, wine (avoid Chianti, sherry), and chocolate.

12. **Suggested Answer:** In Neuroleptic Malignant Syndrome (NMS), the client presents with very rigid muscle tone and fever secondary to severe muscle injury. There may also be altered mental status, joint pain, tachycardia, tachypnea and sweating.

13. **Suggested Answer:** Medications that affect the metabolism, synthesis, or reuptake of serotonin may result in serotonin accumulation and the serotonin syndrome (SES). This syndrome is characterized by mental status changes (confusion, restlessness, anxiety, disorientation), ataxia, myoclonus, tremors, rigidity, hypertension, and autonomic dysfunction). Symptoms usually occur within 2 to 72 hours up to several weeks after beginning the administration of a serotonergic drug and it is treated by discontinuing the drug and providing supportive care.

14. **Answer:** 2
Rationale: Use of long-acting haloperidol decanoate (Haldol Decanoate) by IM injection results in a prolonged duration of action of approximately three weeks. This product should not be confused with the shorter-acting parenteral formulation. This formulation

is often used for clients who do not adhere to conventional therapy.
Cognitive Level: Analysis
Nursing Process Step: Planning
NCLEX: Physiological Integrity: Pharmacological and Parenteral Therapies

15. **Answer:** 2
Rationale: Fluoxetine hydrochloride (Prozac), an SSRI that demonstrates significant an adverse effect of GI disturbances. To reduce nausea, the client should be advised to take the medicine with meals. The other options do not address concerns related to drug side effects of fluoxetine.
Cognitive Level: Application
Nursing Process Step: Implementation
NCLEX: Physiological Integrity: Pharmacological and Parenteral Therapies

16. **Answer:** 3
Rationale: By blocking dopamine, antipsychotic medications produce extrapyramidal side effects, such as restless fidgeting or pacing, motor restlessness and not being able to sit still or lie down quietly. The therapeutic treatment is the administration of anticholinergic agents such as benztropine (Cogentin), trihexyphenidyl (Artane), or procyclidine (Kemadrin). Diphenhydramine (Benadryl), an antihistamine, also may be administered. Zyprexa, Moban, and Mellaril are antipsychotics that could cause these effects.
Cognitive Level: Application
Nursing Process Step: Planning
NCLEX: Physiological Integrity: Pharmacological and Parenteral Therapies

17. **Answer:** 2
Rationale: Although agranulocytosis occurs in only about 1% to 2% of clients taking clozapine, this risk is greater than the risk with standard antipsychotic agents. After the first 6 months, blood counts are drawn biweekly, so the nurse would want to obtain one to determine whether the client is experiencing agranulocytosis or flu. The nurse would provide specific instructions but avoid alarming the client. The other responses by the nurse place the client at risk by ignoring the possibility of agranulocytosis.
Cognitive Level: Application
Nursing Process Step: Implementation
NCLEX: Physiological Integrity: Pharmacological and Parenteral Therapies

18. **Answer:** 1
Rationale: The most common adverse effects of antipsychotic medications include the following: dry mouth, blurred vision, nasal stuffiness, weight gain, difficulty urinating, infection, decreased sweating, increased sensitivity to sunlight, yellowing of the eyes (especially the whites of the eyes), breast enlargement/lactation, skin rash, anhedonia, itchy skin, and constipation.
Cognitive Level: Application
Nursing Process Step: Evaluation

NCLEX: Physiological Integrity: Pharmacological and Parenteral Therapies

19. **Answer:** 1
Rationale: Antidepressant medications can cause orthostatic or postural hypotension, and the nurse will teach the client to change positions slowly, and to dangle the feet at the bedside before getting out of bed in the morning. The client may also take the dose at bedtime to minimize these effects. The other responses do not address the concern of orthostatic hypotension.
Cognitive Level: Application
Nursing Process Step: Implementation
NCLEX: Physiological Integrity: Pharmacological and Parenteral Therapies

20. **Answer:** 3
Rationale: An adequate fluid intake of 2.5 to 3 L daily and sufficient sodium intake are needed to maintain therapeutic drug levels. A normal diet with sufficient sodium intake is also important because sodium depleted states (e.g., decreased sodium intake, sweating, vomiting, diarrhea) all result in increased reabsorption of lithium in the kidney and can lead to rapidly escalating lithium levels and toxicity. Coffee, tea, and cola intake should be limited because of the diuretic effect, and exercise, saunas, and exposure to hot weather should be avoided. Lithium levels are drawn every 3 months or so after the initial stabilization period, during which they are measured every 1 to 2 weeks.
Cognitive Level: Application
Nursing Process Step: Implementation
NCLEX: Physiological Integrity: Pharmacological and Parenteral Therapies

CHAPTER 20

Overview of the Autonomic Nervous System

1. f, e, b, c, a, d
2. reflex arc
3. cholinergic neurons; cholinergic transmission
4. feedback control mechanism
5. smooth muscle, cardiac muscle, and glands of parasympathetic fibers and effector organs of the cholinergic sympathetic fibers
6. ganglia of both parasympathetic and sympathetic fibers, the adrenal medulla, and the skeletal (striated) muscle that is supplied by the somatic motor system
7. parasympathetic
8. sympathetic
9. neurohormonal
10. Nicotinic (N)
11. Muscarinic (M)
12. norepinephrine, epinephrine
13. acetylcholinesterase

Drugs Affecting the Parasympathetic Nervous System and the Neurotransmitter Acetylcholine

1.

```
P A R A S Y M P A T H O M I M E T I C
A N M U S C H O N S Y M P E R G O I I
R T I N D A S Y T A C E T Y L A G S T
A I D A T R O P I N E P A R A R S T Y
C C A C T M U S M A N T I I E C H O L
H H P O S T G A U S Y N T N P A R A O
O O P E R I D U S C A R E D S Y M P H
L L C H I L O P C E R R A I S P I T T
N I C O T I N E A C D R A R S Y N T A
B N P H Y S O T R A N E O E B E T H P
E E I N E R G I I I N D I C D I R E M
T R S C R E A T N S Y M P T Y E A M Y
H G H R O S T A I C H O L A H I C E S
D I A C E T Y L C A N T I C H I N E A
I C M U S C I C O T A C E T P A T A R
R I B E T H A N E C H O L I S Y M T A
E A N T I P A R I C H O L N A N T I P
S R Y Q N E X R N C L V R G S S N Y T
```

2. sympathetic nervous system
3. parasympathetic nervous system
4. muscarinic effects of acetylcholine; anticholinergic
5. plant sources; synthesized; direct-acting; indirect-acting
6. acetylcholine; postganglionic; muscarine
7. Nicotine
8. physostigmine
9. bladder
10. Physostigmine salicylate

11. **Suggested Answer:** Atropine acts by occupying the muscarinic (M) receptor sites, thereby preventing or reducing muscarinic response of acetylcholine. The drug-receptor complex is formed at the neuroeffector junctions of smooth muscle, cardiac muscle, and exocrine glands. Atropine is indicated for the treatment of irritable bowel syndrome, spastic biliary tract disorders, and genitourinary disorders and as an antidote for cholinergic toxicity from excessive amounts of cholinesterase inhibitors, muscarinics, or organophosphate pesticide poisoning. It is also used to treat sinus bradycardia and Parkinson disease, to prevent excessive salivation and respiratory tract secretions (preanesthetic), as an adjunctive medication for peptic ulcers, and for gastrointestinal radiography.

12. **Suggested Answer:** Teach the client to slowly chew one piece of gum for about 30 minutes when the urge to smoke occurs. No more than 30 pieces are to be chewed in a day; the number chewed should be reduced each day over a 2- to 3-month period. Use for more than 3 months is not advised. At 6 months a gradual withdrawal program should be instituted. Nicotine gum may cause damage to dentures, inlays, fillings, and teeth. Client should use sugarless hard candies between doses of gum for oral stimulation and to relieve discomfort. If gum sticks to dental work, discontinue use and consult physician or dentist. Client should not smoke while being treated. Nicotine gum must be used under medical supervision, combined with a supervised program for smoking cessation.

13. **Suggested Answer:** Remove patch from sealed pouch just before application. Remove protective liner from sticky side of patch, and touching this side as little as possible, apply patch to selected skin site. Press patch to skin with palm for about 10 seconds. Fold previously used patch in half with sticky side together and place in newly opened pouch of replacement patch. Throw pouch away. Wash hands immediately.

14. **Answer:** 2

Rationale: If a client experiences adverse effects of cholinergic overstimulation, it will be evidenced by flushing of the skin, headache, severe hypotension, hypothermia, bradycardia, nausea and vomiting, abdominal cramps, bloody diarrhea, shock, or cardiac arrest.

Cognitive Level: Application

Nursing Process Step: Assessment

NCLEX: Physiological Integrity: Pharmacological and Parenteral Therapies

15. **Answer:** 4

Rationale: Anticholinesterase agents (e.g., neostigmine, physostigmine) exert their influence on both muscarinic and nicotinic sites. They are used to treat myasthenia gravis and glaucoma. They are also used postoperatively for urinary retention and GI ileus. Physostigmine salicylate is used for anticholinergic substance toxicity and overdose.

Cognitive Level: Application

Nursing Process Step: Analysis

NCLEX: Physiological Integrity: Pharmacological and Parenteral Therapies

16. **Answer:** 1

Rationale: Neuromuscular blockers do not cause any sedation, are not analgesic, and have no effect on cognition. It is imperative that clients who receive these agents receive respiratory support before administration, because they will cause paralysis of respiratory muscles. Additionally, clients are likely to be quite anxious and must receive sedatives and anxiolytics before and during neuromuscular blocker administration to prevent anxiety and to impair memory of the perioperative period.

Cognitive Level: Application

Nursing Process Step: Implementation

NCLEX: Physiological Integrity: Pharmacological and Parenteral Therapies

17. **Answer:** 3

Rationale: With atropine, the pupil is dilated (mydriasis), and the ciliary muscle (muscle of accommodation) is relaxed (cycloplegia). Pupil dilation may reduce the outflow of aqueous humor, causing a rise in intraocular pressure. This is a hazardous situation for clients with glaucoma, although the usual single therapeutic dose of oral or parenteral atropine has little effect on the eye.

Cognitive Level: Application

Nursing Process Step: Assessment

NCLEX: Physiological Integrity: Pharmacological and Parenteral Therapies

18. **Answer:** 2

Rationale: When low doses of atropine are given or an IV dose is administered slowly, the cardiac rate is temporarily and slightly slowed because of the central action of the drug on the cardiac center in the medulla (paradoxical bradycardia). Larger IV doses given rapidly will block the vagal effect on the sinoatrial node and atrioventricular junction and increase heart rate.

Cognitive Level: Application

Nursing Process Step: Evaluation

NCLEX: Physiological Integrity: Pharmacological and Parenteral Therapies

19. **Answer:** 4

Rationale: For antiemetic or antivertigo effects in adults, a transdermal patch produces an effect for 72 hours. For an antiemetic effect, it should be applied 4 hours before the desired effect is required.

Cognitive Level: Application

Nursing Process Step: Implementation

NCLEX: Physiological Integrity: Pharmacological and Parenteral Therapies

20. **Answer:** 1

Rationale: The client should manage dry mouth with sugarless hard candies or gum, or ice chips and should avoid hazardous activities because dizziness, drowsiness, or abnormal vision (accommodation problems) may occur. The other statements are unrelated to this drug.

Cognitive Level: Application

Nursing Process Step: Implementation

NCLEX: Physiological Integrity: Pharmacological and Parenteral Therapies

CHAPTER 22

Drugs Affecting the Sympathetic (Adrenergic) Nervous System

1. a and c, a, d, d, a, c, a, b
2. inotropic; chronotropic; dromotropic
3. noncompetitive, long-acting antagonists; competitive, short-acting antagonists; ergot alkaloids
4. adrenergic
5. norepinephrine, epinephrine
6. stress, exercise
7. gluconeogenesis, lipolysis
8. dilate
9. extrasystoles, fibrillation
10. vasodilation

11. **Suggested Answer:** Adverse effects of epinephrine include increased nervousness, restlessness, insomnia, tachycardia, tremors, sweating, increased blood pressure, nausea, vomiting, pallor, weakness and, with inhalation devices, bronchial irritation and coughing (with high doses), dry mouth and throat, headaches, and flushing of the face and skin.

12. **Suggested Answer:** Refer to drug monograph in the textbook for complete listing of possible answers.

291

13. **Suggested Answer:** The adverse effects of dobutamine include nausea, headache, angina, respiratory distress, palpitations, increased heart rate and BP, and occasionally premature ventricular beats.

14. **Answer:** 1
Rationale: If the heart rate exceeds 110 beats/min, a slower infusion rate or a temporary discontinuance of the drug will be prescribed. Intended effects of the drug are improved systolic blood pressure and adequate urine output. A one-sided weakness in pedal pulses is more likely because of local pathology than a general systemic drug effect.
Cognitive Level: Analysis
Nursing Process Step: Planning
NCLEX: Physiological Integrity: Pharmacological and Parenteral Therapies

15. **Answer:** 3
Rationale: Observe the client for blanching along the route of the infused vein and for cold, hard swelling around the injection site. The other signs listed indicate thrombophlebitis.
Cognitive Level: Application
Nursing Process Step: Assessment
NCLEX: Physiological Integrity: Pharmacological and Parenteral Therapies

16. **Answer:** 2
Rationale: The expected outcome for ergot alkaloid therapy is that the client will experience diminished headaches or will not experience any headaches without adverse effects of ergot alkaloid therapy. The other signs listed are not relevant, although muscle pain is a sign of ergot toxicity.
Cognitive Level: Application
Nursing Process Step: Evaluation
NCLEX: Physiological Integrity: Pharmacological and Parenteral Therapies

17. **Answer:** 4
Rationale: β_2-adrenergics blockade the appearance of the warning signs and symptoms of acute hypoglycemia (sweating, increased heart rate, and anxiety), which is of concern for clients on insulin. Therefore these agents should be used with caution in such clients. The health problems in the other options of not necessarily of concern, although a history of chronic obstructive pulmonary disorder (COPD) would be cause for cautious use of β blockers.
Cognitive Level: Application
Nursing Process Step: Analysis
NCLEX: Physiological Integrity: Pharmacological and Parenteral Therapies

18. **Answer:** 1
Rationale: If the pulse is slower than 50 beats/min or the rate is irregular, the client should withhold the drug and call the prescriber immediately.
Cognitive Level: Application
Nursing Process Step: Implementation
NCLEX: Physiological Integrity: Pharmacological and Parenteral Therapies

19. **Answer:** 3
Rationale: If the drug is to be discontinued, it is important to reduce the dosage over a 1- to 2-week period.
Cognitive Level: Application
Nursing Process Step: Implementation
NCLEX: Physiological Integrity: Pharmacological and Parenteral Therapies

20. **Answer:** 2
Rationale: Atenolol is cardioselective in that it affects β_1 receptors. The other drugs listed are not cardioselective in that they affect both β_1 and β_2 receptors.
Cognitive Level: Application
Nursing Process Step: Planning
NCLEX: Physiological Integrity: Pharmacological and Parenteral Therapies

CHAPTER 23

Drugs for Specific Dysfunctions of the Central and Peripheral Nervous Systems

1.

```
B A C L O F E N A T S P A S M S I D
B A C Y T R N T R O P S I G N E Y S
I N E O S T I G M I N E F E N S T E
S A N Y I C P D O N A D F E T A I K
E B E N Z D O D A K A E S O P T C L
L E S T E R R A K A T S N R E D I I
E D E M E N T I A D E I N E R D T Z
G E O D O N Z O F E A G T R O L S E
I G R N A W N K A K I N E S I A A P
L O S T A Z E D R U B E B A C I P E
I T O L C Z B A P O N R S E L S S N
N S E L E G E T O L C D A N T I S O
E N T O L C A P O N E R T I A H E D
A K A B E N Z A I T O U P A N T N E
D E A P O D O V E L I G M E N S I C
D O N A A N T I A K A S S E L A G I
T R O P A K A S K I B C H O L K E N
A N T I C H O L I N E S T E R A S E
```

2. Parkinson's disease
3. Myasthenia gravis
4. anticholinergic, dopamine
5. alcohol
6. renal
7. bromocriptine
8. dysphagia, respiratory muscle weakness
9. acetylcholinesterase
10. 30, 45

11. **Suggested Answer:** Answers should include two of the following:

Guanadrel, guanethidine, mecamylamine, trimethaphan: May antagonize action of cholinesterase inhibitor drugs, resulting in increased muscle weakness, respiratory muscle weakness, and difficulty swallowing.

Procainamide: May antagonize action of cholinesterase inhibitor drugs.

Other cholinesterase inhibitors: Serious additive toxicity may result.

12. **Suggested Answer:** With short-term (1- to 3-days' use) or chronic oral intake of dantrolene: mild diarrhea, dizziness, sleepiness, feelings of uncomfortableness or unusual fatigue, muscle weakness (not of respiratory muscles), nausea, or vomiting.

13. **Suggested Answer:** In addition to the nursing management discussed as appropriate to centrally acting skeletal muscle relaxant therapy in general, baclofen requires the following considerations:

- Dosage should be increased gradually.
- A gradual reduction in dosage over a period of 2 weeks is recommended.
- Tell the client that maximum benefit may not be reached for 1 to 2 months.
- Alert the client to possible adverse effects. If orthostatic hypotension is a concern, instruct the client to come to an upright position slowly.
- Administration of baclofen may increase the client's blood glucose levels, requiring an adjustment of insulin dosage during therapy and when baclofen therapy is stopped.
- Older clients are at risk for adverse CNS reactions.
- Clients with epilepsy are at risk for increased seizure activity.
- Monitor the client's clinical state and EEG results during therapy.

14. **Answer:** 1

Rationale: Benztropine is indicated for use as an anti-dyskinetic, for treatment of tremor in Parkinson's disease, and for treatment of drug-induced extrapyramidal symptoms (EPS) associated with typical antipsychotic drug use. It is not intended to affect blood pressure, temperature, or cognition.

Cognitive Level: Analysis

Nursing Process Step: Evaluation

NCLEX: Physiological Integrity: Pharmacological and Parenteral Therapies

15. **Answer:** 3

Rationale: Improvement is usually seen within 2 to 3 weeks, although some clients may require levodopa for up to 6 months to obtain a therapeutic effect. Peak concentration is achieved in 1 to 3 hours. The duration of action is up to 5 hours per dose.

Cognitive Level: Application

Nursing Process Step: Implementation

NCLEX: Physiological Integrity: Pharmacological and Parenteral Therapies

16. **Answer:** 2

Rationale: After treatment is initiated, the client should be observed closely for signs of toxic cholinergic effects. The nurse should keep atropine sulfate and equipment for respiratory support on hand. Tenormin is a β blocker. Calcium gluconate is used to treat tetany, whereas calcium carbonate is an antacid (Tums).

Cognitive Level: Application

Nursing Process Step: Planning

NCLEX: Physiological Integrity: Pharmacological and Parenteral Therapies

17. **Answer:** 4

Rationale: Neostigmine and edrophonium are the two drugs that are used to diagnose myasthenia gravis. Pyridostigmine and ambenonium are used to treat the disease but not for diagnosis. Bromocriptine is an antiparkinson medication.

Cognitive Level: Application

Nursing Process Step: Planning

NCLEX: Physiological Integrity: Pharmacological and Parenteral Therapies

18. **Answer:** 1

Rationale: Tacrine has a higher risk for hepatotoxicity and requires routine testing of serum alanine aminotransferase for liver toxicity. As such, tacrine use has been largely replaced with the other agents in this class.

Cognitive Level: Application

Nursing Process Step: Analysis

NCLEX: Physiological Integrity: Pharmacological and Parenteral Therapies

19. **Answer:** 3

Rationale: The adverse effects of baclofen include transient drowsiness, vertigo, confusion, sleepiness, weakness, and nausea.

Cognitive Level: Application

Nursing Process Step: Assessment

NCLEX: Physiological Integrity: Pharmacological and Parenteral Therapies

20. **Answer:** 2

Rationale: Clients should be taught that mental alertness, judgment, and physical coordination may be affected. Alert clients that alcohol and other CNS depressants will increase the CNS effects of these drugs. Because many clients experience postural hypotension with central-acting skeletal muscle relaxants, they should be cautioned about changing position in keeping with physical limitations.

Cognitive Level: Application

Nursing Process Step: Implementation

NCLEX: Physiological Integrity: Pharmacological and Parenteral Therapies

CHAPTER 24

Overview of the Cardiovascular System

1.

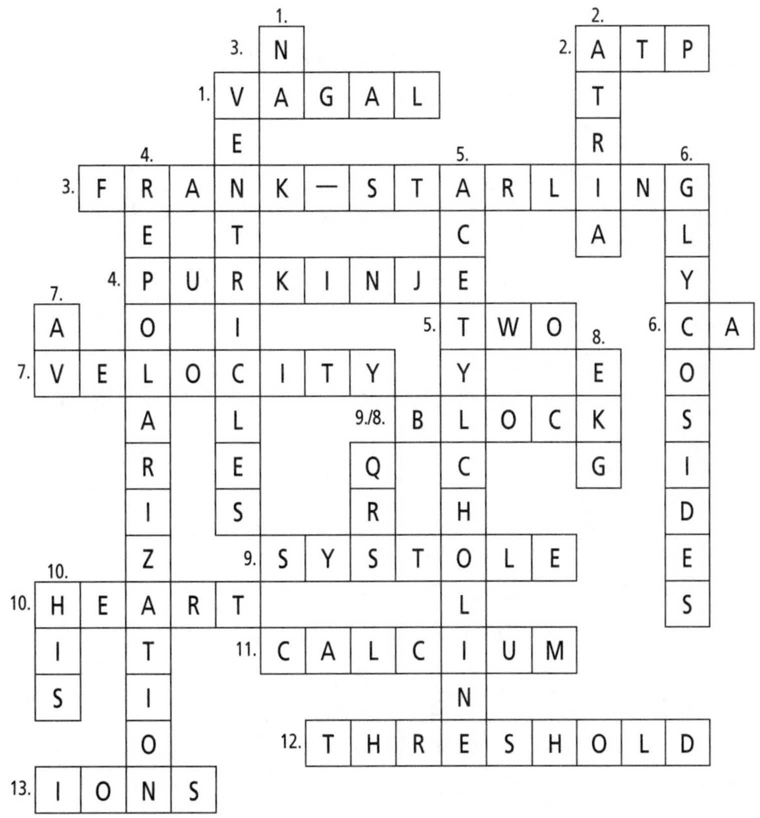

					1.						2.		
			3.	N					2.	A	T	P
		1.	V	A	G	A	L			T	
			E				5.			R		6.
4.	3.	F	R	A	N	K	—	S	T	A	R	L	I	N	G

Crossword puzzle (answer key):

- 1. Across: **VAGAL**
- 2. Across: **ATP**
- 3. Across: **FRANK–STARLING**
- 3. Down: **N E T W O R K**
- 4. Across: **PURKINJE**
- 5. Across: **TWO**
- 6. Across: **CA**
- 7. Across: **VELOCITY**
- 8. Down: **PEG**
- 9. Across: **SYSTOLE**
- 10. Across: **HEART**
- 11. Across: **CALCIUM**
- 12. Across: **THRESHOLD**
- 13. Across: **IONS**

Down entries include: VERTEBRATE, ATRIAL, GLYCOSIDES, AV NODE, POLARIZES, VASCULARIZ, QRS, CHANNEL, SINUS, CA, AUTOMATIC, HIS.

2. electrical charge
3. Depolarization
4. automaticity
5. Conductivity
6. refractoriness
7. Electrocardiograms (ECGs)

8. calcium
9. Cardiac output, stroke volume, heart rate
10. Contractility
11. Preload
12. Afterload

Agents Used in the Treatment of Heart Failure

1.

```
G N C P S F L K O A M R T S Q D W V K X
Y L S E R Z Z L Q W H F O Z X Z H V I K
O S R W E J G K P J A B X W C L B Q L R
O U W V K Y X U A C V L I E R H P E S R
M B P X A H A Y H S Q Z C K R N R Z I U
R Y I O M C X K K C F Z I G J B J Y Z V
J I N E E W J W R M J A T L X Z W Z W V
F H A O C E D X H B G L Y C O S I D E B
G E M Y A H W A L V E C R H D L B M I Y
H N R G P W F Z G Q N P I R J E X C E K
N O I T A L L I R B I F O O Z V C M N O
U N N S O A F D G Z X M U N I X O G I D
R I O U R U V P I N O T R O P I C Y H J
K R N V R U U J M T N A P T X R T D Y Z
T L E S P N N F R D A J E R Y E K T J Q
Q I J J K E X O C O L M B O A I B J Y O
X M Q W U D P Y O N G F A P Z N R O C Q
G M N R R I D I G I T A L I Z A T I O N
W O B R C B D P V Q Q B W C O Z X B Q K
J W W W J B H Y J U Y W J B Y X J Z X W
```

2. Heart failure
3. inotropic
4. chronotropic
5. dromotropic
6. Digitalis
7. positive, negative, negative
8. dose-
9. refractory period, conduction
10. antidote

11. **Suggested Answer:** Answers should include three of the following: potassium loss (through hypokalemia, poor dietary intake, adrenal steroid use, or surgical procedures associated with severe electrolyte disturbances); hypercalcemia; pathologic conditions such as kidney, liver, and severe heart disease.

12. **Suggested Answer:** Instruct client to take digoxin at the same time each day, precisely as prescribed. Do not skip or double a dose if missed. Do not change brand. Inform client that digoxin and Lanoxin are essentially the same drug. If using elixir form, dose should be determined using special dropper. Caution client not to take other medications without prior approval of physician.

Restrict sodium intake to 2 g daily. Report weight gain of 1 or 2 pounds a day; avoid licorice.

Advise client to carry medical identification and to alert health professionals unfamiliar with drug regimen that the drug is being taken.

Teach client how to take pulse before each dose. Dose should be withheld and physician notified if the pulse is below 60 or above 110 and/or is erratic or if client suffers from anorexia, diarrhea, nausea, vomiting, sudden weight gain, or apparent edema. Visual disturbances should be reported.

13. **Suggested Answer:** The adverse effects of inamrinone are infrequent and include nausea, vomiting, abdominal pain, fever, taste alterations, hypotension, dysrhythmias, chest pain, and thrombocytopenia.

The inotropic effects of inamrinone are additive to those of digoxin.

14. **Answer:** 1
Rationale: Serious adverse effects of digoxin include heart block, bradycardia, ventricular fibrillation, and other serious cardiac dysrhythmias, many of which can be more serious in the presence of electrolyte imbalance. Other adverse effects include nausea, vomiting, diarrhea, dizziness, visual disturbances, rash, hallucinations, confusion, dizziness, and delirium.
Cognitive Level: Application
Nursing Process Step: Assessment
NCLEX: Physiological Integrity: Pharmacological and Parenteral Therapies

15. **Answer:** 3
Rationale: With digoxin, heart size is often decreased toward normal. Venous pressure falls, and the pulmonary and systemic congestion and their accompanying signs and symptoms are either diminished or eliminated. Coronary circulation is enhanced, myocardial oxygen demand is reduced, and the supply of oxygen and nutrients to the myocardium is improved.
Cognitive Level: Application
Nursing Process Step: Planning
NCLEX: Physiological Integrity: Pharmacological and Parenteral Therapies

16. **Answer:** 4
Rationale: Beneficial effects of digoxin are correlated with therapeutic serum levels of 0.8 to 2 ng/mL. The client with an elevated level should be assessed for toxicity manifestations.
Cognitive Level: Analysis
Nursing Process Step: Assessment
NCLEX: Physiological Integrity: Pharmacological and Parenteral Therapies

17. **Answer:** 4
Rationale: In the rapid digitalization (loading) method, which is reserved for clients who are in acute distress from heart failure, IV digoxin is given in divided doses in a 24-hour period for the client who has not previously taken digoxin. A common protocol is to administer a total IV dose of 1 mg of digoxin. Digoxin may be prescribed as 0.5 mg IV now and 0.25 mg IV every 6 hours for two doses (for a total of 1 mg).
Cognitive Level: Application
Nursing Process Step: Planning
NCLEX: Physiological Integrity: Pharmacological and Parenteral Therapies

18. **Answer:** 1
Rationale: Common dose-related adverse effects of the digoxin include anorexia, nausea, bradycardia, visual disturbances manifest by yellow vision, stomach pain, and dysrhythmias. A loss of appetite is usually the first sign of toxicity; nausea and vomiting and abdominal distress usually occur several days after the anorexia. Confusion or changes in mental status can

also be related to digoxin use, particularly in the older adult.
Cognitive Level: Application
Nursing Process Step: Assessment
NCLEX: Physiological Integrity: Pharmacological and Parenteral Therapies

19. **Answer:** 3
Rationale: The normal potassium level is 3.5 to 5.1 mEq/L. A fall in potassium serum level enhances the effect of digoxin and the risk of digoxin toxicity. Excess potassium increases the risk of cardiac dysrhythmias. The nurse could safely administer the dose if the client is free from either hypokalemia and hyperkalemia.
Cognitive Level: Analysis
Nursing Process Step: Planning
NCLEX: Physiological Integrity: Pharmacological and Parenteral Therapies

20. **Answer:** 2
Rationale: Clients need to take own pulse before each dose of medication. The dose should be withheld and the prescriber notified if the pulse is below 60 or above 110 beats/min and/or is erratic or if he experiences anorexia, diarrhea, nausea, vomiting, sudden weight gain, or apparent edema. Visual disturbances, such as blurred vision or green or yellow halos around objects, should also be reported to the prescriber. Clients should restrict sodium intake to 2 g or less daily and report a weight gain of 2 pounds a day and should *not* take the oral preparation with meals that have high fiber content because this will reduce absorption.
Cognitive Level: Application
Nursing Process Step: Implementation
NCLEX: Physiological Integrity: Pharmacological and Parenteral Therapies

CHAPTER 26

Antidysrhythmics

1. a, b, g, a, e, c, f, b, f, d
2. Sinus bradycardia
3. Sinus tachycardia
4. ectopic focus
5. Reentry, unidirectional
6. excitability, conduction, contractility
7. Stokes-Adams
8. sodium, potassium
9. refractory
10. tachycardia, fibrillation

11. **Suggested Answer:** When a client is on antidysrhythmic drug therapy with lidocaine, he or she will:
   - Experience effective tissue perfusion related to the therapeutic effect of the antidysrhythmic drug.
   - Not experience injury related to the adverse effects of antidysrhythmic drug therapy.

- Demonstrate adequate knowledge of the antidys-rhythmic drug therapy.
- Report any report any dizziness, chest pain, or shortness of breath to the nursing staff.

12. **Suggested Answer:** Amiodarone is structurally related to thyroid hormone. It increases the refractory period in all cardiac tissues by having a direct effect on the tissues. Amiodarone decreases automaticity, prolongs AV conduction, and decreases the automaticity of fibers in the Purkinje system. It may block potassium, sodium and calcium channels, and a receptors. It has the potential to cause a variety of complex effects on the heart and has serious adverse effects.

13. **Suggested Answer:** Sotalol is a nonselective β-adrenergic blocking agent that prolongs the duration of the action potential, increasing the effective refractory period in atrial, ventricular, and AV junction. Unlike other β-adrenergic blockers, sotalol affects potassium channels rendering this drug effective in the treatment of ventricular dysrhythmia.

14. **Answer:** 1
Rationale: Unlike other antidysrhythmic agents, quinidine is unique because if quinidine is administered to clients with myasthenia gravis, it may increase muscle weakness secondary to its weak curare-like action.
Cognitive Level: Application
Nursing Process Step: Implementation
NCLEX: Physiological Integrity: Pharmacological and Parenteral Therapies

15. **Answer:** 3
Rationale: Procainamide is associated with hypotension on IV administration, and diarrhea, nausea, and vomiting.
Cognitive Level: Application
Nursing Process Step: Assessment
NCLEX: Physiological Integrity: Pharmacological and Parenteral Therapies

16. **Answer:** 2
Rationale: Because electric activities of lidocaine are primarily limited to the ventricular cells, the major use of lidocaine is in abolishing ventricular dysrhythmias. It is not used to treat the other rhythms listed.
Cognitive Level: Application
Nursing Process Step: Planning
NCLEX: Physiological Integrity: Pharmacological and Parenteral Therapies

17. **Answer:** 4
Rationale: A client is given a bolus dose to rapidly attain therapeutic serum concentrations. When the intravenous drip is started, it is important to monitor the prescribed IV rate of flow; lidocaine should not exceed 4 mg/min.
Cognitive Level: Application
Nursing Process Step: Implementation
NCLEX: Physiological Integrity: Pharmacological and Parenteral Therapies

18. **Answer:** 1
Rationale: Acebutolol is indicated for ventricular dysrhythmia because of its ability to suppress ectopic ventricular beats. It is also indicated for hypertension and angina. The adverse effects for acebutolol are similar to other β-adrenergic antagonists. Of major concern are the risks for AV block and bradycardia. As a negative inotrope, its use in clients with heart failure (HF) should generally be avoided.
Cognitive Level: Application
Nursing Process Step: Implementation
NCLEX: Physiological Integrity: Pharmacological and Parenteral Therapies

19. **Answer:** 3
Rationale: A blue-gray coloration of the skin occurs with long-term use (more than 1 year) and affects sun-exposed parts of the body (e.g., face, neck, and arms) and those with fair skin. The other options are not unique adverse effects of this drug.
Cognitive Level: Application
Nursing Process Step: Implementation
NCLEX: Physiological Integrity: Pharmacological and Parenteral Therapies

20. **Answer:** 2
Rationale: Diltiazem interacts with a number of drugs metabolized by cytochrome P450 3A4, including but not limited to amiodarone, cimetidine, digoxin, fluoxetine, ketoconazole, itraconazole, omeprazole, phenytoin, and grapefruit juice. Thus the nurse should avoid administering a dose with grapefruit juice.
Cognitive Level: Application
Nursing Process Step: Implementation
NCLEX: Physiological Integrity: Pharmacological and Parenteral Therapies

CHAPTER 27

Antihypertensives

1.

```
E D I Z A I H T O R O L H C O R D Y H
C A N G N B A R O C L O N H Y P I N D
N I F E G H Y D R A T H I S I D U P A
L O S A I C A P T T H I R N I T R S E
P B A R O R E C E P T O R E D A E R N
A R T A T H Y D R O T A R T Z I T N I
C A T E E P R A Z A S O R O P S I A P
L O S A N C L U L P I T S A R T C R I
O T E N S A R I C L O I C A P R S E D
N T I N I A D S I N N C A R T I D I E
I A Z A N O I S N E T R E P Y H A Z F
D A C T S S A R C L H P R I L A P O I
I N D A C L O P R I I T I N G H A R N
N E V A Z Z H Y D R A L A Z I N E E T
E D I L V A S I L A Z T O C A P E Z R
R E C T O R P T E L I R P O T P A C E
E L O S A R T A N I D H Y D R O P R I
C L O P I L I N E W E P R U S C A P W
C A P L O S E D I S S U R P O R T I N
```

2. arterioles
3. antianginal; antidysrhythmic; antihypertensive
4. peripheral vascular resistance; blood pressure
5. target organ
6. Thiazide
7. spironolactone (Aldactone), triamterene (Dyrenium)
8. ACE inhibitors, ARBs
9. angioedema
10. arterioles, veins
11. **Suggested Answer:** Diuretics and calcium antagonists.

12. **Suggested Answer:** Older adults have increased risk of cardiovascular (CV) morbidity and mortality. Nonpharmacologic means of blood pressure reduction are indicated. Antihypertensive drugs should be started with smaller than usual doses, increased by smaller than usual amounts, and scheduled at less frequent intervals, because older adults are more sensitive to volume depletion and sympathetic inhibition than younger clients. They commonly have impaired CV reflexes, making them more susceptible to hypotension. In clients with isolated systolic hypertension who are treated with antihypertensive drugs, the systolic pressure should be cautiously decreased to 140 to 160 mm Hg. Only if this medication level is tolerated without adverse effects should consideration be given to further lowering the systolic value. The older adult's response to both nonpharmacologic and pharmacologic therapies should be monitored closely.

13. **Suggested Answer:** The typical treatment is to use IV atropine, isoproterenol, norepinephrine, or calcium chloride. An electronic cardiac pacemaker may be necessary.

14. **Answer:** 2

Rationale: JNC VII recommends thiazide diuretics as first-line drug therapy for uncomplicated hypertension. Other drugs used in the management of hypertension include the angiotensin converting enzyme inhibitors (ACE-inhibitors), angiotensin$_2$ receptor blockers (ARBs), α-adrenergic blockers, and calcium channel blockers (CCBs).

Cognitive Level: Application
Nursing Process Step: Analysis
NCLEX: Physiological Integrity: Pharmacological and Parenteral Therapies

15. Answer: 1

Rationale: Clients should be encouraged to take the single daily dose of hydrochlorothiazide in the morning to minimize the effect of increased frequency of urinary frequency on sleep.

Cognitive Level: Application

Nursing Process Step: Implementation

NCLEX: Physiological Integrity: Pharmacological and Parenteral Therapies

16. Answer: 4

Rationale: Alert client to assess ability to undertake physical exertion because of possible activity intolerance related to atenolol's adverse effects of fatigue and weakness. Teach client to check his pulse before he takes his atenolol; if it is less than 50 beats/min to withhold the atenolol and notify his prescriber. He should also alert his prescriber if he experiences any light-headedness, wheezing or shortness of breath, edema, sudden weight gain, or symptoms of depression or sexual dysfunction.

Cognitive Level: Application

Nursing Process Step: Implementation

NCLEX: Physiological Integrity: Pharmacological and Parenteral Therapies

17. Answer: 3

Rationale: The dry cough is an expected adverse effect of Lisinopril therapy that should resolve once the medication dose can be tapered or if the client is switched to another medication. The client should report any sign of infection (e.g., sore throat, fever), which indicates possible neutropenia. Urinary protein determinations are done periodically on the first morning urine; if proteinuria is greater than 1 g/day, the drug regimen should be reevaluated.

Cognitive Level: Application

Nursing Process Step: Analysis

NCLEX: Physiological Integrity: Pharmacological and Parenteral Therapies

18. Answer: 2

Rationale: Like the ACE inhibitors, the ARBs pose the risk for angioedema, which can threaten the airway. Other adverse effects of losartan include headache, tiredness, back or muscle pain, diarrhea, nasal congestion, dizziness, and upper respiratory infection. A dry cough and insomnia are considered rare effects.

Cognitive Level: Application

Nursing Process Step: Planning

NCLEX: Physiological Integrity: Pharmacological and Parenteral Therapies

19. Answer: 4

Rationale: FDA-approved indications for various calcium channel blockers include angina pectoris (bepridil, diltiazem, felodipine, mibefradil, nicardipine, nifedipine, verapamil), dysrhythmias (diltiazem parenteral, verapamil), hypertension (diltiazem, felodipine, isradipine, mibefradil, nicardipine, nifedipine extended-release tablets, verapamil), sub-

arachnoid hemorrhage (nimodipine), and prophylaxis for vascular headaches (flunarizine [Sibelium[CN169]]).

Cognitive Level: Analysis

Nursing Process Step: Analysis

NCLEX: Physiological Integrity: Pharmacological and Parenteral Therapies

20. Answer: 1

Rationale: Calcium channel blockers should be avoided for individuals with systolic heart failure because these agents are negative inotropes.

Cognitive Level: Analysis

Nursing Process Step: Analysis

NCLEX: Physiological Integrity: Pharmacological and Parenteral Therapies

CHAPTER 28

Vasodilators and Blood Viscosity–Reducing Agents

1. d, f, a, c, b, e
2. Stable
3. depression, elevation
4. supply, demand, occlusion
5. headache, vasodilation
6. pain, cramps, weakness
7. flexibility, viscosity
8. GI distress, nausea and vomiting
9. platelet
10. hepatic, renal

11. **Suggested Answer:** Instruct client to place the tablet between upper lip and gum to dissolve and above incisors if food or drink is to be taken within 3 to 5 hours. Caution against using at bedtime, because aspiration is a risk. The tablet may be replaced if it is accidentally swallowed.

12. **Suggested Answer:** To decrease duration and intensity of pain during an attack; to prophylactically decrease frequency of attacks and improve work capacity even though angina may occur; to prevent or delay the onset of myocardial infarction.

13. **Suggested Answer:** It improves microcirculation of ischemic tissues by inhibiting phosphodiesterase, which increases cyclic AMP, and it lowers blood viscosity by decreasing fibrinogen concentration and inhibiting aggregation of RBCs and platelets.

14. **Answer: 2**

Rationale: Flushing and headache are frequent adverse effects caused by the vasodilating effects of nitroglycerin. It often diminishes or disappears over time as the client gets used to the drug. The client does not need a larger dose or a different drug, and this does not indicate atypical hypersensitivity reaction.

Cognitive Level: Analysis

Nursing Process Step: Analysis

NCLEX: Physiological Integrity: Pharmacological and Parenteral Therapies

15. **Answer:** 4

Rationale: Nitroglycerin is a coronary vasodilator that can be used to prevent chest pain during activities that precipitate it. Lopressor is a β-adrenergic blocker with antihypertensive and antianginal effects, but cannot be used on a PRN basis before activity. Pentoxifylline is an antihemorheologic agent used for intermittent claudication, whereas papaverine is a vasodilator that is rarely used today.

Cognitive Level: Application

Nursing Process Step: Implementation

NCLEX: Physiological Integrity: Pharmacological and Parenteral Therapies

16. **Answer:** 3

Rationale: Correct dosing is to take up to three tablets 5 minutes apart as needed until chest pain is relieved. If the client still has pain after three doses, emergency medical services (911) should be called.

Cognitive Level: Application

Nursing Process Step: Evaluation

NCLEX: Physiological Integrity: Pharmacological and Parenteral Therapies

17. **Answer:** 3

Rationale: The patch should not be trimmed because this will alter the rate at which drug is released through the system into the skin. The client needs further information about this point. The other options indicate correct information and therefore additional client teaching is not needed about those points.

Cognitive Level: Application

Nursing Process Step: Evaluation

NCLEX: Physiological Integrity: Pharmacological and Parenteral Therapies

18. **Answer:** 1

Rationale: Nitroglycerin should be stored in a cool, dark, dry location. They should remain in the original brown glass container. The client should not eat or drink while taking the tablet under the tongue, and should use a new supply every 6 months so the tablets do not lose potency.

Cognitive Level: Application

Nursing Process Step: Implementation

NCLEX: Physiological Integrity: Pharmacological and Parenteral Therapies

19. **Answer:** 3

Rationale: Pentoxifylline is indicated as an adjunct to surgery for the treatment of intermittent claudication caused by occlusive arterial disease of the limbs. Femoral popliteal bypass surgery would be such a procedure. The other surgeries are not indications for use of this drug as adjunct therapy.

Cognitive Level: Analysis

Nursing Process Step: Analysis

NCLEX: Physiological Integrity: Pharmacological and Parenteral Therapies

20. **Answer:** 2

Rationale: The most common adverse effect of pentoxifylline is gastrointestinal (GI) upset with abdominal distress, nausea and vomiting. Other adverse effects of pentoxifylline include dizziness and headaches. Rare adverse effects are chest pain and an irregular heart rate. With an overdose the client experiences increased sedation, flushing of the skin, a feeling of faintness, increased excitability, or seizures.

Cognitive Level: Application

Nursing Process Step: Assessment

NCLEX: Physiological Integrity: Pharmacological and Parenteral Therapies

Overview of the Blood

1.

```
         1.                    2.           3.
    1. L  E  U  K  O  C  Y  T  E  S         L
       R                       T            Y        5.
       Y                    2. A  L  B  U  M  I  N
       T           4.          S            P        E
    3. H  E  M  O  G  L  O  B  I  N         H        U
       R           P           S                     T
       O        5. H  C  T                           R
    4. P  L  A  S  M  A              6. F  A  C  T  O  R
       O                       6.                     P
    7. F  I  B  R  I  N     8. A  N  E  M  I  A  10. R  H
       E        7.    8.    B  9.    10.               I
    9. T  H  R  O  M  B  O  C  Y  T  E  S              L
       I        X     L     L     Y                    S
       N        Y     O     O  11. P  L  T
                G     O     T     E
                E     D     S
                N
```

2. Hematocrit
3. 120
4. anemia
5. neutrophils, eosinophils, basophils, lymphocytes, monocytes
6. 150,000, 350,000
7. Fibrinogen
8. Hemostasis
9. intrinsic, extrinsic
10. A, O
11. universal donors
12. negative, positive

7. Heparin
8. Protamine sulfate
9. plasminogen, plasmin
10. 500

11. **Suggested Answer:** apprehension, restlessness, fever, chills, head or back pain, rash, hypotension, nausea and vomiting, dyspnea, cyanosis

12. **Suggested Answer:** Increased risk of bleeding and hemorrhage. Heparin has been administered with fibrinolytic agents to treat an acute coronary arterial occlusion.

13. **Suggested Answer:** Refer to box titled Special Considerations for Older Adults: Anticoagulants.

14. **Answer:** 2
Rationale: Target INR for prevention and treatment of most thromboembolic events is 2.5 (range, 2.0 to 3.0). For individuals with recurrent systemic emboli or mechanical heart valves, goal INR may be as high as 3.0 (range, 2.5 to 3.5), and occasionally higher. INR result reflects warfarin dose administered 36 to 72 hours prior to testing.
Cognitive Level: Analysis
Nursing Process Step: Analysis

CHAPTER 30

Antiplatelets, Anticoagulants, Fibrinolytics, and Blood Components

1. a, b, b, a, a, b, a, b
2. dissolve, extension
3. antiplatelet
4. prostaglandins
5. bone marrow
6. warfarin (Coumadin)

NCLEX: Physiological Integrity: Pharmacological and Parenteral Therapies

15. **Answer:** 4

Rationale: Injection sites should be rotated systematically and this medication is given in the lower abdomen. A 25- to 27-gauge, 3/8- to 5/8-inch needle is used. Bruising could result if aspiration or massaging occurs and are therefore avoided.

Cognitive Level: Application
Nursing Process Step: Implementation
NCLEX: Physiological Integrity: Pharmacological and Parenteral Therapies

16. **Answer:** 1

Rationale: The antidote to warfarin sodium is vitamin K (phytonadione). Protamine sulfate is the antidote to heparin. Argatroban is used for prophylaxis or treatment of thromboembolic events in clients with heparin induced thrombocytopenia. Aminocaproic acid prevents the breakdown of existing clots.

Cognitive Level: Application
Nursing Process Step: Planning
NCLEX: Physiological Integrity: Pharmacological and Parenteral Therapies

17. **Answer:** 3

Rationale: Clients taking anticoagulants should not take aspirin (option 4) or nonsteroidal antiinflammatory drugs (options 1 and 2) without specific health care provider approval because they increase the risk of bleeding. Acetaminophen does not carry this risk.

Cognitive Level: Analysis
Nursing Process Step: Implementation
NCLEX: Physiological Integrity: Pharmacological and Parenteral Therapies

18. **Answer:** 2

Rationale: Fibrinolytic therapy would be contraindicated with severe uncontrolled hypertension (>200 mm Hg systolic and/or >120 mm Hg diastolic) because of the risk of cerebral hemorrhage.

Cognitive Level: Application
Nursing Process Step: Assessment
NCLEX: Physiological Integrity: Pharmacological and Parenteral Therapies

19. **Answer:** 3

Rationale: As administration of a blood product begins, the nurse remains with the client and observe the client closely for reactions for 15 minutes or more while the flow rate is kept at a keep-open rate, because transfusion reactions are more likely to occur within this timeframe.

Cognitive Level: Application
Nursing Process Step: Planning
NCLEX: Physiological Integrity: Pharmacological and Parenteral Therapies

20. **Answer:** 1

Rationale: A febrile nonhemolytic reaction is the most common transfusion reaction. It is a reaction between preformed recipient WBC antibodies directed against transfused WBC in the product or cytokines that accumulate in the blood bag during storage. Antipyretic premedication such as acetaminophen will prevent this reaction.

Cognitive Level: Application
Nursing Process Step: Planning
NCLEX: Physiological Integrity: Pharmacological and Parenteral Therapies

Antihyperlipidemic Drugs

1.

```
C  H  O  L  E  S  T  Y  R  A  M  I  N  E  N
H  O  Z  I  L  A  T  H  E  T  C  H  O  L  I
Y  L  I  P  O  L  O  V  A  H  N  I  A  T  A
L  S  C  L  E  R  E  M  I  E  L  O  B  A  C
O  C  H  O  S  T  Y  N  I  R  G  E  M  G  H
M  I  A  L  I  P  O  P  R  O  T  E  I  N  O
I  G  E  M  S  T  R  A  T  S  I  A  C  I  L
C  L  B  V  A  I  E  R  C  N  I  V  A  L  E
R  O  S  I  S  F  I  B  E  L  I  P  O  C  F
O  T  H  E  R  M  I  C  R  E  O  Z  A  I  I
N  I  T  N  O  P  N  I  A  R  C  H  Y  N  B
S  N  I  T  A  T  S  A  V  O  L  O  S  I  L
L  E  F  I  L  O  S  T  A  S  N  I  C  H  I
G  E  M  F  I  B  R  O  Z  I  L  P  O  R  P
T  E  I  I  P  O  A  T  H  S  S  T  A  R  E
H  Y  P  E  R  L  I  P  I  D  E  M  I  A  M
```

2. metabolic; cholesterol; triglycerides
3. high levels of circulating triglycerides and cholesterol
4. cholesterol and triglycerides; the body cell membranes; the liver
5. lipid compounds; plasma proteins; densities and electrophoretic mobilities
6. cholesterol
7. largest; dense; the small intestine during absorption of a fatty meal
8. large, medium
9. 5, 20
10. myopathy
11. **Suggested Answer:** Answers should include two of the following drugs and their effects:

Oral anticoagulants, coumarins, indanediones: decrease absorption of oral anticoagulants and vitamin K.

Digitalis glycosides, especially digitoxin: half-life of digitalis glycosides and GI absorption may be reduced.

Thiazide diuretics (oral), oral propranolol, oral penicillin G, oral tetracyclines, oral vancomycin: decreased absorption of these medications has been reported.

Thyroid hormones: decreased absorption of thyroid products is reported.

12. **Suggested Answer:** Before initiating clofibrate therapy, advise client to adhere to diet prescribed by physician. Encourage weight reduction and physical exercise. Warn client that a paradoxical rise may occur in 2 or 3 months, but afterward a further decrease is customary. Instruct client to keep clinical appointments. If serum cholesterol and triglyceride levels are not lowered within 3 months, drug therapy is usually discontinued. Advise client to report flu-like symptoms. Instruct individual to check with physician about alcohol intake because its use may be restricted to prevent hypertriglyceridemia.

13. **Suggested Answer:** flatulence, stomach pain, nausea, diarrhea or constipation, headaches

14. **Answer:** 1

Rationale: Most of the HMG-CoA reductase inhibitors such as lovastatin are metabolized by cytochrome P450 3A4 and interact with a number of drugs and foods, including cyclosporine (Neoral, Sandimmune), grapefruit juice, and azole antifungals.

Cognitive Level: Application

Nursing Process Step: Implementation

NCLEX: Physiological Integrity: Pharmacological and Parenteral Therapies

15. **Answer:** 3

Rationale: Liver enzymes should be checked to be sure there is no liver function impairment because active hepatic disease is a contraindication for HMG-CoA reductase inhibitors.

Cognitive Level: Application

Nursing Process Step: Assessment

NCLEX: Physiological Integrity: Pharmacological and Parenteral Therapies

16. **Answer:** 2

Rationale: Niacin is the only B-complex vitamin that is known to have a lipid lowering effect.

Cognitive Level: Application

Nursing Process Step: Implementation

NCLEX: Physiological Integrity: Pharmacological and Parenteral Therapies

17. **Answer:** 4

Rationale: The more common adverse effects of the bile acid sequestering agents include constipation, indigestion, abdominal pain, nausea and vomiting, gas, dizziness, and headache.

Cognitive Level: Application

Nursing Process Step: Assessment

NCLEX: Physiological Integrity: Pharmacological and Parenteral Therapies

18. **Answer:** 1

Rationale: The most obvious adverse effect of niacin is increased feelings of warmth, flushing or red skin on the face and neck. This flushing is common and can be minimized by initiating with very low doses of niacin and slowly increasing doses over the first few weeks or months of therapy.

Cognitive Level: Application

Nursing Process Step: Implementation

NCLEX: Physiological Integrity: Pharmacological and Parenteral Therapies

19. **Answer:** 4

Rationale: Because resins interfere with the absorption of other drugs when taken concurrently, the nurse should administer other drugs 1 hour before or 4 to 6 hours after cholestyramine or colestipol.

Cognitive Level: Application

Nursing Process Step: Planning

NCLEX: Physiological Integrity: Pharmacological and Parenteral Therapies

20. **Answer:** 2

Rationale: Fenofibrate is similar to clofibrate and gemfibrozil. Although its exact mechanism of action is unknown, the active metabolite fenofibric acid is believed to lower triglyceride levels by inhibiting triglyceride synthesis and stimulating the breakdown of triglyceride-rich lipoproteins (VLDL).

Cognitive Level: Analysis

Nursing Process Step: Analysis

NCLEX: Physiological Integrity: Pharmacological and Parenteral Therapies

CHAPTER 32

Overview of the Urinary System

1. a, a, a, e, b, b, c, d, a
2. kidneys, ureters, bladder, urethra
3. homeostasis
4. Glomerular filtration
5. nitrogenous
6. decreased, concentrated
7. hydrogen, ammonia
8. erythropoietin
9. 8, 20
10. urinalysis
11. Creatinine clearance
12. Culture

CHAPTER 33

Diuretics

1. c, a, b, b, a, c
2. hypertension; cirrhosis; nephrotic syndrome; heart failure; electrolyte
3. diuresis, urination
4. Thiazide
5. loop of Henle, loop
6. Osmotic
7. Potassium-sparing
8. carbonic anhydrase, glaucoma, seizures
9. sodium, water
10. ototoxicity

11. **Suggested Answer:** Clients who have renal insufficiency, a history of hyperkalemia, or who are on angiotensin-converting enzyme (ACE) inhibitors, angiotensin receptor blockers (ARBs), potassium sparing diuretics, or potassium supplements should not routinely be encouraged to increase dietary potassium intake because they may be predisposed to hyperkalemia.

12. **Suggested Answer:** Dehydration may be manifested by postural hypotension, confusion, or difficulty in ambulation.

13. **Suggested Answer:** While receiving diuretic therapy, the client will:
    - Regain fluid and electrolyte balance.
    - Remain free of injury related to the effects of diuretic therapy.
    - Effectively manage the diuretic therapy regimen.

14. **Answer:** 2
    Rationale: Mannitol is an osmotic diuretic that is used to manage cerebral edema, which can occur with increased intracranial pressure. It is not used to manage glaucoma, acute renal failure, or renal insufficiency.
    Cognitive Level: Analysis
    Nursing Process Step: Analysis
    NCLEX: Physiological Integrity: Pharmacological and Parenteral Therapies

15. **Answer:** 4
    Rationale: Daily weight (and intake and output) are direct reliable indicators of fluid balance. The other measures are less reliable because they change either more indirectly or more slowly, if at all, with fluid changes in the body
    Cognitive Level: Application
    Nursing Process Step: Assessment
    NCLEX: Physiological Integrity: Pharmacological and Parenteral Therapies

16. **Answer:** 1
    Rationale: A baked potato with skin has approximately 844 mg of potassium. Lima beans have 370 mg per half cup serving; orange juice has 248 mg per half cup serving, and a raw tomato has about 273 mg of potassium.
    Cognitive Level: Application
    Nursing Process Step: Implementation
    NCLEX: Physiological Integrity: Pharmacological and Parenteral Therapies

17. **Answer:** 4
    Rationale: The client should take the medication on arising in the morning so that the diuretic effect is lessened when the client goes to bed at night, and thus reduces the risk of nocturia. The word "best" in the question indicates that one time is preferred over the others, such as mid-morning. Both late afternoon and bedtime dosing increase the risk of nocturia.
    Cognitive Level: Application
    Nursing Process Step: Implementation
    NCLEX: Physiological Integrity: Pharmacological and Parenteral Therapies

18. **Answer:** 3
    Rationale: Spironolactone (Aldactone) is a potassium-sparing diuretic and thus the client should avoid using salt substitutes, which are high in potassium. Options

1 and 2 are loop diuretics, which cause potassium loss, and option 4 is a thiazide diuretic, which also causes potassium loss.
Cognitive Level: Application
Nursing Process Step: Implementation
NCLEX: Physiological Integrity: Pharmacological and Parenteral Therapies

19. **Answer:** 4
    Rationale: HCTZ is a potassium-wasting diuretic and the nurse is alert for hypokalemia as an adverse drug effect. Because the normal potassium level is 3.5-5.1 mEq/L, the nurse would report the low level of 3.2 mEq/L.
    Cognitive Level: Analysis
    Nursing Process Step: Evaluation
    NCLEX: Physiological Integrity: Pharmacological and Parenteral Therapies

20. **Answer:** 2
    Rationale: The client should self-weigh daily on arising on the same scale in similar clothing and report any overnight 2 pound increase to the prescriber.
    Cognitive Level: Application
    Nursing Process Step: Implementation
    NCLEX: Physiological Integrity: Pharmacological and Parenteral Therapies

CHAPTER 34

Uricosuric Drugs

1. d, c, a, e, b
2. metabolic; acute pain; swelling; tenderness
3. hyperuricemia; uric acid
4. deposits of uric acid or urates which form in cartilage
5. hypoxanthine, xanthine, xanthine, uric acid
6. uric acid
7. phagocytosis, leukocytes
8. aspirin
9. alopecia
10. prevent, relieve

11. **Suggested Answer:** To end the acute gouty attack as soon as possible; to prevent recurrence of acute gouty arthritis; to prevent formation of uric acid stones in the kidneys; to reduce or prevent disease complications that result from sodium urate deposits in joints and kidneys.

12. **Suggested Answer:** It inhibits secretion of weak organic acids at both the proximal and the distal renal tubules in the kidneys.

13. **Suggested Answer:** You should have designed a sheet or card, using the drug interactions in the probenecid monograph in the textbook, rewording and simplifying the information in lay-person's terms.

14. **Answer:** 4

Rationale: The peak effect of colchicine for relief of pain and inflammation is reached in 1 to 2 days, but the reduction of swelling may require 3 days or more.

Cognitive Level: Application

Nursing Process Step: Planning

NCLEX: Physiological Integrity: Pharmacological and Parenteral Therapies

15. **Answer:** 3

Rationale: When prescribed for acute gout, colchicine is discontinued as soon as the pain of the acute episode is relieved, the maximum dose is reached, or diarrhea, nausea, vomiting, or stomach pain occur. The other options are not indicators for stopping colchicine therapy.

Cognitive Level: Application

Nursing Process Step: Implementation

NCLEX: Physiological Integrity: Pharmacological and Parenteral Therapies

16. **Answer:** 3

Rationale: The reduction of uric acid to a normal range occurs in 1 to 3 weeks, whereas a decrease in the frequency of acute gout attacks may require several months of drug therapy. To ensure that the client's uric acid level has been affected by the drug, the nurse should schedule the client for a lab draw in 3 weeks; the 1-week time frame may be too narrow and the others are too early or late.

Cognitive Level: Application

Nursing Process Step: Planning

NCLEX: Physiological Integrity: Pharmacological and Parenteral Therapies

17. **Answer:** 1

Rationale: A high fluid intake (80 to 96 ounces daily to produce 2 L of urine) and alkalinization of the urine are necessary to lessen the risk of stone formation and sludging of the tubules with urates. Allopurinol should be administered with food to minimize GI distress. Increased intake of B vitamins is unnecessary.

Cognitive Level: Application

Nursing Process Step: Implementation

NCLEX: Physiological Integrity: Pharmacological and Parenteral Therapies

18. **Answer:** 4

Rationale: Probenecid lowers serum levels of uric acid by competitively inhibiting the reabsorption of urate at the proximal renal tubule, thus increasing the urinary excretion of uric acid. It has no antiinflammatory action or analgesic effects, and does not decrease the production of uric acid.

Cognitive Level: Application

Nursing Process Step: Analysis

NCLEX: Physiological Integrity: Pharmacological and Parenteral Therapies

19. **Answer:** 3

Rationale: Probenecid is contraindicated for clients who are at increased risk of uric acid renal calculi formation or urate nephropathy, such as clients undergoing cancer chemotherapy or radiation therapy or those with moderate to severe renal function impairment. Its use is carefully considered in clients with blood dyscrasias, a history of uric acid kidney stones, or mild renal function impairment, because these conditions may be exacerbated. There is no risk related to chronic obstructive pulmonary disease.

Cognitive Level: Analysis

Nursing Process Step: Analysis

NCLEX: Physiological Integrity: Pharmacological and Parenteral Therapies

20. **Answer:** 2

Rationale: Sulfinpyrazone is excreted by the kidneys, so the nurse should be most careful in monitoring the client with a history of renal insufficiency.

Cognitive Level: Analysis

Nursing Process Step: Analysis

NCLEX: Physiological Integrity: Pharmacological and Parenteral Therapies

Drug Therapy for Renal System Dysfunction

1.

```
A C K S D A X E D Q Q Q R Y Y
S N O I T N E V R E T N I A E
T N W S D T E X Q F H G H H A
O G S Y A N Q J W K G K R P P
R X H L L A E N O T I R E P A
D Q L A N E R Y U K E W T L C
L G N I S R U N G K W B M N U
X R Z D A B K Q N L I F C T X
H Z X O E J R W Z T C I E E J
H N B M U A B F A I L U R E F
H B E E L U C H R O N I C L D
C D S H N M A U D E V D U H C
T R G A E A Z O T E M I A T R
B N X C M S S D P E D A W V E
F A K C P I R O B U B G M S A
O P N X N L E D Y P Y N X G T
Y X B G E T Y Q R D P O G Q I
G S Q V I H R O D U D S R Z N
V M C N D T T V N U G I O A I
V G F R A R E Z D C O S T U N
U X Q N O I T A U L A V E S E
```

2. decline; 5
3. irreversible
4. urea in the blood
5. hemodialysis; peritoneal dialysis; organ transplantation
6. electrolytes; wastes; osmosis; diffusion; filtration
7. creatinine, blood urea nitrogen
8. Hemodialysis, diffusion, ultrafiltration
9. 0.5, 1.2, 5, 20
10. unchanged, metabolites

11. **Suggested Answer:** Most common: increasing weakness, fatigue, lethargy. GI signs: anorexia, GI distress, nausea, vomiting, thirst, weight loss. Paresthesias, peripheral neuropathy, seizures, and neuromuscular irritability may also occur. On examination, the client may appear pale and dehydrated and have an increased respiratory rate and uremic breath. Hypertension with retinopathy, cardiac hypertrophy, pulmonary edema, or pericarditis may often be present.

12. **Suggested Answer:** The nurse would use layman's terms to tell the client the following information: Epoetin alfa is a glycoprotein chemically identical to human erythropoietin. It is indicated for treatment of

anemia associated with renal failure and severe anemia associated with AIDS. Epoetin alfa has the same biologic action as the endogenous hormone; it stimulates erythropoiesis in the bone marrow and also induces the release of reticulocytes from bone marrow. Because endogenous erythropoietin is manufactured mainly in the kidneys, anemia resulting from chronic renal failure is caused by inadequate production of the hormone.

13. **Suggested Answer:** Drug dosage may be decreased (dosage reduction method) while maintaining the usual interval, or if the dosage is the usually prescribed dose, the interval between doses is lengthened (interval extension method). Usually the dosage reduction method is preferred for drugs that require a constant blood therapeutic level.

14. **Answer:** 4
Rationale: Nephrotoxic agents such as aminoglycoside antibiotics (tobramycin, gentamicin) are toxic to the renal tubule, leading to a condition known as acute tubular necrosis or ATN. The other types of antibiotics do not share this grave concern, although doses may be reduced as needed with renal disease based on individual client needs.
Cognitive Level: Analysis
Nursing Process Step: Implementation
NCLEX: Physiological Integrity: Pharmacological and Parenteral Therapies

15. **Answer:** 2
Rationale: The goal of therapy with calcium acetate is to maintain serum phosphate concentrations below 6 mg/dL without precipitating severe hypercalcemia.
Cognitive Level: Analysis
Nursing Process Step: Evaluation
NCLEX: Physiological Integrity: Pharmacological and Parenteral Therapies

16. **Answer:** 1
Rationale: The most common adverse effect of calcium acetate is constipation. This can be prevented by eating foods acceptable on the renal diet that are high in fiber and by increasing activity as tolerated. Fluids cannot be encouraged because they are commonly restricted in renal failure (option 2). Reducing intake of milk and milk products may help control calcium levels but are unrelated to constipation. Nighttime driving is unrelated to the question.
Cognitive Level: Analysis
Nursing Process Step: Implementation
NCLEX: Physiological Integrity: Pharmacological and Parenteral Therapies

17. **Answer:** 3
Rationale: Sevelamer is a polymer that binds phosphate in the GI tract. It results in decreased absorption of dietary phosphate. Sevelamer is recommended for clients with elevated calcium and phosphate levels. In such circumstances, its use avoids hypercalcemia

associated with calcium salts, and reduces the potential for calcium phosphate deposits in tissue.
Cognitive Level: Analysis
Nursing Process Step: Analysis
NCLEX: Physiological Integrity: Pharmacological and Parenteral Therapies

18. **Answer:** 4
Rationale: The blood pressure should be monitored for hypertension because the resultant increase in hematocrit from epoetin increases blood viscosity and peripheral vascular resistance, leading to a rise in blood pressure.
Cognitive Level: Application
Nursing Process Step: Implementation
NCLEX: Physiological Integrity: Pharmacological and Parenteral Therapies

19. **Answer:** 3
Rationale: Epoetin is administered IV or subcutaneously; often it is given IV because there is IV access with hemodialysis. Each single-dose vial of epoetin should be used to administer one dose only because the injection contains no preservative. Unused portions of the drug should be discarded. The nurse should not shake the vial; shaking may denature the substance and render it biologically inactive. The nurse should not mix epoetin with other medications.
Cognitive Level: Application
Nursing Process Step: Implementation
NCLEX: Physiological Integrity: Pharmacological and Parenteral Therapies

20. **Answer:** 1
Rationale: The nurse should perform neurologic assessments periodically for premonitory signs of the risk of seizures, particularly during the first 90 days of therapy and at times when the hematocrit rises rapidly. The other assessments are more routine in nature.
Cognitive Level: Analysis
Nursing Process Step: Planning
NCLEX: Physiological Integrity: Pharmacological and Parenteral Therapies

CHAPTER 36

Overview of the Respiratory System

1. d, f, e, c, a, b
2. Respiration
3. oxygen
4. mucociliary blanket
5. 100
6. bronchoconstriction
7. epinephrine
8. phosphodiesterase
9. rhythmicity, fourth ventricle
10. oxygen, carbon dioxide, hydrogen ions
11. carbon dioxide
12. bicarbonate, carbon dioxide or carbonic acid

Bronchodilator, Antiasthmatic, and Mucolytic Drugs

1. h, g, d, a, b, e, c, f
2. contraction, edema, inflammation, hypersecretion
3. one, two, one, two
4. caffeine, theophylline, theobromine
5. degranulation, histamine, bronchoconstriction
6. chronic pulmonary diseases
7. methylxanthines
8. theophylline
9. antiinflammatory
10. inhalation

11. **Suggested Answer:** Bronchodilation and pulmonary decongestion; loosening of secretions; topical applications of steroids; moistening, cooling, or heating of inspired air

12. **Suggested Answer:** Start within 10 to 12 hours after ingestion of overdose for most benefit, but it is still beneficial if started within the first 24 hours. Support client through gastric lavage, induced emesis, or other appropriate therapies. Monitor liver function studies and plasma acetaminophen concentrations for potential hepatotoxicity. Monitor the client with knowledge deficit or a high risk for self-harm.

13. **Suggested Answer:**
    (1) Fully insert canister into shell, remove cap, and shake.
    (2) Exhale fully.
    (3) Place mouthpiece over the tongue in the mouth. Close lips tightly and press top of canister firmly, simultaneously inhaling deeply through the mouth (with some models, mouthpiece should be held 1 or 2 inches from open mouth).
    (4) Hold breath and inhale as long as possible.
    (5) Release pressure, remove inhaler, and breathe slowly. Wait 1 full minute before administering second puff. Repeat steps.

14. **Answer:** 2
Rationale: Concurrent use of drugs with cardiac stimulant properties (e.g., sympathomimetics-options 1 and 4, MAO inhibitors-option 3, tricyclic antidepressants) may increase the potential for tachycardia or dysrhythmias. α-adrenergic blockers (e.g., propranolol) will blunt the effect of albuterol.
Cognitive Level: Analysis
Nursing Process Step: Analysis
NCLEX: Physiological Integrity: Pharmacological and Parenteral Therapies

15. **Answer:** 4
Rationale: Inhaled albuterol has an onset of action between 5 and 15 minutes, a peak effect in 1 to 1.5 hours after two inhalations, and a duration of action of 3 to 6 hours.
Cognitive Level: Application

Nursing Process Step: Implementation
NCLEX: Physiological Integrity: Pharmacological and Parenteral Therapies

16. **Answer:** 1
Rationale: Ipratropium is indicated for maintenance therapy (not for acute episodes) in clients with COPD (chronic bronchitis or emphysema). It is not utilized at all for acetaminophen overdose; acetylcysteine is the drug for this purpose.
Cognitive Level: Application
Nursing Process Step: Analysis
NCLEX: Physiological Integrity: Pharmacological and Parenteral Therapies

17. **Answer:** 3
Rationale: Inhaled corticosteroids such as Fluticasone (Flovent) can increase the risk of oral/pharyngeal candidiasis. Typical instructions are to have the client rinse the mouth after use to reduce this risk. The other medications listed are bronchodilators and do not carry the risk of candidiasis.
Cognitive Level: Application
Nursing Process Step: Implementation
NCLEX: Physiological Integrity: Pharmacological and Parenteral Therapies

18. **Answer:** 2
Rationale: The therapeutic serum levels for bronchodilator effects with theophylline are usually between 10 and 20 mg/L. Because there can be some variation shown in research results, the nurse should always monitor the client's clinical response.
Cognitive Level: Analysis
Nursing Process Step: Evaluation
NCLEX: Physiological Integrity: Pharmacological and Parenteral Therapies

19. **Answer:** 4
Rationale: Recombinant human DNase or dornase alfa (Pulmozyme) is used to increase expectoration in cystic fibrosis. Cystic fibrosis is a respiratory disease associated with thick secretions caused by an accumulation of DNA from degenerating neutrophils and inflammation. Asthma, emphysema, and chronic bronchitis are other respiratory conditions commonly managed by bronchodilators, corticosteroids, and other antiinflammatory medications.
Cognitive Level: Comprehension
Nursing Process Step: Analysis
NCLEX: Physiological Integrity: Pharmacological and Parenteral Therapies

20. **Answer:** 2
Rationale: Clients with asthma often have multiple inhalers prescribed, such as ipratropium (Atrovent), an anticholinergic; beclomethasone (Vanceril), a corticosteroid; and albuterol (Ventolin), a β$_2$ agonist. If the prescriber has not given specific dosing instructions, generally the order of administration to obtain optimal drug effects is as follows:

- The β agonist is used first to open the airways.
- The anticholinergic agent is administered.
- The corticosteroid is administered.

Cognitive Level: Application
Nursing Process Step: Implementation
NCLEX: Physiological Integrity: Pharmacological and Parenteral Therapies

CHAPTER 38

Oxygen and Miscellaneous Respiratory Agents

1. d, e, b, f, a, c
2. arterial blood oxygen saturation
3. hypoxia; brain
4. COPD; hypercapnia
5. increased respiratory rate; oxygen therapy
6. colorless; odorless; tasteless; life
7. colorless; odorless; respiration; circulation; central nervous system
8. opioid, depressant
9. sodium reabsorption
10. inflammatory, alveolocapillary

11. **Suggested Answer:** Nasal catheter; nasal cannula; oxygen mask; simple face mask; partial rebreathing mask; nonrebreathing mask; Ventimask

12. **Suggested Answer:** Advise client to: maintain dental hygiene and checkups; ease dry mouth with ice, sugarless gum, or hard candy; use caution driving or operating hazardous equipment; report symptoms of blood dyscrasias; avoid ingestion of alcohol or CNS depressants. As prophylaxis for motion sickness, the drug must be taken 30 minutes to 1 or 2 hours before effect is needed. These drugs interfere with allergy skin tests.

13. **Suggested Answer:** The intermittent use of hyperbaric oxygen is controversial in the treatment of infections caused by *Clostridium perfringens, C. septicum,* or *C. histolyticum*—anaerobic bacilli that produce gas gangrene. It is believed that increased oxygen pressure in the tissue may exert an inhibitory effect on the enzyme systems of these bacteria. Hyperbaric oxygen has also been used in certain circulatory disturbances, such as air or gas embolism, decompression sickness, carbon monoxide and cyanide poisoning, and exceptional blood loss. It has also been used in certain local circulatory disturbances such as necrotizing soft-tissue infections; acute traumatic ischemia, crush injury, and compartment syndrome; compromised (ischemic) grafts and flaps; radiation necrosis; refractory osteomyelitis; and enhancement of healing in selected problem wounds.

14. **Answer:** 3
Rationale: A nonrebreathing mask is designed to fit tightly over the face and is usually made of rubber with a reservoir bag and a nonrebreathing valve. On inhalation, oxygen flows into the bag and mask, and the one-way valve prevents exhaled air from flowing back into the bag. The expired air instead escapes through the one-way flap valve in the mask. The concentration of oxygen is 80% to 100%, and the flow is adjusted to keep the reservoir bag fully inflated. This type of mask is used for short-term therapy, such as counteracting smoke inhalation.
Cognitive Level: Application
Nursing Process Step: Planning
NCLEX: Physiological Integrity: Pharmacological and Parenteral Therapies

15. **Answer:** 4
Rationale: Nurses caring for premature infants in incubators must be constantly aware of the danger of retrolental fibroplasia (retinopathy of prematurity). This is a vascular proliferative disease of the retina that occurs in some premature infants who have received high concentrations of oxygen at birth.
Cognitive Level: Application
Nursing Process Step: Implementation
NCLEX: Physiological Integrity: Pharmacological and Parenteral Therapies

16. **Answer:** 1
Rationale: The expected outcome of oxygen therapy is that the client will have adequate gas exchange as evidenced by a respiratory rate of 12 to 20 breaths/min or a rate in keeping with the client's baseline and blood gas values: Pao_2 greater than 60 mm Hg, $Paco_2$ 35 to 45 mm Hg, and pH 7.35 to 7.45.
Cognitive Level: Analysis
Nursing Process Step: Evaluation
NCLEX: Physiological Integrity: Pharmacological and Parenteral Therapies

17. **Answer:** 2
Rationale: The client or caregiver should check the system daily, including proper function of the equipment, prescribed flow rates, remaining liquid or compressed gas content, and backup supply to meet the client's needs. The supplier's name and phone number need to be in a handy place for reordering or in case of emergency. To avoid fire hazards, the client and family should not smoke or use an open flame in the room where and when the oxygen is on. Electrical appliances, such as razors and electric blankets, should not be used in the vicinity of the administration of the oxygen. No oil (Vaseline, hair oils, body oils), wool blankets, or flammable liquids (alcohol) should be used in the area. "No smoking" signs should be posted as reminders. The local fire department should be alerted to the presence of oxygen tanks in the house.
Cognitive Level: Application
Nursing Process Step: Implementation
NCLEX: Physiological Integrity: Pharmacological and Parenteral Therapies

18. Answer: 3

Rationale: Benzonatate is indicated for the symptomatic treatment of a nonproductive cough. The other options listed are not indications for use of this drug.

Cognitive Level: Application

Nursing Process Step: Evaluation

NCLEX: Physiological Integrity: Pharmacological and Parenteral Therapies

19. Answer: 4

Rationale: The *most common* adverse effects with diphenhydramine include sedation and antimuscarinic effects, including dry mouth, urinary retention, and constipation. Other effects include increased appetite, diarrhea, blurred vision, and thickened bronchial secretions.

Cognitive Level: Application

Nursing Process Step: Implementation

NCLEX: Physiological Integrity: Pharmacological and Parenteral Therapies

20. Answer: 1

Rationale: The client should blow the nose before delivering the spray and aim spray away from nasal septum (aim for inner corner of the eye). If the client experiences blocked nasal passages, he/she may use a topical decongestant just prior to the nasal corticosteroid, but because of congestive rebound they should only be used for 3 to 5 days. It may be 3 weeks before experiencing optimal benefits. Clients should also avoid immunizations while taking nasal corticosteroids because of a lack of immunologic response or possible neurologic hazard.

Cognitive Level: Application

Nursing Process Step: Implementation

NCLEX: Physiological Integrity: Pharmacological and Parenteral Therapies

CHAPTER 39

Overview of the Gastrointestinal Tract

1. a, c, b, f, d, h, e, c, e, g, d, e
2. mechanical; chemical; digestion
3. swallowing
4. dysphagia
5. food bolus; GI tract; band contraction
6. inflammation; gallstones
7. mouth; anus
8. muscular, glandular
9. Systemic, nutritional, mechanical
10. retrosternal pain, heartburn, swallowing
11. food, 2 to 6
12. cytochrome P450

CHAPTER 40

Drugs Affecting the Gastrointestinal Tract

1. c and b, d, a, a, b
2. topical, systemically
3. antimuscarinic (anticholinergic)
4. lower esophageal sphincter (LES)
5. proton pump
6. hydrochloric acid, increase
7. peptic, antibacterials, proton pump inhibitors
8. diarrhea, constipation
9. nonsteroidal antiinflammatory drugs
10. amylase, trypsin, lipase, cystic fibrosis, chronic pancreatitis

11. **Suggested Answer:** Store out of reach in a safe area, preferably a locked cabinet. Use of mouthwash by children is not recommended because children often swallow the mouthwash rather than expectorate it.

12. **Suggested Answer:** Administer oral form 30 minutes before meals and at bedtime; administer IV injections slowly over 1 to 2 minutes; infusions should not be for a period of less than 15 minutes. Keep solutions of parenteral dosage for 48 hours after dilution; protect from light; discard unused portions after 48 hours. Do not give in combination with drugs having extrapyramidal side effects. Extrapyramidal side effects may be seen at therapeutic doses and are more likely to occur in children and young adults.

13. **Suggested Answer:** Diarrhea, headache

14. **Answer:** 1

Rationale: The nurse should administer antacids 1 hour before or 2 hours after other drugs, such as digoxin, tetracyclines, phenothiazines, and all enteric-coated medications. For a client receiving an antacid dose at 09:00, the digoxin should be either at 08:00 or anytime from 11:00 on during the day.

Cognitive Level: Application

Nursing Process Step: Planning

NCLEX: Physiological Integrity: Pharmacological and Parenteral Therapies

15. **Answer:** 2

Rationale: The adult dosage of sucralfate for the treatment of a duodenal ulcer is 1 g four times daily, 1 hour before each meal and at bedtime. Thus the doses would be scheduled around the meal delivery schedule for the nursing unit ideally.

Cognitive Level: Application

Nursing Process Step: Planning

NCLEX: Physiological Integrity: Pharmacological and Parenteral Therapies

16. Answer: 3

Rationale: Scopolamine transdermal is recommended for use in adults only. In the United States, the product is a four-layered film that releases 0.5 mg of scopolamine over a 3-day period. It is applied on the skin behind the ear, usually 4 hours before the antiemetic effect is desired.

Cognitive Level: Application

Nursing Process Step: Implementation

NCLEX: Physiological Integrity: Pharmacological and Parenteral Therapies

17. Answer: 4

Rationale: Ursodiol is used to treat (dissolve) gallstones in selected clients. As such, the client should experience decreased or absence of biliary colic and abdominal discomfort. It is not used to treat GERD, diarrhea, or nausea and vomiting.

Cognitive Level: Application

Nursing Process Step: Planning

NCLEX: Physiological Integrity: Pharmacological and Parenteral Therapies

18. Answer: 1

Rationale: With sulfasalazine, there are related drugs that have cross-sensitivity, such as sulfonamides, furosemide, thiazide diuretics, sulfonylureas, or carbonic anhydrase inhibitors. The nurse should assess the client for allergy to any of these, which could increase the risk of hypersensitivity to sulfasalazine.

Cognitive Level: Application

Nursing Process Step: Implementation

NCLEX: Physiological Integrity: Pharmacological and Parenteral Therapies

19. Answer: 2

Rationale: Antidiarrheal products have a warning stating that they are not to be used for longer than 2 days, not to be used if a fever is present, and not to be used in infants or children under 3 years of age. For adults and children 12 years of age and older, the dosage of Lomotil is 1 to 2 tablets PO three or four times daily. The prescriber may modify these instructions.

Cognitive Level: Analysis

Nursing Process Step: Evaluation

NCLEX: Physiological Integrity: Pharmacological and Parenteral Therapies

20. Answer: 1

Rationale: Cimetidine is associated with stronger antimuscarinic properties than the other H_2 blockers. Properties include constipation, confusion and dry mouth, which are more problematic in older clients with renal insufficiency. For this reason, the client will probably benefit more from a drug that has fewer of these effects.

Cognitive Level: Analysis

Nursing Process Step: Analysis

NCLEX: Physiological Integrity: Pharmacological and Parenteral Therapies

CHAPTER 41

Overview of the Eye

1. e, c, a, f, b, d
2. receptor; vision
3. anterior; transparent; light
4. constriction; miosis
5. dilation; mydriasis
6. shape; in sharp focus
7. transparency; opaque; cataract
8. Parasympathetic
9. canals, Schlemm
10. rods, cones
11. Blinking
12. lacrimal canaliculi

CHAPTER 42

Ophthalmic Drugs

1. d, a, e, b, c
2. abnormally elevated intraocular pressure (IOP); irreversible blindness
3. glaucoma; accommodative esotropia (crossed eyes)
4. enzymatic destruction of acetylcholine; inactivating cholinesterase
5. primary, secondary, congenital
6. solution, ointment
7. Contact lenses
8. cross-contamination
9. 30, 60, inner canthus
10. intraocular pressure, aqueous humor

11. **Suggested Answer:** Deficient knowledge deficit related to new ophthalmic drug regimen; anxiety related to possible decrease in or loss of vision; altered comfort related to ophthalmic disorder; risk for injury related to impaired vision

12. **Suggested Answer:** The procedure is the same except that the ointment is expressed directly into the exposed conjunctival sac from the inner to outer canthus with a small individual tube. Have the client close his or her eye; gently massage the eye to distribute the medication.

13. **Suggested Answer:** Bradycardia, syncope, low blood pressure, asthmatic attack, heart failure, hallucinations, loss of appetite, headaches, nausea, weakness, depression

14. **Answer:** 3

Rationale: Once opened, most eye medications have a limited life (3 months or the end of the current illness). If stored longer, the medication is more likely to become contaminated and lead to an infection of the eye.

Cognitive Level: Application

Nursing Process Step: Evaluation

NCLEX: Physiological Integrity: Pharmacological and Parenteral Therapies

15. **Answer:** 4

Rationale: Allergic reactions, burning on instillation, and conjunctivitis are the most common adverse effects. A small risk for Stevens-Johnson syndrome is possible, particularly in clients who are immunocompromised.

Cognitive Level: Application
Nursing Process Step: Assessment
NCLEX: Physiological Integrity: Pharmacological and Parenteral Therapies

16. **Answer:** 3

Rationale: Ophthalmic corticosteroids are indicated for the treatment of allergic and inflammatory ophthalmic disorders of the conjunctiva, cornea, and anterior segment of the eye. Although these drugs will reduce inflammation, they can also increase the risk for infection.

They are not used for pyogenic (pus-producing) inflammations of the eye because corticosteroids decrease defense mechanisms and reduce resistance to pathogenic organisms. Corticosteroid therapy is not recommended for minor corneal abrasions. Steroids may actually increase ocular susceptibility to fungal, viral, or tuberculosis infection. Cataracts and chronic open-angle glaucoma may be worsened.

Cognitive Level: Application
Nursing Process Step: Analysis
NCLEX: Physiological Integrity: Pharmacological and Parenteral Therapies

17. **Answer:** 1

Rationale: Anticholinesterase drugs inhibit destruction of acetylcholine by activating cholinesterase, promoting pupil constriction (miosis) and ciliary muscle contraction (accommodation). The irreversible anticholinesterase drugs (echothiophate [Phospholine Iodide] and isoflurophate [Floropryl]) form stable complexes with cholinesterase and thus irreversibly impair the destructive function of the enzyme. The cholinesterase inhibitors are usually reserved for clients who respond inadequately to the first-line agents, such as β blockers, cholinergics (pilocarpine), and sympathomimetics (dipivefrin).

Cognitive Level: Analysis
Nursing Process Step: Analysis
NCLEX: Physiological Integrity: Pharmacological and Parenteral Therapies

18. **Answer:** 2

Rationale: Systemic effects can be minimized by applying pressure for 30 seconds to one minute over the inner canthus next to the nose. This prevents systemic absorption through the tear duct.

Cognitive Level: Application
Nursing Process Step: Implementation
NCLEX: Physiological Integrity: Pharmacological and Parenteral Therapies

19. **Answer:** 2

Rationale: Local anesthetics are used to prevent pain during surgical procedures (removal of sutures and foreign bodies) and tonometry examinations. The local anesthetics have a rapid onset (within 20 seconds) and last for 15 to 20 minutes. Classic agents include tetracaine and proparacaine.

Cognitive Level: Application
Nursing Process Step: Implementation
NCLEX: Physiological Integrity: Pharmacological and Parenteral Therapies

20. **Answer:** 3

Rationale: Fluorescein is a nontoxic, water-soluble dye that is used as a diagnostic aid. When applied to the cornea, corneal lesions or ulcers are stained a bright green, and foreign bodies appear to be surrounded by a green ring. Ketotifen and levocabastine are used to treat allergic conjunctivitis, whereas lodoxamide is used to treat conjunctivitis and other eye disorders.

Cognitive Level: Application
Nursing Process Step: Planning
NCLEX: Physiological Integrity: Pharmacological and Parenteral Therapies

CHAPTER 43

Overview of the Ear

1. a, c, b, b, c
2. thin, transparent partition of tissue; auditory canal; middle ear
3. middle ear; nasopharynx; the individual swallows, chews, yawns, or moves the jaw
4. malleus; incus; stapes; sound waves
5. cochlea
6. external, middle, inner
7. tympanic membrane
8. bony labyrinth
9. membranous labyrinth
10. infections, earwax
11. otitis media
12. otosclerosis, Meniere

CHAPTER 44

Drugs Affecting the Ear

1. c, a, b, d
2. topical, external auditory canal
3. swimmer's ear
4. cerumen, tympanic membrane
5. ototoxicity
6. tympanic membrane
7. fluoroquinolone
8. Glycerin, mineral, olive
9. hygiene, health
10. warmed

11. **Suggested Answer:** Burning, redness, rash, swelling, or other signs of topical irritation that were not present before the start of therapy.

12. **Suggested Answer:**
    (1) Assess (a) hearing and symptoms, (b) that ear canal is clear and that tympanic membrane is intact, (c) for improper hygiene or practices.
    (2) Run warm water over bottle or immerse it in warm water.
    (3) Let an irritable child get comfortable. Cleanse any drainage and position affected ear upward.
    (4) In children 3 years or younger, gently pull pinna slightly down and back to instill drops. In older children and adults, hold pinna up and back. Gently massage area immediately anterior to the ear to facilitate entry.
    (5) Instruct client to remain on his or her side for 5 minutes, using a cotton pledget if desired. Alert client to the hazard of temporary impaired hearing related to therapy.

13. **Suggested Answer:** Serum levels of some drugs may be monitored. Monitor client's ability to hear by observing cues and noting client's comments on hearing ability. Report indications of increased hearing loss to the prescriber. When given IV, aminoglycosides should be administered over 30 to 60 minutes to avoid high peak levels. Instruct clients to report tinnitus or any other hearing impairment immediately.

14. **Answer:** 4
Rationale: Hydrocortisone is a corticosteroid that will reduce inflammation and pain that accompanies otitis externa. It does not affect cerumen production or density, or reduce bacteria or hearing loss.
Cognitive Level: Analysis
Nursing Process Step: Evaluation
NCLEX: Physiological Integrity: Pharmacological and Parenteral Therapies

15. **Answer:** 1
Rationale: Tinnitus and hearing loss can occur with damage to the cochlea of the ear from ototoxic drugs. Vertigo and ataxia indicate damage to the vestibular portion of the ear, whereas headache is an unrelated finding.
Cognitive Level: Application
Nursing Process Step: Assessment
NCLEX: Physiological Integrity: Pharmacological and Parenteral Therapies

16. **Answer:** 1
Rationale: The instillation of eardrops requires knowledge of anatomic structure across the life span; the shape of the auditory canal of a young child is different from that of an adult. To instill eardrops in children 3 years of age or younger, gently pull the pinna of the ear slightly down and back. In older children and adults, hold the pinna up and back.
Cognitive Level: Analysis

Nursing Process Step: Evaluation
NCLEX: Physiological Integrity: Pharmacological and Parenteral Therapies

17. **Answer:** 2
Rationale: The client should lie on the side with the affected ear up for 5 minutes after instillation of eardrops. Antibiotics are used as scheduled, not as needed for pain. The client can gently massage the area immediately anterior to the ear before instillation to facilitate entry of eardrops into the auditory canal. The symptoms should not worsen temporarily.
Cognitive Level: Application
Nursing Process Step: Implementation
NCLEX: Physiological Integrity: Pharmacological and Parenteral Therapies

18. **Answer:** 3
Rationale: Carbamide peroxide and glycerin is a formulation used to treat build-up of cerumen or earwax. Options 1 and 2 are used for "swimmer's ear" while option 4 is used as an antiinflammatory and antipruritic.
Cognitive Level: Application
Nursing Process Step: Implementation
NCLEX: Physiological Integrity: Pharmacological and Parenteral Therapies

19. **Answer:** 4
Rationale: The hearing loss induced by ethacrynic acid is often irreversible, whereas the hearing loss induced by the other drugs listed is often reversible.
Cognitive Level: Analysis
Nursing Process Step: Analysis
NCLEX: Physiological Integrity: Pharmacological and Parenteral Therapies

20. **Answer:** 3
Rationale: Aminoglycosides can cause ototoxicity that is both cochlear (with hearing loss) or vestibular (with problems regarding balance). Other antibiotics of concern are clarithromycin, erythromycin, and vancomycin.
Cognitive Level: Application
Nursing Process Step: Analysis
NCLEX: Physiological Integrity: Pharmacological and Parenteral Therapies

CHAPTER 45

Overview of the Endocrine System

1. See Figure 45-1 in the textbook.
2. Hormones
3. steroid, amino acids
4. negative feedback
5. urine, bile
6. receptors, specificity
7. hypothalamus
8. thyroxine (T4), triiodothyronine (T3), and calcitonin
9. iodine
10. calcium

11. glucocorticoids (cortisol), mineralocorticoids (primarily aldosterone), androgens (primarily dehydroepiandrosterone)

12. Insulin

CHAPTER 46

Drugs Affecting the Pituitary

1.

```
E A A N T E R I O R C C J M R I Y I H
L C M B P R W O S A O D P K I X P L U
E T J I U C H O L N D I O U N X I M M
C H S T E S W L F K W A S L S V T E A
T O F T L Y E U J K A B T S I E U R T
R R V N F R S Q U R R E E O P I I T R
O M H P G I U L K I F T R M I X T A O
L O R I O I S C R S I E I A D V A M P
Y N C N F M Z C H J S S O T U R R O E
T E N I R C O D N E M J R O S M Y S F
E B S G I G A N T I S M L S L Z R M X
S N U R S I N G O N A D O T R O P I N
E N I S S E R P O S A V O A C K J M F
K X G R K W U B Y A N X V T H C W Q O
W E X Z U S A T T I E J N I R J M X X
D I C X D S I C G P V Y E N A A X M O
```

2. growth
3. Somatrem and somatropin
4. somatomedin-C, insulin-like
5. growth, thyrotropin, adrenocorticotropin, follicle-stimulating, luteinizing, and prolactin.
6. vasopressin, oxytocin
7. epiphyses, benzyl alcohol
8. growth, glucagon, and insulin
9. water reabsorption, collecting ducts

10. nocturnal enuresis

11. **Suggested Answer:** Most frequent: pain at injection site (usually with tannate dosage form). Less frequent: stomach gas and pain, diarrhea, dizziness, increased pressure for bowel evacuation, nausea, vomiting, tremors, sweating, pallor.

12. **Suggested Answer:** Obtain baseline data from bone age determinations, thyroid function studies, and anti–growth hormone antibody; monitor periodically. Pain and swelling have occurred at the site of injection. After several months of therapy, antibodies to somatrem may be formed in some clients. These rarely reduce the response to therapy. Monitor for signs of hypothyroidism. Dilute for parenteral use with 1 to 5 mL diluent provided. Do not shake vial; rotate gently until clear. Do not use cloudy solution. Store in refrigerator. Advise client to visit endocrinologist regularly.

13. **Suggested Answer:** Hepatitis and AIDS as a result of shared needles and syringes

14. **Answer:** 1
Rationale: Excessive doses may produce gigantism in children, an abnormal condition characterized by excessive size and stature. Rarely, it can lead to hypothyroidism (options 2 and 4). Hypoglycemia can be a long-term effect (option 3).
Cognitive Level: Application
Nursing Process Step: Evaluation
NCLEX: Physiological Integrity: Pharmacological and Parenteral Therapies

15. **Answer:** 2
Rationale: Pegvisomant (Somavert) is an antagonist of growth hormone used on a restricted basis to treat acromegaly. It is not used to treat dwarfism, diabetes insipidus, or syndrome of inappropriate ADH.
Cognitive Level: Application
Nursing Process Step: Assessment
NCLEX: Physiological Integrity: Pharmacological and Parenteral Therapies

16. Answer: 4

Rationale: Norditropin comes in cartridge form for use only in the NordiPen delivery system for easy subcutaneous administration. Refrigerate but protect from freezing.

Optimal dosing is often achieved when the drug is administered at bedtime. Physiologic release is more normally simulated as a result of pituitary release of GH during the first 45 to 90 minutes after the onset of sleep.

Cognitive Level: Application
Nursing Process Step: Implementation
NCLEX: Physiological Integrity: Pharmacological and Parenteral Therapies

17. Answer: 3

Rationale: Vasopressin (Pitressin) is used to treat diabetes insipidus and for treatment of GI hemorrhage, including bleeding esophageal varices. It is also used as part of cardiac resuscitation protocols for cardiac asystole, and may be slightly more effective for this indication compared with epinephrine. It is not used for heart failure or cerebrovascular accident, and could worsen a hypertensive crisis.

Cognitive Level: Application
Nursing Process Step: Analysis
NCLEX: Physiological Integrity: Pharmacological and Parenteral Therapies

18. Answer: 2

Rationale: The client should experience a decreased urinary output, increased urine osmolality and specific gravity, decreased thirst, and resolution of dehydration. Decreased urine specific gravity indicates that drug therapy has not been effective.

Cognitive Level: Application
Nursing Process Step: Evaluation
NCLEX: Physiological Integrity: Pharmacological and Parenteral Therapies

19. Answer: 2

Rationale: With desmopressin therapy, the client or caregiver should be instructed to withhold the medication and report symptoms of water intoxication (e.g., weight gain, headache, confusion, and drowsiness). The other responses do not address this adverse effect.

Cognitive Level: Application
Nursing Process Step: Analysis
NCLEX: Physiological Integrity: Pharmacological and Parenteral Therapies

20. Answer: 3

Rationale: An anticipated effect is reduction in urine output to counteract the effects of diabetes insipidus. The changes in vitals signs or blood glucose are not intended effects of the drug.

Cognitive Level: Analysis
Nursing Process Step: Evaluation
NCLEX: Physiological Integrity: Pharmacological and Parenteral Therapies

CHAPTER 47

Drugs Affecting the Parathyroid and Thyroid Glands

1. a, c, b, a, a, d, b, b, b, c, a
2. primary hyperparathyroidism
3. Levothyroxine (T4)
4. antithyroid; thyroid release from hyperfunctioning thyroid gland
5. hypothyroidism
6. surgical risks, cardiac disease, older adult
7. decreased, increased
8. neoplasms, bone metastasis
9. excretion, resorption
10. antithyroid, radioiodine, surgery

11. **Suggested Answer:** Vitamin D and calcium supplements. Calcitriol is an active metabolite form of vitamin D.

12. **Suggested Answer:** Zoledronic acid (Zometa) is indicated for the treatment of hypercalcemia and bone metastasis of solid tumors.

13. **Suggested Answer:** Instruct client in appropriate methods for disposal of urine and feces. If client is discharged but radiation precautions are still necessary, ensure that the client receives specific instruction. If the client received dosage of ^{131}I for hyperthyroidism or thyroid carcinoma, these 48- to 72-hour precautions may include the following: avoiding close contact with others, especially children; not kissing anyone or sharing others' eating or drinking utensils; washing sink and tub after use; using and washing clothes, towels, and linens separately.

14. Answer: 2

Rationale: The adverse effects of calcitonin as a parenteral dosage form are flushing or a tingling sensation of the face, ears, hands, and feet; gastric distress, anorexia, nausea, and vomiting; and pain or swelling at the injection site. To reduce the nausea or flushing adverse effects, bedtime administration is suggested, or a reduction in dosage may be required. The other actions would be of no benefit.

Cognitive Level: Application
Nursing Process Step: Implementation
NCLEX: Physiological Integrity: Pharmacological and Parenteral Therapies

15. Answer: 4

Rationale: Etidronate (Didronel) is a bisphosphonate. The bisphosphonates are incorporated into bone to inhibit normal and abnormal resorption of bone primarily by decreasing activity of osteoclasts. Among the bisphosphonates, etidronate is unique in also reducing osteoblastic activity as well.

Cognitive Level: Application
Nursing Process Step: Implementation
NCLEX: Physiological Integrity: Pharmacological and Parenteral Therapies

16. **Answer:** 3

Rationale: Alendronate must be administered with water only in the fasting state on arising, and no other food or drink should be administered for at least 30 minutes. Clients must remain in the upright position for at least 30 minutes after dosing to minimize the risk for esophageal ulcers.

Cognitive Level: Application

Nursing Process Step: Evaluation

NCLEX: Physiological Integrity: Pharmacological and Parenteral Therapies

17. **Answer:** 1

Rationale: An overdose of thyroid products results in hyperthyroidism—alterations in appetite and menstrual periods, elevated temperature, diarrhea, hand tremors, increased irritability, leg cramps, increased nervousness, tachycardia, irregular heart rate, increased sensitivity to heat, chest pain, respiratory difficulties, increased sweating, vomiting, weight loss, and insomnia. The general signs of an underdose or hypothyroidism are dysmenorrhea, ataxia, coldness, dry skin, constipation, lethargy, headaches, drowsiness, tiredness, weight gain, and muscle aching.

Cognitive Level: Application

Nursing Process Step: Implementation

NCLEX: Physiological Integrity: Pharmacological and Parenteral Therapies

18. **Answer:** 4

Rationale: Cholestyramine (Questran) or colestipol (Colestid) may bind thyroid hormones, delaying or decreasing their absorption from the GI tract. A 4- to 5-hour interval is recommended between the administrations of these drugs.

Cognitive Level: Application

Nursing Process Step: Planning

NCLEX: Physiological Integrity: Pharmacological and Parenteral Therapies

19. **Answer:** 3

Rationale: To prevent radiation contamination of others/environment, the nurse instructs the client in the need to use disposable utensils and the appropriate methods for disposing of urine and feces (e.g., double-flushing the toilet, washing hands after using the toilet) until radiation precautions are no longer needed. To avoid exposure to the radioactive products of the iodine, the nurse wears rubber gloves when giving ^{131}I to clients and when disposing of their excreta. Disposal meal trays are used to prevent exposure of others to radiation via the standards meal tray. As a general measure, the client needs to increase the fluid intake to 2500 mL daily to enhance excretion of the isotope.

Cognitive Level: Application

Nursing Process Step: Implementation

NCLEX: Physiological Integrity: Pharmacological and Parenteral Therapies

20. **Answer:** 2

Rationale: The adverse effects of the thioamide derivatives include a loss of taste, nausea, vomiting, dizziness, skin rash, fever, and other signs of infection secondary to leukopenia or agranulocytosis.

Cognitive Level: Application

Nursing Process Step: Implementation

NCLEX: Physiological Integrity: Pharmacological and Parenteral Therapies

CHAPTER 48

Drugs Affecting the Adrenal Cortex

1. d, a, f, c, b, e
2. hormones; glucocorticoids; mineralocorticoids
3. dark/light, sleep/wakefulness
4. Cortisol
5. antiinflammatory
6. cholesterol, adrenal cortex
7. corticotropin-releasing, adrenocorticotropic
8. epinephrine, norepinephrine
9. sodium
10. addisonian

11. **Suggested Answer:** Answers should include any three of the following: antiinflammatory action; maintenance of normal blood pressure; carbohydrate and protein metabolism; fat metabolism; thymolytic, lympholytic, and eosinopenic actions; stress effects.

12. **Suggested Answer:**
GI: abdominal pains, black tarry stools (GI bleeding)
Immune: lowers resistance to infections; may also mask symptoms of infections
Musculoskeletal: hip or shoulder pain; muscle cramping or pain; increased weakness; muscle weakness; bone pain

13. **Suggested Answer:** Use antiadrenals cautiously in clients undergoing stress such as surgery, infection, trauma, and acute illness. Do not administer to clients with recent exposure to chickenpox and herpes zoster. Do not give to pregnant women. Older clients may be more sensitive to the drug's CNS effects. Obtain baseline lying and standing blood pressures, serum electrolyte levels, thyroid function studies, and AST (SGOT) concentrations.

14. **Answer:** 3

Rationale: When a shorter-acting agent (e.g., cortisone or hydrocortisone) is used as replacement therapy, the drug should be scheduled according to the normal endogenous secretion of corticosteroid in the body; give two-thirds of the dose in the morning and one-third in the evening.

Cognitive Level: Application

Nursing Process Step: Planning
NCLEX: Physiological Integrity: Pharmacological and Parenteral Therapies

15. **Answer:** 1
Rationale: The adverse effects of the glucocorticoids include euphoria, increased appetite, insomnia, restlessness, anxiety, gas, hyperpigmentation, hypotension, headache, hirsutism, lowered resistance to infections, visual disturbances (cataracts), increased urination or thirst, and decreased growth in children.
Cognitive Level: Application
Nursing Process Step: Assessment
NCLEX: Physiological Integrity: Pharmacological and Parenteral Therapies

16. **Answer:** 2
Rationale: Glucocorticoids may elevate serum glucose levels (both during therapy and after, if the glucocorticoid is stopped). The normal serum glucose level is 7-110 mg/dL. The sodium and potassium levels are at the upper and lower ends or normal, respectively. The elevated BUN (8-22 mg/dL) is not related to the effects of this drug.
Cognitive Level: Analysis
Nursing Process Step: Evaluation
NCLEX: Physiological Integrity: Pharmacological and Parenteral Therapies

17. **Answer:** 3
Rationale: Adverse effects that affect body image include abdominal distention, acneiform eruptions, fat deposits on upper back ("buffalo hump"), fluid retention, hirsutism, hyperpigmentation, loss of muscle mass, lupus erythematosus–like lesions, petechiae and ecchymosis, purpura, round face ("moon face"), striae, thin fragile skin, thinning of extremities, thickening of torso, and weight gain.
Cognitive Level: Application
Nursing Process Step: Implementation
NCLEX: Physiological Integrity: Pharmacological and Parenteral Therapies

18. **Answer:** 3
Rationale: Most clients receiving glucocorticoids should follow a high-potassium, low-sodium diet to counter the potassium-depleting and sodium-retaining effects of the drug. To minimize peptic ulceration, clients should limit intake of alcohol, caffeine, aspirin, and other gastric irritants.
Cognitive Level: Application
Nursing Process Step: Implementation
NCLEX: Physiological Integrity: Pharmacological and Parenteral Therapies

19. **Answer:** 2
Rationale: Aminoglutethimide is indicated for the treatment of Cushing's syndrome associated with adrenal carcinoma, ectopic adrenocorticotropic hormone tumors, or adrenal gland hyperplasia.
Cognitive Level: Application
Nursing Process Step: Analysis

NCLEX: Physiological Integrity: Pharmacological and Parenteral Therapies

20. **Answer:** 1
Rationale: The expected outcome of fludrocortisone therapy is that the client does not show any signs of Addison disease, fluid volume deficit, other signs and symptoms of mineralocorticoid insufficiency, or any adverse effects of fludrocortisone therapy. The client remains compliant with the medication regimen, institutes a low sodium, high potassium diet and states reportable adverse symptoms prescriber.
Cognitive Level: Analysis
Nursing Process Step: Evaluation
NCLEX: Physiological Integrity: Pharmacological and Parenteral Therapies

CHAPTER 49

Drugs Affecting Conditions of the Pancreas

1. b, a, a, b, b, b, a
2. insulin; glucagon
3. glycogenolysis; gluconeogenesis
4. carbohydrate, deficiency, resistance
5. endogenous
6. 40, 90
7. diet, exercise, medication
8. free fatty acids
9. dehydration, electrolyte
10. slow, deep, carbon dioxide

11. **Suggested Answer:** Mark first injection site with spot bandage and give future injections around bandage. Imagine circle as a clock, administering injections at 12, 3, 6, and 9 o'clock points before starting new circle more than an inch away from previous sites. Administer five injections per circle.

12. **Suggested Answer:** Answers should include any of the following: 3 glucose tablets, 4-oz orange juice, 6-oz regular soda, 6- to 8-oz 2% fat or skim milk, 6 to 8 Life-Savers, 3 graham cracker squares, 6 jelly beans, 2 tablespoons raisins, 1 small (2-oz) tube of cake frosting

13. **Suggested Answer:** They enhance the release of insulin from beta cells in the pancreas, decrease liver glycogenolysis and gluconeogenesis, and increase the sensitivity to insulin in body tissues. Therefore they reduce blood glucose concentration in persons with a functioning pancreas.

14. **Answer:** 3
Rationale: Regular insulin is usually given approximately 15 to 30 minutes before meals.
Cognitive Level: Application
Nursing Process Step: Planning
NCLEX: Physiological Integrity: Pharmacological and Parenteral Therapies

319

15. **Answer:** 2

Rationale: Alcohol promotes hypoglycemia and blocks the formation, storage, and release of glycogen. It may also interact with many other drugs, including oral hypoglycemic agents such as chlorpropamide. Cocaine and marijuana may lead to hyperglycemia, whereas morphine has no direct effect on blood glucose.

Cognitive Level: Application

Nursing Process Step: Analysis

NCLEX: Physiological Integrity: Pharmacological and Parenteral Therapies

16. **Answer:** 3

Rationale: When mixing insulins, first inject air (equal to the volume of the dose to be withdrawn) into the vial of NPH insulin, which is cloudy. Then inject air into the vial of the regular insulin. Keep the needle in the vial, and draw the regular insulin into the syringe first to prevent contaminating regular insulin vial with the NPH insulin. Then return to the NPH vial and withdraw the dose of NPH insulin. Vials should be rolled gently in the hands to mix.

Cognitive Level: Application

Nursing Process Step: Implementation

NCLEX: Physiological Integrity: Pharmacological and Parenteral Therapies

17. **Answer:** 1

Rationale: Metformin is contraindicated in clients at risk for renal insufficiency as it may increase the risk for lactic acidosis. The other conditions are not reasons for withholding this type of drug therapy.

Cognitive Level: Analysis

Nursing Process Step: Analysis

NCLEX: Physiological Integrity: Pharmacological and Parenteral Therapies

18. **Answer:** 2

Rationale: The most common adverse effect of the sulfonylureas is hypoglycemia. Others are diarrhea or constipation, dizziness, gas, anorexia, headache, nausea, vomiting, or abdominal distress. Less common adverse effects are photosensitivity or rash. Rare adverse effects, include respiratory difficulties, espe-

cially in persons with cardiac problems and heart failure; sedation; muscle cramping; seizures; edema of the face, hands, or ankles; comatose state, increased weakness (antidiuretic effect); pruritus, jaundice, light-colored stools, dark urine (impairment of liver function); or increased fatigue, sore throat, increased temperature, increased bleeding or bruising (blood dyscrasias).

Cognitive Level: Application

Nursing Process Step: Implementation

NCLEX: Physiological Integrity: Pharmacological and Parenteral Therapies

19. **Answer:** 1

Rationale: The most serious adverse effect of this class of drugs is hepatotoxicity which can potentially be life-threatening. Although rare, hepatotoxicity may occur. Liver function should be monitored for clients receiving drugs in this class. Fluid retention is a troublesome adverse effect of rosiglitazone and may contribute to heart failure in some clients. Headache, muscle and back pain, upper respiratory tract infection, and anemia are also possible.

Cognitive Level: Analysis

Nursing Process Step: Implementation

NCLEX: Physiological Integrity: Pharmacological and Parenteral Therapies

20. **Answer:** 2

Rationale: Instruct the client and family about the symptoms of hypoglycemia and the importance of ingesting some form of sugar when symptoms first occur, such as orange juice, honey, syrup, hard candy, sugar cubes, or milk. If glucagon is necessary, teach the family and the client how to mix the drug and how to inject it properly. A standard insulin syringe may be used for injection unless the dose is greater than the capacity of the syringe. The injection should be made at a 90-degree angle instead of the usual subcutaneous approach. Advise the client and family to keep supplies on hand and check the expiration dates frequently.

Cognitive Level: Application

Nursing Process Step: Implementation

NCLEX: Physiological Integrity: Pharmacological and Parenteral Therapies

Overview of the Male and Female Reproductive Systems

1.

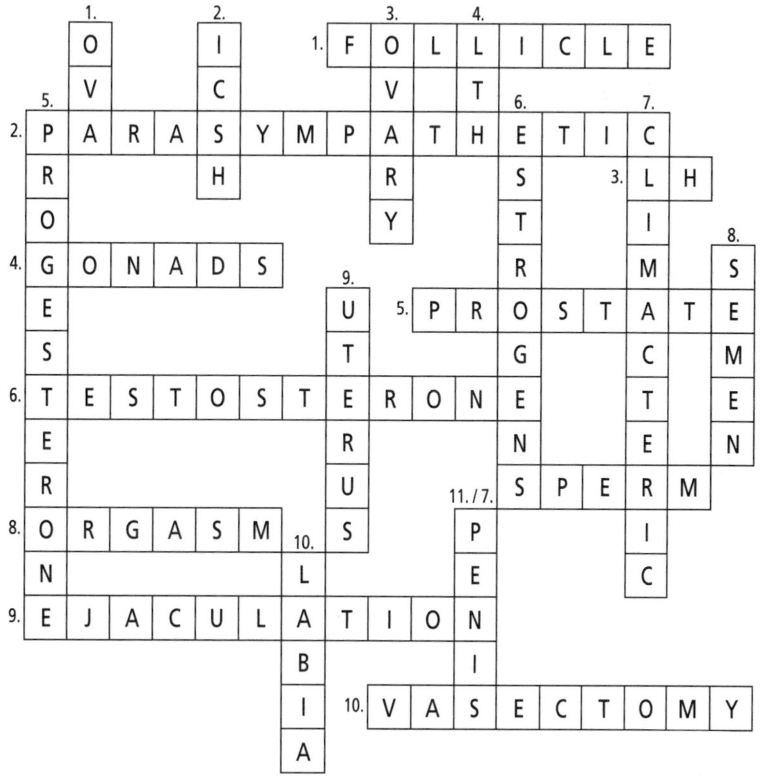

Crossword puzzle (solution):

```
          1.        2.             3.   4.
          O         I        1. F  O  L  L  I  C  L  E
     5.   V         C           V     T   6.           7.
  2. P  A  R  A  S  Y  M  P  A  T  H  E  T  I  C
     R         H              R        S      3. L  H
     O         Y              Y        T         I
                                       R        M      8.
  4. G  O  N  A  D  S      9.           R        M      S
     E                        U     5. P  R  O  S  T  A  T  E
     S                        T        G        C      M
  6. T  E  S  T  O  S  T  E  R  O  N  E        T      E
     E                        R        N        E      N
     R                        U    11./7. S  P  E  R  M
  8. O  R  G  A  S  M   10.    S        P        I
     N                   L              E        C
  9. E  J  A  C  U  L  A  T  I  O  N
                         B              I
                         I    10. V  A  S  E  C  T  O  M  Y
                         A
```

2. ovaries, fallopian, uterus, vagina
3. testes, seminal, prostate, bulbourethral, penis
4. follicle-stimulating
5. Luteinizing
6. Ovulation
7. psychologic, local sexual
8. parasympathetic
9. Bartholin, lubricant
10. Testosterone
11. vas deferens
12. menopause, male climacteric

8. menotropins
9. vasomotor, menopause
10. thromboembolic, cancers

11. **Suggested Answer:** C, A, A, A, A, A, C, A, A, A, A, A and C

12. **Suggested Answer:** Advise couples to have frequent intercourse at or around the time that ovulation is anticipated, usually approximately 7 days (range, 5 to 10 days) after the last dose of clomiphene to enhance fertilization. If the medication is to start on day 5, count the first day of the menstrual period as day 1. Advise the client that taking the medication at the same time every day maintains drug levels and helps in remembering the daily dose. Advise the client to take a missed dose as soon as possible. If the dose is not remembered until it is time for the next dose, both should be taken together. If more than one dose is missed, consult the prescriber.

13. **Suggested Answer:** The most commonly reported adverse effects of urofollitropin in women are ovarian cysts or ovarian enlargement, and severe pelvic pain as a result of severe ovarian hyperstimulation

CHAPTER 51

Drugs Affecting Women's Health and the Female Reproductive System

1. c, b, f, d, g, a, e
2. luteinizing, follicle-stimulating, anterior pituitary
3. hypogonadism
4. endometriosis, central precocious puberty
5. premature ovulation
6. chorionic gonadotropin
7. cryptorchidism, hypogonadism

syndrome (OHS). Pain and redness at the injection site can be noted with all formulations in both men and women. Other effects include severe stomach pain, bloating, decreased urination, severe nausea, vomiting or diarrhea, weight gain, swelling of the lower extremities, breathing difficulties, skin rash, elevated temperature, and chills.

14. **Answer:** 1
Rationale: The nurse would alert the client to the symptoms of hypersensitivity reaction (e.g., hives, wheezing, and dyspnea), and indicate that these are to be reported immediately. Other adverse effects include pain or inflammation at the injection site, and multiple pregnancies.
Cognitive Level: Application
Nursing Process Step: Implementation
NCLEX: Physiological Integrity: Pharmacological and Parenteral Therapies

15. **Answer:** 3
Rationale: Nafarelin is administered nasally, with maximum serum levels reported in 10 to 40 minutes. It has a half-life of 3 hours and a maximum effect within 1 month. The dosage for endometriosis is one nasal spray of 200 mcg in one nostril in the morning and one spray in the other nostril at night. It is usually administered for a period of 6 months.
Cognitive Level: Application
Nursing Process Step: Implementation
NCLEX: Physiological Integrity: Pharmacological and Parenteral Therapies

16. **Answer:** 3
Rationale: Ganirelix is used to inhibit premature LH increase in women receiving controlled ovarian hyperstimulation. An appropriate goal is that the client will conceive without experiencing adverse effects of the drug. Others include that the client will effectively manage the therapeutic regimen, including administering subcutaneous injections appropriately, medication compliance, stating reportable symptoms to prescriber, undertaking supportive interventions to the drug, and will collaborate with health care providers for monitoring and treatment.
Cognitive Level: Application
Nursing Process Step: Planning
NCLEX: Physiological Integrity: Pharmacological and Parenteral Therapies

17. **Answer:** 4
Rationale: Estrogens are contraindicated in women who are pregnant (because of risk of fetal malformation), have a history of coronary artery disease, thromboembolic events or have a history of estrogen dependent neoplasms. Estrogens should be avoided unless the benefit outweighs risk for clients who smoke, have a family history of breast cancer, history of gallstones, hypertension, heart failure, hypercalcemia or hypertriglyceridemia, or who are breastfeeding.
Cognitive Level: Application
Nursing Process Step: Analysis

NCLEX: Physiological Integrity: Pharmacological and Parenteral Therapies

18. **Answer:** 2
Rationale: Smoking increases the incidence of serious adverse effects with estrogen therapy, particularly in women older than age 35 years.
Cognitive Level: Application
Nursing Process Step: Implementation
NCLEX: Physiological Integrity: Pharmacological and Parenteral Therapies

19. **Answer:** 2
Rationale: The patch should be applied to the trunk below the waist on clean, dry, intact skin without hair. The sites should be rotated to prevent application to any site more frequently than every 7 days. It should not be applied to the breasts or to the waistline, where clothing might cause the patch to become loose. Scopolamine patches are placed behind the ear.
Cognitive Level: Application
Nursing Process Step: Evaluation
NCLEX: Physiological Integrity: Pharmacological and Parenteral Therapies

20. **Answer:** 1
Rationale: The tablets are taken at the same time each day, preferably in association with another daily routine (e.g., brushing of teeth, cleansing of face in the morning or at night). The client should keep an extra month's supply on hand and rotate the packages on a regular basis. The client who is beginning to use oral contraceptives should use a barrier method of birth control for the first cycle until the body adjusts to the medication. If she misses a dose for 1 day of the 21-day schedule, she should take it as soon as she remembers. If she does not remember until the next day, tell her to take the missed tablet and the regularly scheduled one together.
Cognitive Level: Application
Nursing Process Step: Implementation
NCLEX: Physiological Integrity: Pharmacological and Parenteral Therapies

CHAPTER 52

Drugs for Labor and Delivery

1. d, e, a, b, c
2. pharmacokinetics
3. uterus
4. oxytocics, tocolytics
5. milk ejection
6. dinoprostone
7. Preterm labor
8. contractions, delivery, 48, 72
9. indomethacin
10. maternal-fetus, gestational

11. **Suggested Answer:** Most frequent: nausea or vomiting, mostly after IV administration. Less frequent:

diarrhea, dizziness, tinnitus, increased sweating, confusion. Dose-related effect: abdominal cramping.

12. **Suggested Answer:** Check the pulse before boluses are delivered, keep prefilled syringes cool and protected from light when stored, and protect the pump from moisture and from being dropped. Also review proper disposal of used syringes and infusion sets.

13. **Suggested Answer:** Excess fluid volume (pulmonary edema); altered comfort related to headache, or nausea and vomiting; impaired skin integrity related to rash; anxiety (restlessness, nervousness, emotional lability); the collaborative problems of increased cardiac output (tachycardia), which could result in angina, myocardial infarction, and cardiac dysrhythmias and hepatitis.

14. **Answer:** 3
Rationale: The adverse effects of parenteral oxytocin include nausea, vomiting, tachycardia, and an irregular heart rate. It may occasionally cause fetal bradycardia, dysrhythmias, neonatal jaundice, postpartum excessive bleeding and, rarely, hematoma in the pelvic area. Prolonged therapy may result in water intoxication and possible maternal death because of its slight antidiuretic effects.
Cognitive Level: Application
Nursing Process Step: Assessment
NCLEX: Physiological Integrity: Pharmacological and Parenteral Therapies

15. **Answer:** 1
Rationale: An oxytocin infusion should be discontinued at any sign of uterine hyperactivity or fetal distress (such as drop in fetal heart rate). The dosage is titrated for each client depending on maternal and fetal response. The other options are not necessarily reasons to terminate the infusion.
Cognitive Level: Application
Nursing Process Step: Evaluation
NCLEX: Physiological Integrity: Pharmacological and Parenteral Therapies

16. **Answer:** 3
Rationale: The adverse effects include nausea, vomiting, diarrhea, dizziness, tinnitus, increased sweating, confusion, hypertension, chest pain and, rarely, respira-

tory difficulties, pruritus, cold hands or feet, leg weakness, and pain in the arms, legs, or lower back.
Cognitive Level: Application
Nursing Process Step: Implementation
NCLEX: Physiological Integrity: Pharmacological and Parenteral Therapies

17. **Answer:** 1
Rationale: Ritodrine is indicated to prevent and treat uncomplicated premature labor in pregnancies of 20 or more weeks' gestation.
Cognitive Level: Application
Nursing Process Step: Analysis
NCLEX: Physiological Integrity: Pharmacological and Parenteral Therapies

18. **Answer:** 4
Rationale: Early signs and symptoms of hypermagnesemia: bradycardia, diplopia, flushing, headache, hypotension, nausea, vomiting, shortness of breath, slurred speech, and weakness.
Cognitive Level: Application
Nursing Process Step: Assessment
NCLEX: Physiological Integrity: Pharmacological and Parenteral Therapies

19. **Answer:** 3
Rationale: Dinoprostone is indicated to promote cervical ripening prior to labor induction. A suppository formulation has been used as part of protocols to terminate pregnancy.
Cognitive Level: Application
Nursing Process Step: Planning
NCLEX: Physiological Integrity: Pharmacological and Parenteral Therapies

20. **Answer:** 2
Rationale: Bromocriptine (Parlodel) directly inhibits the release of prolactin from the anterior pituitary gland, resulting in the suppression of lactation. It may indirectly reduce breast discomfort but this is not the primary intended effect. It is not used for postpartum hemorrhage or pain.
Cognitive Level: Application
Nursing Process Step: Evaluation
NCLEX: Physiological Integrity: Pharmacological and Parenteral Therapies

CHAPTER 53

Drugs Affecting the Male Reproductive System

1.

```
U T K P N I I B G E G C C O D I B I L
T B A V R R D P F N E I U Y V L S W Y
P S S R G G Z H C C I T F Q F B S W O
T Q J Z C R H M N A S S E S S M E N T
H A C F N O E K U P E A R N S L N A M
T Q H S L Y V C U I D L W U H Q I A D
V R A B P L Z B P N I P J Q N F Z I E
J C F D R M E A N D R O G E N S Z T P
L U C J O R L N A I E E E K H M I S R
E P D H T M L E Y C T N C Z R E D A E
M R O Y E X M M S A S I I N E R J M S
I O N N I Q X I P T A T D P A E Q O S
D S T I N D Q A C I N N U C C X C I
W T Y H V J S U X O I A U R T T S E O
O A X S D B T T Z N F O A R I I X N N
Y T B L D D O X V S C U J N O O V Y K
T E S T O S T E R O N E I X N N A G O
F U J A I A M P Y R S D B G S S Q Y K
O V O U Z O O H Y P O G O N A D I S M
```

2. Androgens
3. virilism
4. benign prostatic hypertrophy
5. Testosterone
6. anabolic
7. III
8. anticoagulant, hypoglycemic
9. neck, urethra, retention, bacteriuria
10. hesitancy, frequency, and nocturia

11. **Suggested Answer:** Treatment of androgen deficiency; treatment of delayed male puberty when not induced by a pathologic condition; treatment of breast carcinoma; anemia.

12. **Suggested Answer:** Disturbed self-concept; excess fluid volume; altered comfort related to nausea, vomiting, and abdominal pain; disturbed sleep pattern; potential complications of erythrocytosis, hepatic impairment, hypercalcemia, and polycythemia.

13. **Suggested Answer:** Decreased libido, impotence, decreased amount of ejaculate.

14. **Answer:** 1
Rationale: Oxandrolone is an androgen that can cause polycythemia as an adverse effect, leading to increased hemoglobin and hematocrit. It could also lead to increased LDLs (hypercholesterolemic effect). Androgens may decrease blood glucose concentrations, and these although these drugs are metabolized in the liver, they do not reduce liver enzymes.
Cognitive Level: Application
Nursing Process Step: Assessment
NCLEX: Physiological Integrity: Pharmacological and Parenteral Therapies

15. **Answer:** 4
Rationale: The matrix type of patch is adhered to the scrotum and may be removed for swimming, bathing, or sexual activity. In contrast, the reservoir type of patch is placed on the abdomen, back, thighs, or upper arms and is not removed for those activities.
Cognitive Level: Application
Nursing Process Step: Implementation
NCLEX: Physiological Integrity: Pharmacological and Parenteral Therapies

16. Answer: 3

Rationale: Priapism (persistent, abnormal penile or clitoral erection) is an indication of excessive dosing of the androgen and temporary withdrawal of the drug is indicated. Complications of testosterone therapy include accelerated bone maturation, altered glucose regulation, fluid retention, aggressive behavior, anxiety, elevated LDL and reduced HDL cholesterol, and liver injury.

Cognitive Level: Application

Nursing Process Step: Implementation

NCLEX: Physiological Integrity: Pharmacological and Parenteral Therapies

17. Answer: 2

Rationale: Serious complications of testosterone therapy include accelerated bone maturation leading to epiphyseal closure, altered glucose regulation, fluid retention, aggressive behavior, anxiety, elevated LDL and reduced HDL cholesterol, and liver injury.

Cognitive Level: Application

Nursing Process Step: Implementation

NCLEX: Physiological Integrity: Pharmacological and Parenteral Therapies

18. Answer: 4

Rationale: The androgens are used to treat breast carcinoma; palliative or secondary treatment for inoperable metastatic breast cancer in postmenopausal women who have previously responded well to hormone therapy. Androgens are rated Category X, which means that their use is contraindicated in pregnant or lactating females. This client should understand this rating because of her age and possible reproductive status.

Cognitive Level: Application

Nursing Process Step: Implementation

NCLEX: Physiological Integrity: Pharmacological and Parenteral Therapies

19. Answer: 3

Rationale: Finasteride does not cure benign prostatic hyperplasia, but helps to control it, and it takes at least 6 months for its full effect to occur in relieving symptoms.

Cognitive Level: Application

Nursing Process Step: Implementation

NCLEX: Physiological Integrity: Pharmacological and Parenteral Therapies

20. Answer: 1

Rationale: A baseline assessment prior to finasteride therapy includes liver function studies, prostatic status, and an evaluation of urinary elimination pattern. The others are unnecessary.

Cognitive Level: Application

Nursing Process Step: Planning

NCLEX: Physiological Integrity: Pharmacological and Parenteral Therapies

CHAPTER 54

Drugs Affecting Sexual Behavior

1. d, c, e, f, a, b
2. Sexuality
3. psychological and physiologic
4. psychological, social, and physiologic
5. libido
6. clinical depression, chronic disease, medication
7. erectile dysfunction
8. penile erection
9. psyche, autonomic
10. female, masculinize

11. **Suggested Answer:** Depression is often associated with diminished sexual interest, drive, and activity, and the drugs used to treat depression often compound the negative effects on sexual function. Although antidepressants generally elevate mood and thus increase sexuality, they can cause impotence and have an adverse effect on sexual behavior. Although monoamine oxidase (MAO) inhibitors may be used as antihypertensives and antidepressants, the impotence that can result may be caused by their tendency to block peripheral ganglionic nerve transmission. The selective serotonin reuptake inhibitors are also known to decrease libido and sexual function.

12. **Suggested Answer:**

Antidepressants, antihypertensives: impotence
Diuretics, H_2 receptors: impotence, gynecomastia
Antianxiety drugs, alcohol, barbiturates: impotence, decreased sexual activity

13. **Suggested Answer:** Gaining understanding and acceptance of feelings about one's own sexuality; being open to clients' discussions; allowing clients to hold any belief or sexual practice that is not overtly harmful; recognizing that it is probably impossible to be truly comfortable with all clients or topics; keeping current with constantly changing data about drugs with potential for causing sexual dysfunction; being able to identify and interpret client cues about problems dealing with sexuality; discussing clients' medication with them; consulting with prescriber when adverse effects appear and suggesting alternate forms, if feasible; listening with sensitivity to expressed feelings that may attend body image changes.

14. **Answer:** 1

Rationale: The major contraindication to the use of sildenafil is concurrent nitrate therapy (including the use of amyl nitrate, sublingual or topical nitroglycerin, and oral nitrate derivatives like isosorbide mono- and di-nitrates), which can result in severe hypotension. Concurrent use with other drugs that lower blood pressure (e.g., antihypertensives) may also result in additive hypotension.

Cognitive Level: Analysis

Nursing Process Step: Analysis

NCLEX: Physiological Integrity: Pharmacological and Parenteral Therapies

15. **Answer:** 2

Rationale: While taking tadalafil or other phosphodiesterase type 5 inhibitors, the client should avoid drugs and foods that inhibit cytochrome P450 3A4 activity (e.g., grapefruit juice, azole antifungals, macrolide antimicrobials, and many other drugs) because they may result in excessive effects.

Cognitive Level: Application

Nursing Process Step: Implementation

NCLEX: Physiological Integrity: Pharmacological and Parenteral Therapies

16. **Answer:** 3

Rationale: The pediatric formulation of alprostadil is indicated for temporary control of patent ductus arteriosus in neonates. The other options are not indications for this drug.

Cognitive Level: Application

Nursing Process Step: Analysis

NCLEX: Physiological Integrity: Pharmacological and Parenteral Therapies

17. **Answer:** 4

Rationale: Vardenafil should not be used if possible with indinavir, itraconazole, ketoconazole or ritonavir, because these could lead to elevated vardenafil levels. If they must be used, the maximum dose of vardenafil recommended with these drugs is 2.5 mg.

Cognitive Level: Application

Nursing Process Step: Evaluation

NCLEX: Physiological Integrity: Pharmacological and Parenteral Therapies

18. **Answer:** 2

Rationale: Penile pain is the most common complaint with the injection and urethral pellets. Urethral burning is also noted with pellet use. Other effects include hypertension, headache, prolonged erection and penile edema.

Cognitive Level: Application

Nursing Process Step: Implementation

NCLEX: Physiological Integrity: Pharmacological and Parenteral Therapies

19. **Answer:** 4

Rationale: Concurrent use of amyl nitrite with phosphodiesterase type 5 inhibitors (e.g., sildenafil [Viagra]) may result in significant hypotension and is absolutely contraindicated. The other substances may not be effective but pose no specific risks because of drug interactions.

Cognitive Level: Application

Nursing Process Step: Implementation

NCLEX: Physiological Integrity: Pharmacological and Parenteral Therapies

20. **Answer:** 4

Rationale: Drugs such as morphine, heroin, cocaine, marijuana, lysergic acid diethylamide (LSD) are also used by some as aphrodisiacs. For some, these agents can enhance the enjoyment of the sexual experience under certain circumstances, but individual response is often not predictable. These agents have no particular properties that specifically increase sexual potency; instead they tend to affect the user according to expectations. Thus the user's state of mind and the amount consumed contribute considerably to the effect achieved.

Cognitive Level: Application

Nursing Process Step: Implementation

NCLEX: Physiological Integrity: Pharmacological and Parenteral Therapies

---

CHAPTER 55

Principles of Antineoplastic Chemotherapy

1. d, f, a, e, c, b
2. pharmacologic, radiation, surgery
3. cytotoxic, hormonal, antiangiogenesis, biologic response
4. rapidly dividing, cell cycle
5. DNA
6. cervix, endometrium
7. cell cycle–nonspecific
8. receptors, enzyme,
9. stomatitis, diarrhea, malabsorption
10. Resistance

11. **Suggested Answer:**
    GI tract: nausea, vomiting, anorexia, diarrhea
    Bone marrow: bone marrow suppression
    Hair follicles: alopecia (hair loss)
    Mouth: stomatitis (inflammation of the mouth)

12. **Suggested Answer:** *Constipation:* addition to diet of high-fiber foods and prune juice, 1 to 2 tablespoons of bran, 8 to 10 glasses of fluid daily, and/or hot lemon water in the morning.
    Alopecia: assure client that hair will begin to grow back in 6 to 8 weeks, although it may be a different texture or color.
    Stomatitis: good oral hygiene; small, frequent servings of cold or room-temperature, bland, nonirritating foods. Choice of mouthwash depends on status of client's lesions.

13. **Suggested Answer:** They should be handled with gloves, emptied directly into toilet, washed with

326

detergent and water without splashing with the rinse water discarded directly into toilet, and the toilet flushed three times.

14. **Answer:** 3

Rationale: Because hot foods have been reported to contribute to nausea, foods should be served at room temperature or cooler. Resting for 1 to 2 hours after eating is advised, because activity can slow the digestive process. Some clients have reduced desire for red meat or other protein foods because they are most commonly perceived as bitter tasting. Because protein is essential for good nutrition (greater than 1 g/kg of body weight), alternative sources for red meat should be pursued. Cold cooked turkey, fish, eggs, and dairy products may be suitable substitutes. The biggest meal of the day should be planned for the time the client is usually hungriest, even if that time is early morning or midnight.

Cognitive Level: Application

Nursing Process Step: Implementation

NCLEX: Physiological Integrity: Pharmacological and Parenteral Therapies

15. **Answer:** 1

Rationale: Foods that are high in potassium (to replace losses from diarrhea) and that usually do not worsen diarrhea should be encouraged; these include bananas, apricot or pear nectar, red meat (if tolerated), saltwater fish, boiled or mashed potatoes, and orange juice. The client should avoid foods that may cause gas and cramping, such as cabbage, beans, and highly spiced foods or irritating foods, such as alcohol. Foods that decrease tone of the lower esophageal sphincter, including coffee, wine and chocolate, may also contribute to nausea or gastric distress. Hot, spicy foods should be avoided because they increase peristalsis. Reducing high-fiber foods in the diet (e.g., raw fruits and vegetables, popcorn, bran, and whole grain cereals and bread) may help to control diarrhea. A low-residue, high-protein, high-calorie diet is recommended.

Cognitive Level: Application

Nursing Process Step: Implementation

NCLEX: Physiological Integrity: Pharmacological and Parenteral Therapies

16. **Answer:** 2

Rationale: Clients with low platelet counts (normal 150,000-400,000/mm^3) are at increased risk for bleeding. Avoid taking rectal temperatures and administering vaginal douches, rectal suppositories or enemas to such clients. Protective care for these clients might include the administration of stool softeners and the use of soft-bristled toothbrushes, electric razors, and the use of nail file rather than nail clippers. Avoid flossing. Use oral preparations of analgesics and other medications to avoid the tissue damage resulting from IM injections; however, avoid aspirin and NSAID use because of the risk for prolonged bleeding.

Cognitive Level: Application

Nursing Process Step: Planning

NCLEX: Physiological Integrity: Pharmacological and Parenteral Therapies

17. **Answer:** 4

Rationale: The risk for infection is increased when there is bone marrow depression. Antipyretics (e.g., aspirin, NSAIDs, and acetaminophen) are typically avoided so as not to mask fever, which may be the only indication of infection. Use strict aseptic (handwashing) technique during contact with the client, who should also be protected from persons harboring harmful microorganisms. Clients with granulocytopenia should receive topical antibiotics for abrasions and scratches. Caution the client to avoid crowds and individuals with infectious diseases (e.g., colds, influenza, chickenpox, measles) and pet excreta including fish tanks. Avoid exposure to fresh fruit, vegetables, flowers, and live plants.

Cognitive Level: Application

Nursing Process Step: Implementation

NCLEX: Physiological Integrity: Pharmacological and Parenteral Therapies

18. **Answer:** 1

Rationale: *Impaired oral mucous membranes* following antineoplastic therapy may be xerostomia (dryness of the mouth), stomatitis (an inflammatory condition of the mouth) or mouth ulcers. In both instances, the client reports a burning sensation before tissue changes, and a sensitivity to heat, cold and salty and spicy foods. The goal is to provide nutritional intake with minimum discomfort. Small, frequent servings of foods that are cold or at room temperature, bland, and nonirritating are best tolerated by the client. Remove dentures to prevent further irritation. Avoid the use of commercial mouthwash products containing alcohol, lemon/glycerin swabs, or hydrogen peroxide combinations to minimize irritation. Use sugar-free gum or sugar-free candies to stimulate salivation.

Cognitive Level: Application

Nursing Process Step: Evaluation

NCLEX: Physiological Integrity: Pharmacological and Parenteral Therapies

19. **Answer:** 4

Rationale: Clients, even those who experience only thinning of the hair, need assurance that the hair will begin to grow back in approximately 3 to 5 months after the last antineoplastic treatment, although it may have a different texture or color. Because the hair may be more fragile, the client should avoid permanents, hair coloring, curling irons or electric rollers until the regrowth is long enough to have had 2 haircuts. Clients who are purchasing a wig are advised to do so before therapy begins when their energy levels are still high.

Cognitive Level: Application

Nursing Process Step: Planning

20. **Answer:** 4

Rationale: The kidneys are at risk for injury because of the nephrotoxicity of some antineoplastic drugs and their effectiveness. There may be direct damage to the glomerulus and nephron and/or precipitation of metabolites. Alert the oncologist if the BUN is greater than 22 mg/dL and/or the serum creatinine is greater than 2 mg/dL.

Cognitive Level: Analysis

Nursing Process Step: Implementation

NCLEX: Physiological Integrity: Pharmacological and Parenteral Therapies

CHAPTER 56

Antineoplastic Chemotherapy Agents

1. d, g, a, f, b, e, c
2. Antineoplastic
3. Fluorouracil
4. Mechlorethamine
5. Doxorubicin
6. Vinblastine, vincristine
7. Interferon
8. Paclitaxel
9. nitrogen mustard
10. hematocrit, platelet, WBC

11. **Suggested Answer:** c, a, b, d

12. **Suggested Answer:** Apply topical cooling via the following steps:
    (1) Cooling of site to client tolerance for 24 hours.
    (2) Elevate and rest extremity for 24 to 48 hours, then resume normal activity as tolerated.
    (3) If pain, erythema, and/or swelling persist beyond 48 hours, discuss with the physician the need for consultation with surgeon.

13. **Suggested Answer:** Wear two pairs of gloves when cleaning up an antineoplastic drug spill. Wash hands before and after. Wear a mask and eye protection if the medication is powdered. Place the spilled substance in a plastic bag. Wipe up the remainder with a damp cloth and also place in the plastic bag. Seal the bag and place it inside of a second bag, and seal the second bag. Label it BIOHAZARD and send it for disposal by incineration.

14. **Answer:** 4

Rationale: Cisplatin causes many of the typical adverse effects of chemotherapeutic drugs. Other symptoms to watch for are a loss of taste and numbness or tingling in the fingers, toes, or face, indicating peripheral neuropathy. The drug should be discontinued at the first indication of this, because it may be irreversible. Ototoxicity is another relatively unique adverse effect.

Cognitive Level: Application

Nursing Process Step: Assessment

NCLEX: Physiological Integrity: Pharmacological and Parenteral Therapies

15. **Answer:** 4

Rationale: Doxorubicin carries a risk of cardiotoxicity, so this client should be carefully monitored for signs of heart failure if this drug is used for chemotherapy. The other drugs listed are not likely to cause cardiac adverse effects, although they may cause pulmonary effects.

Cognitive Level: Analysis

Nursing Process Step: Planning

NCLEX: Physiological Integrity: Pharmacological and Parenteral Therapies

16. **Answer:** 2

Rationale: Leucovorin is used with methotrexate (a folic acid type of antimetabolite) to preserve normal cells and reduce adverse drug effects. The other drugs listed are other cancer chemotherapy agents that have no protective function.

Cognitive Level: Application

Nursing Process Step: Planning

NCLEX: Physiological Integrity: Pharmacological and Parenteral Therapies

17. **Answer:** 1

Rationale: Bone marrow suppression is the major adverse effect of vincristine. Vincristine may also induce anorexia, nausea and vomiting, rash, autonomic toxicity (abdominal cramping, constipation, bed-wetting, orthostatic hypotension, lack of sweating, and increased, decreased or painful urination), hyperuricemia, a progressive neurotoxicity (blurred or double vision, difficulty in walking, drooping eyelids, headache, jaw pain, numbness and pain in the fingers and toes, weakness), and SIADH secretion.

Cognitive Level: Application

Nursing Process Step: Assessment

NCLEX: Physiological Integrity: Pharmacological and Parenteral Therapies

18. **Answer:** 3

Rationale: The adverse effects of paclitaxel include severe allergic reactions that may be prevented by pretreatment with a steroid and an H_1 and H_2 antagonist; other adverse effects include bone marrow suppression, peripheral neuropathy, muscle pain, alopecia, and gastric distress.

Cognitive Level: Application

Nursing Process Step: Planning

NCLEX: Physiological Integrity: Pharmacological and Parenteral Therapies

19. **Answer:** 1

Rationale: Tamoxifen (Nolvadex) is believed to bind to estrogen receptors in breast cancer cells and act as a competitive inhibitor of estrogen. It is effective for tumors that contain high concentrations of estrogen receptors. It is also an estrogen agonist in the liver, which has desirable effects on serum lipids in postmenopausal women; it also helps to preserve bone mineral density, which may decrease the risk for osteoporosis in these women.

Cognitive Level: Comprehension
Nursing Process Step: Analysis
NCLEX: Physiological Integrity: Pharmacological and Parenteral Therapies

20. **Answer:** 2
Rationale: Fluid intake at 3000 mL daily before treatment and for 72 hours following cyclophosphamide treatment is needed to ensure frequent voiding, including at least once during the night; this minimizes the risk of hemorrhagic cystitis and promotes the excretion of uric acid. It is also best to administer cyclophosphamide early in the day so that most of the drug's metabolites have been excreted before bedtime; this prevents continued contact of the metabolites with the bladder mucosa. The drug should be discontinued at the first sign of hemorrhagic cystitis.

Cognitive Level: Application
Nursing Process Step: Implementation
NCLEX: Physiological Integrity: Pharmacological and Parenteral Therapies

CHAPTER 57

Overview of Infections, Inflammation, and Fever

1. See Fig. 57-1 in the textbook, which provides an overview of heat loss and heat gain mechanisms.
2. Infection, injury, toxin, antigen-antibody
3. Inflammation
4. bacteremia
5. antimicrobial
6. Neutrophils, monocytes (macrophages), lymphocytes
7. complement, permeability, lysis
8. hypothalamus; production; loss
9. E prostaglandins
10. Salicylates

11. **Suggested Answer:** *Fever of unknown origin* (FUO) is described as a temperature greater than 103°F that is recorded daily for more than 2 weeks in a client with an uncertain diagnosis after a week's evaluation in a hospital setting. Most clients with FUO are later found to have an infection, neoplasm, or connective tissue disease.

12. **Suggested Answer:** Bacteriostatic agents inhibit bacterial growth, which allows the host's defense mechanisms additional time to remove the invading microorganisms. In contrast, bactericidal agents cause bacterial cell death and lysis. Antibacterial agents may be divided into bacteriostatic (e.g., sulfonamides) and bactericidal (e.g., penicillins) categories. However, such categorization is not always valid or reliable, because the same antimicrobial agent may have either effect depending on the dose administered, the concentration achieved at its site of action, and the particular species of bacteria.

13. **Suggested Answer:** Teach that these drugs should never be taken without medical supervision and should be taken in strict accordance with physicians' prescriptions. Allergic clients should be taught to protect themselves from future exposure. Special administration considerations, expected effects, and adverse effects can be described on drug sheets for clients to refer to at home, with a telephone number to call when questions arise. Caution clients that occasionally these drugs will interfere with results of home lab testing kits.

14. **Answer:** 1
Rationale: Hypersensitivity is a state of altered reactivity in which the body reacts with an exaggerated immune response. Such responses may include rash, fever, urticaria with pruritus, chills, generalized erythema, anaphylaxis, and Stevens-Johnson syndrome. The other symptoms are found with the original diagnosis of pneumonia.

Cognitive Level: Application
Nursing Process Step: Assessment
NCLEX: Physiological Integrity: Pharmacological and Parenteral Therapies

15. **Answer:** 3
Rationale: The treatment of allergic reactions includes the use of antihistamines and epinephrine, which block or counteract the effects of the vasoactive mediators of allergy, and the use of corticosteroids, which may reduce tissue injury and edema in the inflammatory response. The use of steroids is controversial in the face of systemic infection because of their prolonged inhibition of normal host defense responses.

Cognitive Level: Application
Nursing Process Step: Planning
NCLEX: Physiological Integrity: Pharmacological and Parenteral Therapies

16. **Answer:** 2
Rationale: *Clostridium difficile* infection of the colon manifests with diarrhea. White patches in the oral cavity or itching in the vaginal area signs of candidiasis. A sore throat is nonspecific.

Cognitive Level: Application
Nursing Process Step: Assessment
NCLEX: Physiological Integrity: Pharmacological and Parenteral Therapies

17. **Answer:** 4
Rationale: The expected outcome of antimicrobial therapy is a decrease in the severity or a disappearance of the clinical and laboratory manifestations of infection. Redness, heat, edema, and pain with local infections should decrease. Temperature, heart rate, respiratory rate, and WBC count should return to normal (5,000-10,000/mm^3), and appetite and a sense of well-being should improve. Purulent drainage, if present, should decrease in amount and change to a more normal appearance and consistency.

Cognitive Level: Analysis
Nursing Process Step: Evaluation

329

18. **Answer:** 1

Rationale: Extracellular volume excess may result from administering multiple doses of IV drugs, each of which is diluted in 100 mL of saline, to a client with heart failure. Edema, pulmonary congestion (crackles) with subsequent shortness of breath, and an increase in body weight indicate the presence of extracellular volume excess. The pulse would increase with volume excess, not decrease. The client would be at risk for hyperglycemia if 5% dextrose in water were used as the solution.

Cognitive Level: Application

Nursing Process Step: Assessment

NCLEX: Physiological Integrity: Pharmacological and Parenteral Therapies

19. **Answer:** 3

Rationale: Cultures are ordered if an area of suspected infection is found. If there is an order to give an antimicrobial agent before an infective source is determined, obtain cultures before administering the first dose of the drug ordered. The nurse could then complete other interventions, such as assessing the client's allergies, performing a baseline assessment (including symptoms of infection), and obtaining the medication.

Cognitive Level: Application

Nursing Process Step: Implementation

NCLEX: Physiological Integrity: Pharmacological and Parenteral Therapies

20. **Answer:** 2

Rationale: The nurse should remain with the client for the first 30 minutes of the dose to observe for an immediate allergy reaction. Family history is less important than personal history of allergy. Penicillin is an antibiotic, not an antiviral agent.

Cognitive Level: Application

Nursing Process Step: Implementation

NCLEX: Physiological Integrity: Pharmacological and Parenteral Therapies

CHAPTER 58

Antibacterials

1. See Figure 3-19 in the textbook.
2. Specimen, cultures
3. Antibacterials
4. bacteria, fungi, yeasts, superinfection
5. food, drugs
6. evenly, 24-hour
7. 15
8. β-lactam ring
9. 8, enamel, discoloration
10. aminoglycosides

11. **Suggested Answer:** The peak and trough determine the pharmacokinetics of an antibiotic and help determine dosage and intervals of administration.

12. **Suggested Answer:** The significant adverse effects for oral doses include nausea, vomiting, and taste alterations. Less often or rarely, adverse effects with parenteral administration include ototoxicity and nephrotoxicity. Reported after bolus or too-rapid drug injection is "red-neck syndrome," a response that results in histamine release and chills, fever, tachycardia, pruritus, rash, or a red face, neck, upper body, back, and arms. It can be minimized by the slow infusion of vancomycin over 60 to 120 minutes.

13. **Suggested Answer:** Parenteral metronidazole is administered by slow IV infusion. It may be administered continuously or intermittently over a 1-hour period. If administered concurrently with a primary IV, the primary IV should be discontinued while the metronidazole is infused.

14. **Answer:** 1

Rationale: The use of cephalosporins is contraindicated if a client had a history of hypersensitivity to cephalosporins, penicillin, penicillin derivatives, or penicillamine. In clients with uncertain history, use caution because the possibility of a cross-reaction is 2% to 10%. The other antibiotics listed do not exhibit cross-sensitivity to cephalosporins.

Cognitive Level: Application

Nursing Process Step: Assessment

NCLEX: Physiological Integrity: Pharmacological and Parenteral Therapies

15. **Answer:** 2

Rationale: Alcohol is not recommended with cefamandole, cefoperazone, or cefotetan. An increase in acetaldehyde in the blood may result, producing a disulfiram (Antabuse)–type reaction (e.g., stomach pain, nausea, vomiting, headaches, low blood pressure, tachycardia, respiratory difficulties, increased sweating, or flushing of the face). Clients should avoid the use of alcoholic beverages, medications containing alcohol, or IV alcohol solutions during the administration of these drugs and for 3 days afterward.

Cognitive Level: Application

Nursing Process Step: Implementation

NCLEX: Physiological Integrity: Pharmacological and Parenteral Therapies

16. **Answer:** 4

Rationale: Reported after bolus or too-rapid drug injection of vancomycin is "red-neck syndrome," a response that results in histamine release and chills, fever, tachycardia, pruritus, rash, or a red face, neck, upper body, back, and arms. It results from excessive speed of infusion and can be minimized by the slow infusion of vancomycin over 60 to 120 minutes. The significant adverse effects for oral doses include nausea, vomiting, and taste alterations. Less often or rarely, adverse effects with parenteral administration include ototoxicity and nephrotoxicity.

Cognitive Level: Application

Nursing Process Step: Assessment

NCLEX: Physiological Integrity: Pharmacological and Parenteral Therapies

17. **Answer:** 3

Rationale: GI symptoms are the most commonly reported adverse effect with erythromycin and its salts. Oral and/or vaginal candidiasis and, less commonly, hypersensitivity and hepatotoxicity have also been reported. Erythromycin in high doses has been associated with prolonged QT interval on ECG.

Cognitive Level: Application

Nursing Process Step: Implementation

NCLEX: Physiological Integrity: Pharmacological and Parenteral Therapies

18. **Answer:** 3

Rationale: Administer clindamycin capsules with a full glass of water or with meals to prevent esophageal ulceration. The other responses do not address this concern.

Cognitive Level: Application

Nursing Process Step: Implementation

NCLEX: Physiological Integrity: Pharmacological and Parenteral Therapies

19. **Answer:** 1

Rationale: Administer fluoroquinolones with a full glass of water and ensure that the client maintains a urinary output of at least 1200 to 1500 mL daily (for adults) to minimize the occurrence of crystalluria. Enoxacin or norfloxacin are to be taken on an empty stomach; ciprofloxacin, lomefloxacin, ofloxacin, and sparfloxacin may be taken either with or without food.

Cognitive Level: Application

Nursing Process Step: Evaluation

NCLEX: Physiological Integrity: Pharmacological and Parenteral Therapies

20. **Answer:** 3

Rationale: The major adverse effects of aminoglycosides, including tobramycin, are nephrotoxicity and ototoxicity. Nephrotoxicity would be evidenced in high blood urea nitrogen (BUN) levels and serum creatinine levels (0.5-2.0 mg/dL). The elevated sodium and decreased albumin levels are not related to this drug. The elevated blood cell count could be related to the original infection.

Cognitive Level: Analysis

Nursing Process Step: Assessment

NCLEX: Physiological Integrity: Pharmacological and Parenteral Therapies

CHAPTER 59

Antifungal and Antiviral Drugs

1. b, j, g, i, h, a, d, f, c, e
2. fungi
3. candidiasis, candidiasis
4. immunocompromised
5. Viruses
6. mammalian, enzyme
7. antiretrovirals
8. resistance
9. blood, blood products
10. nonnucleoside reverse transcriptase

11. **Suggested Answer:** Advise client to complete essential dental work before starting therapy with amphotericin B or to delay it until completing course of drug to avoid gingival bleeding and delayed healing. Teach appropriate oral hygiene, including gentle use of soft toothbrushes and floss and avoidance of toothpicks. Advise client to alert staff at first indication of pain at IV site.

12. **Suggested Answer:** Nausea, myalgia, insomnia, severe headache, bone marrow suppression

13. **Suggested Answer:** Administer on empty stomach. Tablets should not be swallowed whole but thoroughly chewed, crushed, or dissolved in water. Dissolve in at least 30 mL of water, stir, and have client swallow it immediately.

14. **Answer:** 3

Rationale: Amphotericin B is associated with both infusion related reactions, and significant risk for renal injury. Regular monitoring of renal function (creatinine and blood urea nitrogen) and electrolytes is required with amphotericin B therapy.

Cognitive Level: Application

Nursing Process Step: Assessment

NCLEX: Physiological Integrity: Pharmacological and Parenteral Therapies

15. **Answer:** 1

Rationale: A client with heart failure (HF) or ventricular dysfunction should not receive itraconazole because it has negative inotropic effects and poses a risk for edema and worsening heart failure. Hypersensitivity to itraconazole or other azole antifungal agents would be another contraindication for use of the drug.

Cognitive Level: Analysis

Nursing Process Step: Implementation

NCLEX: Physiological Integrity: Pharmacological and Parenteral Therapies

16. **Answer:** 2

Rationale: Valacyclovir is indicated for the treatment of herpes zoster (shingles) caused by VZV and herpes genitalis in immunocompetent persons. When compared to acyclovir, valacyclovir is reported to be more significant in reducing the pain and postherpetic neuralgia associated with herpes zoster in persons older than 50 years of age. Valacyclovir has not been studied in children, immunocompromised individuals, or persons with disseminated zoster.

Cognitive Level: Application

Nursing Process Step: Analysis

NCLEX: Physiological Integrity: Pharmacological and Parenteral Therapies

17. **Answer:** 2

Rationale: For RSV infection in children, this drug is administered by oral inhalation via a Vivatek small-particle aerosol generator, with a ribavirin concentration of 20 mg/mL in the reservoir. It is administered over 12 to 18 hours per day for 3 to 7 days.

Cognitive Level: Application

Nursing Process Step: Planning

NCLEX: Physiological Integrity: Pharmacological and Parenteral Therapies

18. **Answer:** 4

Rationale: Amantadine is indicated for the prevention and treatment of influenza A and for treatment of Parkinson's disease and drug-induced, extrapyramidal reactions.

Cognitive Level: Application

Nursing Process Step: Assessment

NCLEX: Physiological Integrity: Pharmacological and Parenteral Therapies

19. **Answer:** 3

Rationale: It is important to comply with the medication regimen, take the drugs at evenly spaced times and not miss doses. The client may need to use a written drug regimen for the 24 hours and an alarm clock to assist in maintaining compliance. Stress the importance of not taking more medication than prescribed. Increasing drug dosage will not help; instead it leads to greater drug toxicities. The client should not discontinue the antiviral medication without consulting with the prescriber. Many drugs have discomforting adverse effects but may be managed with changes of dosages, schedules, antiemetics, or other palliative measures. Because many of the antivirals have serious drug interactions with a number of drugs, the client should not take other medications, even over-the-counter (OTC) medications, without checking with the prescriber.

Cognitive Level: Analysis

Nursing Process Step: Evaluation

NCLEX: Physiological Integrity: Pharmacological and Parenteral Therapies

20. **Answer:** 1

Rationale: The most serious acute onset adverse effect observed with indinavir is nephrolithiasis, and has been noted in up to 29% of pediatric and 12% of adult clients. Other adverse effects of indinavir include nausea, vomiting, gastric distress, diarrhea, headache, dizziness, fatigue, fever, flu-like syndrome, and chest pain. As with other protease inhibitors, indinavir is associated with metabolic changes, including fat redistribution, elevated cholesterol and triglyceride levels, and increased risk for type 2 diabetes mellitus.

Cognitive Level: Application

Nursing Process Step: Implementation

NCLEX: Physiological Integrity: Pharmacological and Parenteral Therapies

Other Antimicrobial Drugs and Antiparasitic Drugs

1.

```
D J G R U H D S I S O L U C R E B U T Y
L W N X D D G I P A T H O G E N E S I S
I M I H R Y P F Z R M P I T G I R S G X
Y K S W V D Y X M A L A R I A P V I T Z
O Y R V J V T L W T I R C A F M E S O X
L T U E T I S A R A P N E P U A D A X L
A E N I U Q O R O L H C O Y R F I I O F
M F O E R Y T H R O C Y T I C I M N P O
E A T R C O M M U N I T Y O N R A O L W
B S F N P H Y D D G E C E R S S N M A O
I M L B V N I H A B F C H P E I O S U X
A M I N O S A L I C Y L A T E Y Z H M X
S I L Y E N D P D U H Q E S Q J A C O T
I F Y A S K U L Z R C T L G D P R I S B
S U S E Z C Q P R E G N A N C Y R I T
G E N E D U C A T I O N K A U R P T S K
J A S U O T A M O L U N A R G S M F A K
H E L M I N T H S M R O W N I P L N D V
D L D W L T S K S G V Q S A T E D B B Q
Q O G F V L J Y K J F O B L J G Z K G B
```

2. parasitic
3. bite, blood transfusion, needles
4. Quinine, cinchona
5. 1, 4
6. Tuberculosis, acid-fast
7. lungs, extrapulmonary
8. coughs, sneezes
9. 1 to 3, 8 to 12
10. Hansen

11. **Suggested Answer:** Transmitted by airborne droplets, not by objects. Sharing an enclosed environment with an infected person creates high risk of developing this infection.

12. **Suggested Answer:** Encourage compliance with full course of drug. Regular visits and periodic eye examinations are necessary. Report vision changes promptly. Do not use alcohol and oral antacids with isoniazid. Drug may produce false-positive test results with copper sulfate tests. Clients should use other urine glucose tests.

13. **Suggested Answer:** The adverse effects of dapsone include hypersensitivity, hemolytic anemia, and methemoglobinemia.

14. **Answer:** 1
Rationale: Chloroquine is indicated for the prevention and treatment of malaria for the four strains of plasmodium. Quinine is no longer used often because of its adverse effect profile, and pyrazinamide and ethambutol are used to treat tuberculosis.
Cognitive Level: Application
Nursing Process Step: Planning
NCLEX: Physiological Integrity: Pharmacological and Parenteral Therapies

15. **Answer:** 2
Rationale: Significant drug interactions can occur when mefloquine is given with quinidine or quinine. Concurrent use may result in an increased risk of sinus bradycardia, prolonged Q-T intervals, or cardiac arrest. The other medications listed (a β blocker, ACE inhibitor, and calcium channel blocker, respectively) do not cause these interactive effects.
Cognitive Level: Analysis
Nursing Process Step: Planning
NCLEX: Physiological Integrity: Pharmacological and Parenteral Therapies

16. Answer: 3

Rationale: The most serious adverse effect associated with isoniazid is hepatic injury and on rare occasions, has been fatal. Other adverse effects of isoniazid include gastric distress, anorexia, nausea, vomiting, weakness, and peripheral neuritis. Neuritis risk may be reduced with concurrent use of pyridoxine 50 mg PO daily.

Cognitive Level: Application
Nursing Process Step: Implementation
NCLEX: Physiological Integrity: Pharmacological and Parenteral Therapies

17. Answer: 2

Rationale: Clients should be educated about the ability of rifampin to produce a red/orange color to urine, saliva, tears and sweat. The most serious risk with rifampin is hepatotoxicity, although this risk appears significantly lower than with isoniazid. Other adverse effects of rifampin include gastric distress, hypersensitivity, and a flu-like syndrome.

Cognitive Level: Application
Nursing Process Step: Implementation
NCLEX: Physiological Integrity: Pharmacological and Parenteral Therapies

18. Answer: 4

Rationale: The most serious adverse effect of ethambutol is optic neuritis, which requires regular ophthalmologic evaluations with its use. Other adverse effects of ethambutol include gastric distress, confusion, disorientation, and headache.

Cognitive Level: Application
Nursing Process Step: Assessment
NCLEX: Physiological Integrity: Pharmacological and Parenteral Therapies

19. Answer: 4

Rationale: The second-line drugs used to treat TB are typically reserved for drug-resistant cases. These include aminosalicylic acid (PAS), capreomycin, cycloserine, ethionamide, and the aminoglycoside streptomycin. The other drugs listed are first line agents.

Cognitive Level: Application
Nursing Process Step: Analysis
NCLEX: Physiological Integrity: Pharmacological and Parenteral Therapies

20. Answer: 1

Rationale: Dapsone is contraindicated with clients who are hypersensitive to either this drug or sulfonamides. The other drugs do not pose this risk.

Cognitive Level: Application
Nursing Process Step: Assessment
NCLEX: Physiological Integrity: Pharmacological and Parenteral Therapies

CHAPTER 61

Overview of the Immunologic System

1. b; c; d, a, b; c; d, b, a, b, c; d, a; c; d, b
2. B, T, polymorphonuclear leukocytes
3. thymus, body
4. cytotoxic T cells, helper T cells, suppressor T cells
5. interleukin-2
6. first, second
7. Antibodies
8. IgG, complement
9. IgE, mast, basophils
10. humoral
11. passive
12. animal, preservative, antibiotic

CHAPTER 62

Serums, Vaccines, and Other Immunizing Agents

1. P, P, A, A, P, A, P, A, P, A, P, A
2. skin, mucous membranes
3. Active immunity
4. Passive immunity
5. herd immunity
6. microbes, antibodies
7. Toxoids
8. Sera, antitoxins
9. acetaminophen, rest, acetaminophen, sponge baths
10. anaphylactic, 30

11. **Suggested Answer:** Relative safety and merits of immunization versus risk of disease itself should be discussed. Client and/or family should be told that repeat immunization is usually not contraindicated when records are unclear. Unimmunized parents should be identified and probably immunized before their children, especially when TOPV is administered.

Noncompletion of an immunization series may occasionally be prevented if vaccinees or parents know that interruption makes no difference to eventual antibody levels. Copy of schedule enhances compliance. Teach parents or vaccinees to keep careful written records and bring them to each appointment.

12. **Suggested Answer:** Be aware that a crying, wriggling baby or child presents a challenging moving target for injection and therefore must be restrained temporarily. This can often be accomplished just as effectively in the warmth and security of another's arms (parent's arms, if feasible) rather than on a hard table surface. For children old enough to understand, taking out the needle and syringe and explaining that "this may hurt for only a minute" *just* before the actual injection will lessen the fear of pain.

13. **Suggested Answer:** Assess for general contraindications to immunization:
- Current acute or severe febrile illness
- Immunosuppressive therapy in progress or an immunodeficient state
- Recent immune serum globulin (ISG), plasma, or blood transfusions
- Certain malignancies that leave the client susceptible to infection (e.g., leukemias, lymphomas)
- Simultaneous administration of another single live virus, unless proved safe
- Prior unusual or allergic reaction to the same vaccine or a similar vaccine
- Allergy to antibiotics in the vaccine, thimerosal as a preservative, or other constituents

14. **Answer:** 1

Rationale: Local swelling or redness at the injection site is among the most commonly reported adverse effects. Others include drowsiness, irritability, fever, and gastrointestinal (GI) complaints. The pertussis component may increase the likelihood for an encephalopathic or anaphylactic syndrome (including high fever, hypotension/unresponsive state, or seizures), but this risk is probably reduced with the acellular formulation. Infants with inconsolable crying beyond 3 hours should be evaluated for this syndrome as well.

Cognitive Level: Application

Nursing Process Step: Implementation

NCLEX: Physiological Integrity: Pharmacological and Parenteral Therapies

15. **Answer:** 2

Rationale: The nasal formulation of the influenza-virus vaccine (FluMist) is a live vaccine and must be avoided in both immunocompromised individuals and those who have contact with them for a period of 21 days after administration. Influenza virus vaccine live, intranasal contains live attenuated influenza viruses that replicate in the nasopharynx of the recipient and are shed in respiratory secretions. As such, a number of individuals, including health care workers, should not receive the nasal formulation as it may put immunocompromised contacts at risk for the disease. Its use is also limited to otherwise healthy individuals who are between the age of 18 and 49 years.

Cognitive Level: Analysis

Nursing Process Step: Planning

NCLEX: Physiological Integrity: Pharmacological and Parenteral Therapies

16. **Answer:** 4

Rationale: The child with cystic fibrosis has no contraindication to MMR vaccine. Contraindications include pregnancy, prior hypersensitivity to the product, hypersensitivity to egg or egg protein, immunocompromised status or clients receiving immunosuppressant therapy, and clients with tuberculosis.

Cognitive Level: Application

Nursing Process Step: Planning

NCLEX: Physiological Integrity: Pharmacological and Parenteral Therapies

17. **Answer:** 2

Rationale: Hypersensitivity to the inactivated poliovirus vaccine or to any ingredients in the vaccine (including neomycin, streptomycin or polymyxin B) are reasons for avoiding use. Use should be delayed for clients with febrile illness.

Cognitive Level: Application

Nursing Process Step: Analysis

NCLEX: Physiological Integrity: Pharmacological and Parenteral Therapies

18. **Answer:** 2

Rationale: A client's tetanus immunization status must be assessed any time a traumatic wound (especially a puncture wound) is encountered. A booster dose of tetanus toxoid may be in order if the client has not been fully immunized within the past 10 years or if the wound is contaminated and an immunization is older than 5 years of age.

Cognitive Level: Application

Nursing Process Step: Assessment

NCLEX: Physiological Integrity: Pharmacological and Parenteral Therapies

19. **Answer:** 3

Rationale: Because of the risk of anaphylaxis after any immunization, ask parents to keep the baby in the immediate area for up to half an hour for observation of any developing adverse reactions. Be alert for the early symptoms of such a reaction—hives, shock-like appearance, confusion, and hypotension.

Cognitive Level: Application

Nursing Process Step: Implementation

NCLEX: Physiological Integrity: Pharmacological and Parenteral Therapies

20. **Answer:** 1

Rationale: Most products lose their potency at temperatures higher than $35.6°F$ to $46.4°F$ ($2°C$ to $8°C$). Therefore most immunization agents should be stored in a medical refrigerator and replaced immediately after use. They should not be stored near a heat source, on a windowsill, or on a refrigerator door shelf because of unpredictable temperatures.

Cognitive Level: Application

Nursing Process Step: Planning

NCLEX: Physiological Integrity: Pharmacological and Parenteral Therapies

CHAPTER 63

Immunosuppressants and Immunomodulators

1. c, a, b, d
2. Acquired
3. immunosuppression
4. macrophages, cytokines
5. immunotherapy, condition

335

6. chicken pox, herpes zoster
7. opportunistic
8. medical
9. live viral
10. lifelong

11. **Suggested Answer:** It is believed that HIV is a retrovirus that has ribonucleic acid (RNA) in its core. After it binds to CD4+ T-lymphocyte receptor cells, it releases its RNA into the cytoplasm. Reverse transcriptase assists in transcribing the HIV RNA into viral deoxyribonucleic acid (DNA) strands in host body. Thereafter, activation of this DNA results in production of viral substances that infect other CD4+ T-lymphocyte cells. The CD4+ helper cells are destroyed by the virus, which leads to AIDS.

12. **Suggested Answer:** Refer to *Nursing Management: The Immunosuppressed Client* for complete list of possible answers.

13. **Suggested Answer:** Increased hair growth and trembling. With long-term therapy: dose-dependent nephrotoxicity, severe hypertension, lymphomas and other lymphoproliferative-type disorders, gingival hyperplasia.

14. **Answer:** 2
Rationale: When administering the oral solution, use the calibrated measuring device supplied by the manufacturer. Because cyclosporine is a mixture of alcohol and vegetable oil and has an unpleasant taste, mix the Sandimmune oral solution thoroughly with milk, chocolate milk, or orange juice or the Neoral oral solution with apple juice or orange juice at room temperature, and administer it at once. Use a glass container to prevent adherence, and rinse with additional juice or milk to ensure that the entire dose is taken. Wipe the measuring device dry; do not wash it after use.
Cognitive Level: Application
Nursing Process Step: Implementation
NCLEX: Physiological Integrity: Pharmacological and Parenteral Therapies

15. **Answer:** 3
Rationale: Alert the client not to drink grapefruit juice or eat grapefruit; it inhibits the metabolism of cyclosporine, resulting in toxic blood levels of the drug.
Cognitive Level: Application
Nursing Process Step: Implementation
NCLEX: Physiological Integrity: Pharmacological and Parenteral Therapies

16. **Answer:** 4
Rationale: CBCs should be performed weekly during the first month, twice a month for the next 2 to 3 months and monthly thereafter. Notify the prescriber if the leukocyte count is less than 3000/mm³ or if platelets are less than 100,000/mm³; therapy will be reinstituted at reduced dosages when these counts reach an acceptable level, usually after 7 to 10 days.
Cognitive Level: Application
Nursing Process Step: Implementation

NCLEX: Physiological Integrity: Pharmacological and Parenteral Therapies

17. **Answer:** 1
Rationale: The first-dose effect of muromonab-CD3 consists of light-headedness, elevated temperature, chills, nausea, vomiting, diarrhea, headache, dyspnea, chest pain, and tremors and trembling. These effects may be repeated to a lesser degree after the second dose but are rarely encountered with later doses.
Cognitive Level: Application
Nursing Process Step: Implementation
NCLEX: Physiological Integrity: Pharmacological and Parenteral Therapies

18. **Answer:** 1
Rationale: Mycophenolate is given within 72 hours of transplantation. Administer oral doses on an empty stomach, 1 hour before or 2 hours after meals. If the meal is at 08:00, the dose should be given at 07:00 or from 10:00 until an hour before the next meal.
Cognitive Level: Application
Nursing Process Step: Planning
NCLEX: Physiological Integrity: Pharmacological and Parenteral Therapies

19. **Answer:** 3
Rationale: The use of tacrolimus is contraindicated for clients with hypersensitivity to the drug or to HCO-60 polyoxyl hydrogenated castor oil (which is contained in the injection solution).
Cognitive Level: Application
Nursing Process Step: Planning
NCLEX: Physiological Integrity: Pharmacological and Parenteral Therapies

20. **Answer:** 4
Rationale: Because of the risk of anaphylaxis after any immunization, be alert for the early symptoms—hives, shock-like appearance, confusion, and hypotension. Teach clients or their parents how to recognize and differentiate between anticipated side effects and serious adverse reactions. Acetaminophen may be taken for the not uncommon aches, local pain and swelling, or mild temperature elevations, which may occur within 24 hours.
Cognitive Level: Analysis
Nursing Process Step: Assessment
NCLEX: Physiological Integrity: Pharmacological and Parenteral Therapies

---

CHAPTER 64

Overview of the Integumentary System

1. See Figure 64-1 in the textbook.
2. skin, integument
3. epidermis
4. melanin
5. epidermis, diffusion
6. dermis

336

Answer Key   Copyright © 2006, 2001 Mosby, Inc. All rights reserved.

7. Sebaceous
8. eccrine, sweat
9. apocrine
10. loss, conservation
11. fluid, electrolytes, fat, vitamin D, absorption
12. emotional, depression

CHAPTER 65

Dermatologic Drugs

1. b, e, c, b, a, d, f, c, a, c, b, f, e, e, d, e, d
2. physical, personal, family, drug, laboratory, biopsy
3. basal cell, trunk
4. Rosacea
5. weeping, oozing
6. protective, drying
7. sore, wet, elbow, knee
8. oatmeal, starch, gelatin
9. Emollients
10. protectants

11. **Suggested Answer:** Baths, soaps, solutions and lotions, cleansers, emollients, skin protectants, wet dressings and soaks, rubs, liniments

12. **Suggested Answer:** Impaired skin integrity; altered comfort related to pain, burning, or itching of affected areas; risk for infection related to open skin areas; self-care deficits related to location of affected areas; deficient knowledge deficit related to new or altered dermatologic therapy; disturbed self-concept related to perceived and actual disfigurement of affected areas

13. **Suggested Answer:** A skin reaction that makes the client uncomfortable or has an unsightly appearance may be because of a drug sensitivity, allergy, infection, emotional conflict, genetic disease (e.g., atopic eczema, psoriasis), hormonal imbalance, or degenerative disease. Sometimes the cause is unknown.

14. **Answer:** 2
Rationale: The client should apply sunscreen and limit exposure on overcast or cloudy days. Very little UV radiation is blocked by cloud cover, although the infrared radiation that contributes to the sensation of heat is usually reduced. This heat reduction might give a false sense of security against sunburn. Clients should also use a sunscreen SPF of at least 12 to 30 daily, apply the sunscreen to exposed areas 15 to 30 minutes before sun exposure, and reapply every 2 hours or after activity that could result in removal of sunscreen, such as excessive sweating, swimming, or towel drying.
Cognitive Level: Analysis
Nursing Process Step: Evaluation
NCLEX: Physiological Integrity: Pharmacological and Parenteral Therapies

15. **Answer:** 3
Rationale: Instruct the client to use a finger cot or rubber glove when applying the ointment to prevent autoinoculation to other sites. It is applied as soon as symptoms of herpes infection begin. Advise an annual or more frequent Papanicolaou (Pap) smear, because women with herpes genitalis are more likely to develop cervical cancer. Advise the client to avoid sexual activity if either partner has active lesions.
Cognitive Level: Application
Nursing Process Step: Implementation
NCLEX: Physiological Integrity: Pharmacological and Parenteral Therapies

16. **Answer:** 2
Rationale: Topical corticosteroids are generally indicated for the relief of inflammatory and pruritic dermatoses, including those of atopic dermatitis. Conditions that would be worsened by the application of topical corticosteroids include acne vulgaris, ulcers, scabies, warts, molluscum contagiosum, fungal infections, balanitis.
Cognitive Level: Application
Nursing Process Step: Analysis
NCLEX: Physiological Integrity: Pharmacological and Parenteral Therapies

17. **Answer:** 2
Rationale: Review the client's medication regimen. Isotretinoin should not be used concurrently with acitretin, oral tretinoin, or vitamin A, because additive toxic effects may result. The other responses are incorrect.
Cognitive Level: Application
Nursing Process Step: Implementation
NCLEX: Physiological Integrity: Pharmacological and Parenteral Therapies

18. **Answer:** 3
Rationale: Because mafenide and its metabolite are strong carbonic anhydrase inhibitors, acidosis (metabolic) may occur and is usually compensated by hyperventilation. Observe the client carefully for any signs of respiratory alkalosis. If rapid or labored respirations occur, the ointment should be washed off the wound.
Cognitive Level: Application
Nursing Process Step: Planning
NCLEX: Physiological Integrity: Pharmacological and Parenteral Therapies

19. **Answer:** 2
Rationale: Lindane is used to treat both scabies and lice infestations in adults and children over the age of one month when other therapies are not effective or tolerated. Permethrin is used to treat scabies in adults and children. Crotamiton is indicated for the treatment of scabies in adults. Malathion is used to treat pediculosis in adults and children older than the age of 2 years.
Cognitive Level: Application

Nursing Process Step: Analysis
NCLEX: Physiological Integrity: Pharmacological and Parenteral Therapies

20. **Answer:** 4
Rationale: Monitor for signs and symptoms of infection (e.g., cellulitis, pneumonia, abscess, sepsis, bronchitis, gastroenteritis, aseptic meningitis, Legionnaire disease, vertebral osteomyelitis). Obtain monthly platelet counts to determine if thrombocytopenia develops. WBCs increase with therapy and take about 8 weeks to normalize following the discontinuation of efalizumab therapy. Psoriasis lesions should begin to diminish by week 4.
Cognitive Level: Application
Nursing Process Step: Assessment
NCLEX: Physiological Integrity: Pharmacological and Parenteral Therapies

CHAPTER 66

Debriding Agents

1. c, d, b, e, a
2. Cleansing, debridement, dressing
3. cleansing
4. moisture, pressure ulcers
5. debilitated, comatose, immobilized, paralyzed
6. Vacuum-assisted closure
7. causes, nutrition, pressure, friction
8. stage, wound bed
9. osteomyelitis
10. -ase

11. **Suggested Answer:** General ones include delayed healing; increased risk of bacterial infection; allergic or sensitivity reactions. With collagenase: transient erythema. With fibrinolysin and desoxyribonuclease: allergic reactions in persons sensitive to bovine sources, mercury compounds, or chloramphenicol. With sutilains: mild transient pain, local paresthesia, bleeding, transient dermatitis.

12. **Suggested Answer:**
Stage I or II: silicone spray, transparent or hydrocolloidal dressing
Stage III: wet to moist dressings, enzymatic debridement, hydrocolloidal dressing
Stage IV: wet to moist dressings, enzymatic debridement, surgical debridement

13. **Suggested Answer:**
    - Change position frequently (every 1 to 2 hours day and night) for pressure relief.
    - Maintain a clean, dry, and wrinkle-free bed.
    - Provide active and passive exercise to increase muscle and skin tone and to improve vascularity, or use a whirlpool for hydrotherapy.
    - Position the client with pillows and pads; do not exceed a 30-degree elevation of the head.
    - Use hydrofloat devices, silica gel pads, polystyrene, and convoluted foam pads and heel protectors to reduce pressure.
    - Use an alternating pressure mattress pad covered with one layer of sheet to promote circulation and to reduce the occurrence of tissue ischemia.
    - Provide meticulous skin hygiene, with frequent inspections for abnormal alterations.
    - Keep skin dry and clear of urine and fecal contamination, because maceration from moisture promotes tissue breakdown and predisposes to infection.
    - Maintain nutritional support for a positive nitrogen balance, tissue turgor, and adequate fluid intake with 3800 to 4600 cal/24 hours and a diet high in protein, vitamins, minerals, and trace elements.

14. **Answer:** 3
Rationale: Saline solutions are considered safe and effective in cleaning most pressure ulcers. Unless prescribed by the practitioner, avoid the use of povidone-iodine, iodophor, Dakin's solution, acetic acid, and hydrogen peroxide, as they may be cytotoxic (e.g., toxic to fibroblasts) and interfere with the granulation process.
Cognitive Level: Application
Nursing Process Step: Planning
NCLEX: Physiological Integrity: Pharmacological and Parenteral Therapies

15. **Answer:** 4
Rationale: Proteolytic enzymes are used for chemical debridement; they digest or liquefy necrotic tissue. Their use is appropriate for uninfected necrotic sites and for clients unable to tolerate surgical intervention. The enzyme preparation should be discontinued when granulation tissue is evident or if bleeding occurs during gentle cleansing.
Cognitive Level: Analysis
Nursing Process Step: Assessment
NCLEX: Physiological Integrity: Pharmacological and Parenteral Therapies

16. **Answer:** 4
Rationale: A transient erythema has been reported as a cutaneous reaction on the wound surface or the area adjacent to the lesion. Applying a protectant (e.g., zinc oxide paste) may prevent this reaction around the lesion. Nitrofurazone inactivates collagenase and the other substances will not help.
Cognitive Level: Application
Nursing Process Step: Implementation
NCLEX: Physiological Integrity: Pharmacological and Parenteral Therapies

17. **Answer:** 1
Rationale: Cleanse the wound area of debris by gentle irrigation with sterile normal saline. Pat the ulcer dry with a sterile gauze pad. If infection is present, apply a topical antibacterial agent (e.g., neomycin, bacitracin-polymyxin B solution or powder) directly to the

ulcer surface before the collagenase. Collagenase should be applied once daily.

Cognitive Level: Application

Nursing Process Step: Implementation

NCLEX: Physiological Integrity: Pharmacological and Parenteral Therapies

18. **Answer:** 3

Rationale: The average time for complete debridement of dermal ulcers and decubiti with collagenase is approximately 11 days. This time permits debridement of necrotic tissue and the establishment of granulation tissue. The other timeframes are not the average.

Cognitive Level: Application

Nursing Process Step: Implementation

NCLEX: Physiological Integrity: Pharmacological and Parenteral Therapies

19. **Answer:** 3

Rationale: Obtain the client's sensitivity history, because allergic reactions have been observed in clients who are sensitive to bovine source materials or mercury compounds (thimerosal, a mercury derivative, is used as a preservative in the ointment base of Elase).

Cognitive Level: Application

Nursing Process Step: Assessment

NCLEX: Physiological Integrity: Pharmacological and Parenteral Therapies

20. **Answer:** 2

Rationale: Flexible hydroactive dressings and granules are available as a sheet dressing. They provide local management of venous stasis ulcers, ulcers secondary to arterial insufficiency, diabetes mellitus, trauma, pressure ulcers, and superficial wounds. The granule form is for the local management of exudating dermal ulcers in association with the dressings. The use of flexible hydroactive dressings should be avoided with the following dermal conditions: tissue of muscle, tendon, or bone; ulcers with infection (tuberculosis, syphilis, or deep fungal infections); and active vasculitis (periarteritis nodosa, systemic lupus erythematosus, and cryoglobulinemia).

Cognitive Level: Analysis

Nursing Process Step: Analysis

NCLEX: Physiological Integrity: Pharmacological and Parenteral Therapies

CHAPTER 67

Vitamins and Minerals

1.

Vitamin	Other names or chemical names
A	retinal, the carotenes
B_1	thiamine
B_2	riboflavin
B_3	niacin
B_6	pyridoxine
B_9	folic acid
B_{12}	cyanocobalamin
C	ascorbic acid, sodium ascorbate
D	calcifediol, Calcitriol, dihydrotachysterol, or ergocalciferol
E	α-tocopherol

2. fluids, regular, balanced
3. atherosclerosis, cancer, osteoporosis
4. Vitamins
5. 170, carbohydrate
6. food, dietary supplements
7. fractures, bone density
8. Homocystinemia
9. age, health
10. A, D

11. **Suggested Answer:** Recommended daily allowance; the amount of a nutrient that is recommended each day in the diet to promote health.

12. **Suggested Answer:** Alert client that iron preparations cause black stools, which are medically insignificant. However, client should report other symptoms of internal blood loss. Instruct client to maintain diet rich in sources of iron such as liver, green leafy vegetables, potatoes, dried peas and beans, dried fruit, and enriched flour, bread, and cereals.

13. **Suggested Answer:** The general nursing diagnosis for clients with vitamin and mineral deficiencies is imbalanced nutrition: less than body requirements. Depending on the type and severity of the deficiency and the nature of the signs and symptoms, other nursing diagnoses or collaborative problems are also relevant.

14. **Answer:** 4

Rationale: Vitamin A deficiency results in night blindness, xerophthalmia, keratomalacia, and skin lesions.

Cognitive Level: Application

Nursing Process Step: Assessment

NCLEX: Physiological Integrity: Pharmacological and Parenteral Therapies

15. **Answer:** 1

Rationale: Increased bleeding (e.g., ecchymoses, hematuria, gastrointestinal bleeding) is a symptom of vitamin K deficiency. It can be treated with increased intake of vitamin K by dietary supplement or by increasing intake of liver or green leafy vegetables.

Cognitive Level: Analysis

Nursing Process Step: Assessment

NCLEX: Physiological Integrity: Pharmacological and Parenteral Therapies

16. **Answer:** 2

Rationale: The administration of vitamin D is contraindicated in clients with hypercalcemia, hypervitaminosis D, malabsorption syndrome, or abnormal sensitivity to the toxic effects of vitamin D.

Cognitive Level: Application

Nursing Process Step: Implementation

NCLEX: Physiological Integrity: Pharmacological and Parenteral Therapies

17. **Answer:** 3

Rationale: Thiamine is used to prevent and treat thiamine deficiencies that can result in beriberi or Wernicke encephalopathy. It is routinely used for clients with nutritional deficiencies (e.g., recent history of alcohol abuse) prior to administration of carbohydrates (e.g., IV dextrose solutions).

Cognitive Level: Application
Nursing Process Step: Analysis
NCLEX: Physiological Integrity: Pharmacological and Parenteral Therapies

18. **Answer:** 4

Rationale: Cyanocobalamin is used to treat pernicious anemia (caused by a lack of intrinsic factor) and to prevent and treat vitamin B_{12} deficiency caused by malabsorption or strict vegetarianism. Vitamin B_{12} deficiency can lead to macrocytic megaloblastic anemia and irreversible neurologic damage.

Cognitive Level: Application
Nursing Process Step: Analysis
NCLEX: Physiological Integrity: Pharmacological and Parenteral Therapies

19. **Answer:** 2

Rationale: Ascorbic acid is used to prevent and treat vitamin C deficiency (scurvy) and, in larger doses, for urine acidification.

Cognitive Level: Application
Nursing Process Step: Implementation
NCLEX: Physiological Integrity: Pharmacological and Parenteral Therapies

20. **Answer:** 3

Rationale: To minimize staining of the flesh, use a separate needle to withdraw the drug from the vial. It is recommended that iron dextran be administered into the muscle mass of the upper outer quadrant of the buttock using the Z-track technique and a 2- to 3-inch, 19- or 20-gauge needle. The preparation should never be injected into the upper arm or any other exposed area because of the possibility that it will stain the skin dark brown.

Cognitive Level: Application
Nursing Process Step: Implementation
NCLEX: Physiological Integrity: Pharmacological and Parenteral Therapies

CHAPTER 68

Fluids and Electrolytes

1. c — e, f — d — a — b — g — e — b, f — a — h
2. Potassium (K+), magnesium (Mg++)
3. Sodium (Na+), chloride (Cl–), bicarbonate (HCO3–)
4. fluids, electrolytes, acid-base
5. 45, 75
6. excess, overhydration
7. thirst, decrease, dryness
8. kidneys, urine
9. osmosis
10. Osmolality
11. **Suggested Answer:** See the table below.

Category	Solution	Use
Hydrating solution	Dextrose 2.5%, 5%, or higher in water; dextrose in 0.2% or 0.5% normal saline	To hydrate or prevent dehydration; to assess kidney status before electrolyte therapy; to help increase diuresis in dehydrated individuals
Isotonic solution	Isotonic chloride; Ringer's injection; lactated Ringer's injection	To replace extracellular fluid losses in which chloride loss ≥ sodium loss; isotonic or normal saline: before and after blood transfusion; isotonic sodium chloride: to treat metabolic alkalosis
Maintenance solution	Plasma-Lyte; Normosol	To replace daily electrolyte and extracellular needs and water; to replace electrolytes and water loss from severe vomiting or diarrhea

12. **Suggested Answer:** c, b, a, c, c, b, c, a

13. **Suggested Answer:** Ensure that only health care providers, fully prepared in electronic infusion device (EID) technology, be authorized to set up, adjust, or remove IV administration sets. Check that infusion is not running when pump is removed. Check or recalculate infusion rate. Apply visible labels to EIDs that do not prevent free flow to alert staff. Limit use of one type of EID to each unit. Use only protected EIDs in critical care units or with critical care drugs.

14. **Answer:** 3

Rationale: Isotonic or normal saline (0.9% sodium chloride) is the preferred agent to be used before and after a blood transfusion as this avoids dextrose related hemolysis of red blood cells.

Cognitive Level: Application
Nursing Process Step: Implementation
NCLEX: Physiological Integrity: Pharmacological and Parenteral Therapies

15. **Answer:** 3
Rationale: Hydrating solutions include various concentrations of dextrose solutions and 0.45% sodium chloride. The other solutions do not contain the correct amount of sodium chloride.
Cognitive Level: Application
Nursing Process Step: Planning
NCLEX: Physiological Integrity: Pharmacological and Parenteral Therapies

16. **Answer:** 4
Rationale: For adults with life-threatening hypokalemia-induced dysrhythmias or those with a serum potassium level less than 2.0 mEq/L, a more concentrated potassium solution (60 mEq/L can be infused at a rate not exceeding 40 mEq/hour) accompanied by continuous cardiac monitoring.
Cognitive Level: Application
Nursing Process Step: Planning
NCLEX: Physiological Integrity: Pharmacological and Parenteral Therapies

17. **Answer:** 3
Rationale: Liquid preparations are generally preferred for oral therapy, and most contain 10, 20, or 40 mEq of potassium/15 mL. These preparations must be diluted with fruit juice or water before ingestion and taken after meals with a full glass of water to minimize GI irritation and mask taste.
Cognitive Level: Application
Nursing Process Step: Implementation
NCLEX: Physiological Integrity: Pharmacological and Parenteral Therapies

18. **Answer:** 2
Rationale: To improve the solubility of calcium carbonate tablets, especially in achlorhydric conditions, it is recommended the tablets be taken with meals, when acid secretion is highest. Avoid taking the tablets on an empty stomach or at night, because acid secretions are minimal at these times.
Cognitive Level: Application
Nursing Process Step: Implementation
NCLEX: Physiological Integrity: Pharmacological and Parenteral Therapies

19. **Answer:** 3
Rationale: Pulmonary edema occurs when the circulatory system is overloaded with fluids and is evidenced by dyspnea on exertion, orthopnea, and coughing. Tachycardia, tachypnea, dependent crackles, neck vein distention, and diastolic (S_3) gallop may be heard. Slow the IV infusion to a "keep open" (KVO, keep vein open) rate to provide access for emergency medications, which also removes the cause of the symptoms. Pulmonary edema is considered to be a medical emergency; the prescriber needs to be notified

as soon as the client's fluid volume excess is noted after safeguarding the client.
Cognitive Level: Analysis
Nursing Process Step: Implementation
NCLEX: Physiological Integrity: Pharmacological and Parenteral Therapies

20. **Answer:** 1
Rationale: A dry, furrowed tongue is a sign of hypertonic dehydration. Vomiting and abdominal cramps are signs of hypotonic dehydration. An increased pulse rate can occur with all forms of dehydration.
Cognitive Level: Application
Nursing Process Step: Evaluation
NCLEX: Physiological Integrity: Pharmacological and Parenteral Therapies

CHAPTER 69

Enteral and Parenteral Nutrition

1. g, f, h, a, d, b, e, c
2. protein/amino acids, carbohydrates, fats, vitamins, minerals
3. lymphocyte, albumin, transferrin
4. Nasogastric, nasoenteric
5. Dumping, osmotic
6. modular, monomeric, oligomeric, polymeric, disease-specific
7. residual volume
8. 10, central venous
9. Hyperglycemia
10. trace elements, minerals

11. **Suggested Answer:** Refer to the section in the chapter on *Nursing Management of Parenteral Nutrition Therapy* for full coverage of possible answers.

12. **Suggested Answer:** Preparation of client and family member should begin 5 to 7 days before discharge. Teach signs of incorrect tube placement and insertion and removal if needed. Written and verbal instructions on possible complications are also necessary. Understanding of procedure, rationale, and expectations of tube feedings can aid in active client participation and greater satisfaction.

13. **Suggested Answer:** Catheter seeding from bloodborne or distant infection; contamination of catheter entrance site during insertion or long-term catheter placement; solution contamination

14. **Answer:** 2
Rationale: Based on current research, the University of Virginia Health System has developed the following guidelines for initiation of enteral nutrition: full strength (all products except 2 cal/mL) at 50 mL/hour and increase by 25 mL every 8 hours to goal rate. A 2.0 cal/mL is started at 25 mL/hour. The final goal rate depends on the client's caloric requirements and GI comfort.

341

Cognitive Level: Application
Nursing Process Step: Planning
NCLEX: Physiological Integrity: Pharmacological and Parenteral Therapies

15. **Answer:** 3
Rationale: Oligomeric formulations are chemically defined formulations that require minimum digestion and produce minimal residue in the colon. These formulations are indicated for clients with partial bowel obstruction, inflammatory bowel disease, radiation enteritis, bowel fistulas, and short bowel syndrome.
Cognitive Level: Comprehension
Nursing Process Step: Planning
NCLEX: Physiological Integrity: Pharmacological and Parenteral Therapies

16. **Answer:** 1
Rationale: Nursing care for the client receiving enteral feeding consists of several interventions. Elevate the head of the bed at least 30 to 45 degrees during and for 1 hour after the feeding to reduce the risk for aspiration. Warm the feeding to room temperature before administering. Record the name, volume, and strength of the formula and duration and rate (mL/hr) of feeding. Monitor intake and output totals daily. Every 8 hours, chart the volume of formula administered separately from water or other oral intake.
Cognitive Level: Application
Nursing Process Step: Implementation
NCLEX: Physiological Integrity: Pharmacological and Parenteral Therapies

17. **Answer:** 1
Rationale: PPN is considered a temporary measure to provide an appropriate nitrogen balance in clients who have mild deficits or are NPO with a slightly elevated metabolic rate, such as when oral food consumption will not be instituted for 5 or more days.

Central hyperalimentation is used primarily for clients with nonfunctioning GI tracts, those that should not use the oral route for more than 7 days, or conditions of short bowel syndrome, acute pancreatitis, enteric or enterocutaneous fistulas, active inflammatory process, GI tract obstruction, major trauma, or burns.
Cognitive Level: Application
Nursing Process Step: Analysis
NCLEX: Physiological Integrity: Pharmacological and Parenteral Therapies

18. **Answer:** 2
Rationale: Blood glucose levels are determined every 6 to 8 hours for hypo/hyperglycemia until the client's glucose is stable and then at least every day. The client in the question should have a blood glucose level measured within 8 hours, or 18:00.
Cognitive Level: Application
Nursing Process Step: Planning
NCLEX: Physiological Integrity: Pharmacological and Parenteral Therapies

19. **Answer:** 3
Rationale: Clients with cardiac insufficiency need to be watched closely for excess fluid volume while undergoing nutritional therapy with parenteral nutrition. This could be evidenced by increasing pulse, intake largely greater than output, weight gain of more than 1 to 2 pounds in 24 to 48 hours, distended neck veins, and crackles in the lungs. A temperature of 99 is insignificant, although a fever could indicate infection.
Cognitive Level: Analysis
Nursing Process Step: Assessment
NCLEX: Physiological Integrity: Pharmacological and Parenteral Therapies

20. **Answer:** 3
Rationale: It is critical to record daily the following data and to notify the prescriber of abnormal values such as blood glucose in excess of 200 mg/100 mL or abnormal serum electrolytes. The sodium and BUN are within normal limits, and the potassium is low (3.5 to 5.1 mEq/L).
Cognitive Level: Analysis
Nursing Process Step: Assessment
NCLEX: Physiological Integrity: Pharmacological and Parenteral Therapies

CHAPTER 70

Antiseptics, Disinfectants, and Sterilants

1. b, f, h, e, a, d, c, g
2. nosocomial, hospital
3. surgical asepsis, medical asepsis
4. autoclaving or steam under pressure
5. 10, spores, hepatitis
6. handwashing
7. therapeutic, tissues, healing
8. Germicides
9. microorganisms, hypersensitivity
10. Triclosan

11. **Suggested Answer:** They may change the structure of the protein of the microbial cell; lower the surface tension of the aqueous medium of the parasitic cell; interfere with some metabolic processes of the microbial cell in such ways as to interfere with the cell's ability to survive and multiply.

12. **Suggested Answer:** Do not bandage or tape areas treated with tincture of iodine; if treated with povidone-iodine, cover dressing may be applied. If irritation develops, wash the skin. Artificially elevated blood glucose determinations have been noted when povidone-iodine swabs were used for skin preparation. Soap and water cleansing of fingertips before skin puncture for blood glucose monitoring by some reagent strips is recommended. Iodophors will stain only starched linen or clothing. Tinctures and solutions of iodine may stain more freely.

13. **Suggested Answer:** Store in tightly capped, amber containers; solutions in containers should be discarded frequently and fresh solutions used. Bubbling action makes hydrogen peroxide useful for removing mucous secretions from equipment. Do not leave paper cups of hydrogen peroxide in client's reach, because it may be mistaken for water. Keep these compounds secured and out of reach of children.

14. **Answer:** 3
Rationale: Hexachlorophene is a toxic agent that can be absorbed through the skin, causing gastric symptoms and central nervous system (CNS) toxicity. Daily topical use on newborns or application several times daily to the skin or vagina in adults has resulted in confusion, diplopia, lethargy, seizures, respiratory arrest, and death. Hexachlorophene is usually not used routinely or recommended for use in bathing infants or pregnant or hypersensitive persons. Dermatitis and photosensitivity have also been reported.
Cognitive Level: Application
Nursing Process Step: Assessment
NCLEX: Physiological Integrity: Pharmacological and Parenteral Therapies

15. **Answer:** 2
Rationale: The expected outcome of silver compound therapy is that the client's mucous membrane will be moist, pink, and intact without drainage or other signs of inflammation or infection.
Cognitive Level: Analysis
Nursing Process Step: Evaluation
NCLEX: Physiological Integrity: Pharmacological and Parenteral Therapies

16. **Answer:** 1
Rationale: Rash, pruritus, and local edema are the most common adverse effects of povidone-iodine. Ingested orally, it is highly toxic and sodium thiosulfate is used as an antidote.
Cognitive Level: Application
Nursing Process Step: Assessment
NCLEX: Physiological Integrity: Pharmacological and Parenteral Therapies

17. **Answer:** 3
Rationale: Hydrogen peroxide topical solution is used to irrigate suppurating wounds and some extensive traumatic wounds, and disinfect soft contact lens. It should be used in areas in which the oxygen can escape and therefore should not be instilled into closed body spaces or abscesses. It is not recommended for use in pressure ulcers, because it and many other antiseptic agents are considered to be cytotoxic to normal tissues.
Cognitive Level: Application
Nursing Process Step: Implementation
NCLEX: Physiological Integrity: Pharmacological and Parenteral Therapies

18. **Answer:** 2
Rationale: As a hand wash, Hibiclens solution is applied, water added, and friction applied for 15 seconds. Skin wounds should be washed gently with Hibiclens and rinsed. For surgical scrubs, a brush or sponge is used to scrub the hands and forearms with approximately 5 mL Hibiclens for 3 minutes without water. After the hands and forearms are rinsed, the washing is repeated for 3 more minutes.
Cognitive Level: Application
Nursing Process Step: Implementation
NCLEX: Physiological Integrity: Pharmacological and Parenteral Therapies

19. **Answer:** 4
Rationale: In view of the highly questionable efficacy of surface-active agents, especially benzalkonium chloride, question an order or a suggestion to use them as antiseptics or disinfectants. Suggest the substitution of an iodophor, alcohol, or other compound.
Cognitive Level: Application
Nursing Process Step: Implementation
NCLEX: Physiological Integrity: Pharmacological and Parenteral Therapies

20. **Answer:** 1
Rationale: Various acids have been used as antiseptics or as cauterizing agents; of these, acetic acid (vinegar) is the most commonly used, especially in community health nursing, because of its practicality, availability, and low cost.
Cognitive Level: Application
Nursing Process Step: Implementation
NCLEX: Physiological Integrity: Pharmacological and Parenteral Therapies

CHAPTER 71

Diagnostic Agents

1.

```
S N O I T A C I D N I  G L R B E G G N G H
D E S S E R P P U S O N U M M I  C N N I U
L R U M B F N E G T N E O R T F Q I D U U
S G P S X Y V T D C M Y I C H A X N Q Y L
M X O C F Y Z A A O T H Z W G F J O B D T
I M K R Q Z B W N N R P Z N K R R I E D R
R L N E C R V X T T E A Y N J G V T M I A
P A Y E B N Q V I R A R R B A B E C B A S
R T D N X X T D H A T G G N U C P N F G O
A O S I W U M W I S M O S Y T E I U L N N
D M R N O Z M D S T E I R I I A N F U O O
I O T G U A M R T C N G O L K D E H S S G
O G C W T R C V A N T N M D A F P I H T R
N R N B V Y S T M D V A U J K F H T I I A
U A S U S A G I I T L T C S S R W N C P
C P I B X Q G W N V L O N G H X I U G S H
L H N X S D R R E G E H P Y J X N Q E A Y
I Y G F S R F K S O F C C A Z A E R P J H
D A Q E X Z F F W G K L E F Q M J U M B G
E U R A D I O P H A R M A C E U T I C A L
S X V I S U A L I Z A T I O N E B H E H
```

2. Diagnostic agents
3. radiograph examinations, radiopaque
4. iodine
5. barium sulfate, hydrosol gum
6. bowel perforations, fistulas
7. angiography
8. scintigraph
9. Radionuclides
10. half-life

11. **Suggested Answer:** Refer to Table 71-4 in the textbook for a complete listing.

12. **Suggested Answer:** Refer to Table 71-2 in the textbook for a complete listing.

13. **Suggested Answer:** Refer to *Intervention* section under *Radiopaque Agents* for answer.

14. **Answer:** 1
Rationale: A client with a history of allergy is at twice the risk of reaction to contrast media although, paradoxically, these are not true hypersensitivity reactions. Obtain an allergy history, and pay particular attention to any previous reactions to contrast media or iodine-containing foods (e.g., shellfish or iodized table salt).
Cognitive Level: Application
Nursing Process Step: Assessment
NCLEX: Physiological Integrity: Pharmacological and Parenteral Therapies

15. **Answer:** 3
Rationale: Barium sulfate may cause constipation if allowed to remain in the colon. For this reason, clients may benefit from a laxative to clear barium from the bowel.
Cognitive Level: Application
Nursing Process Step: Implementation
NCLEX: Physiological Integrity: Pharmacological and Parenteral Therapies

16. **Answer:** 1
Rationale: The most commonly reported adverse effects are nausea or flushing, with feelings of warmth over the abdomen and chest. Rare adverse effects include

cerebral hematomas, hemodynamic alterations, sinus bradycardia, transient ECG changes, ventricular fibrillation, and petechiae.

Cognitive Level: Application
Nursing Process Step: Implementation
NCLEX: Physiological Integrity: Pharmacological and Parenteral Therapies

17. **Answer:** 1
Rationale: Secondary effects of histamine include flushing, dizziness, headache, dyspnea, asthma, urticaria, hypotension or hypertension, tachycardia, gastrointestinal distress, and seizures.
Cognitive Level: Application
Nursing Process Step: Planning
NCLEX: Physiological Integrity: Pharmacological and Parenteral Therapies

18. **Answer:** 3
Rationale: Antigens applied topically or intradermally cause antigen-antibody reactions that may be manifested by a local inflammatory response at the test site. The test site is assessed after a prescribed time interval. A positive response is indicated by the presence of erythema and induration (a firm lump under the skin).
Cognitive Level: Analysis
Nursing Process Step: Evaluation
NCLEX: Physiological Integrity: Pharmacological and Parenteral Therapies

19. **Answer:** 4
Rationale: Clients who are immunosuppressed because of cancer chemotherapy or radiation treatments, malnutrition, debilitation, or congenital or acquired immunodeficiency syndrome (AIDS) may demonstrate no response (anergy) when tested with a prescribed battery of antigen challenges. These clients are extremely vulnerable to infection and may need metabolic support and precautions to avoid infection.
Cognitive Level: Analysis
Nursing Process Step: Analysis
NCLEX: Physiological Integrity: Pharmacological and Parenteral Therapies

20. **Answer:** 3
Rationale: Intradermal injections are commonly administered on the ventral surface of the forearm. Use a tuberculin syringe with a 25- to 27-gauge needle. The dose is 5 U.S. units, or 0.05 mL. Inject intradermally with the needle nearly parallel to the skin surface, making certain that the needle does not penetrate deeper into subcutaneous tissue. Stop inserting the needle as soon as the tip of the needle, with its bevel up, has entered the skin but is still visible. Inject the antigen with steady pressure. A correctly administered intradermal injection will immediately raise a small, colorless bleb or lump.
Cognitive Level: Application
Nursing Process Step: Implementation
NCLEX: Physiological Integrity: Pharmacological and Parenteral Therapies

CHAPTER 72

Poisons and Antidotes

1. d, a, e, b, f, c
2. poisons; action, effects; detection; diagnosis, treatment
3. relatively small; death; serious bodily harm
4. clusters of signs associated with common drug poisonings or overdoses
5. emetic; bittersweet
6. opioid emetic; reflex action of the vomiting center in the brainstem
7. washing out of the stomach
8. emesis; lavage; an absorbent
9. organophosphate intoxication; Salivation; Lacrimation; Urination; Defecation; Gastrointestinal distress; Emesis
10. central nervous system, irritation, aspirated

11. **Suggested Answer:** Attain quick assessment and history to determine extent of impairments or particular susceptibilities. Observe vital signs and level of consciousness.
Implementation may include turning, deep breathing, coughing, suctioning, and auscultation to demonstrate need for chest radiograph, suctioning, tracheostomy, endotracheal intubation, blood gas determinations, supplemental oxygen, and a respirator/ventilator.
Position victim to prevent aspiration; attend mouth care promptly after emesis. Moderate amounts of plain water by mouth may dilute or effectively inactivate many ingested poisons.

12. **Suggested Answer:** Activated charcoal should not be used in cases of intestinal obstruction or GI perforation. It is not effective for management of acid or alkali, cyanide, organic solvent, iron, ethanol, methanol, or lithium poisonings.

13. **Suggested Answer:** Antidotes work by any of the following mechanisms: (1) antagonizing or stimulating receptor sites that have been rendered hyperfunctional or dysfunctional by the poison, (2) interfering with enzyme inhibition, (3) administering the product of metabolism that has been interfered with, (4) inhibiting the biotransformation of a substance to a poisonous metabolite, (5) giving an agent that inactivates the toxic product, (6) chelation (forming highly stable complexes, tying up the substance—usually a heavy metal such as iron), and (7) producing immunotherapy—the use of antidrug antibodies to bind and inactivate drugs (e.g., severe digoxin poisoning reversed with sheep digoxin-specific antibodies).

14. **Answer:** 2
Rationale: *Grade I.* The individual is asleep but is easily aroused and reacts to painful stimuli. Deep tendon reflexes are present, pupils are normal and reactive, ocular movements are present, and vital signs are stable.
Grade II. Pain response is absent, deep tendon reflexes are depressed, pupils are slightly dilated but reactive, and vital signs are stable.

Grade III. Deep tendon and pupillary reflexes are absent, and vital signs are stable.

Grade IV. Respiration and circulation are depressed.

Cognitive Level: Application

Nursing Process Step: Assessment

NCLEX: Physiological Integrity: Pharmacological and Parenteral Therapies

15. **Answer:** 2

Rationale: The proper management of poisoning includes the following:

- Call poison control immediately for any event in which toxicity is suspected or possible. Do not wait for symptoms to appear.
- Always call the poison control center before undertaking treatment.
- Never induce vomiting unless you are instructed to do so.
- Do not rely on the label's antidote information, because it may be out of date. Instead call poison control.
- If you need to go to an emergency department, take the tablets, capsules, container, and/or label with you.

Cognitive Level: Application

Nursing Process Step: Implementation

NCLEX: Physiological Integrity: Pharmacological and Parenteral Therapies

16. **Answer:** 4

Rationale: Induction of vomiting is contraindicated in the following situations: infants up to 1 year of age; mental status changes or obtunded states in which excessive sedation or comatose state may occur; seizure activity; absent gag and cough reflexes; presence of hematemesis; ingestion of substances inducing seizures, sharp objects (e.g., glass, nails) along with the toxic substance, CNS poisons which produce sedation (numerous agents) or require rapid removal by lavage (e.g., camphor, strychnine), or irritants which may cause further injury on emesis or if aspirated (acids, alkalis, or petroleum distillates, such as kerosene, gasoline, or paint thinner).

Cognitive Level: Application

Nursing Process Step: Analysis

NCLEX: Physiological Integrity: Pharmacological and Parenteral Therapies

17. **Answer:** 1

Rationale: Opioids cause constricted, pinpoint pupils. Antihistamines and cocaine cause pupil dilation. Salicylates do not affect pupil size.

Cognitive Level: Application

Nursing Process Step: Analysis

NCLEX: Physiological Integrity: Pharmacological and Parenteral Therapies

18. **Answer:** 3

Rationale: Possible antidotes to cyanide include amyl nitrate, methylene blue, and sodium thiosulfate.

Cognitive Level: Application

Nursing Process Step: Planning

NCLEX: Physiological Integrity: Pharmacological and Parenteral Therapies

19. **Answer:** 2

Rationale: Edetate calcium disodium (Versenate) or deferoxamine are antidotes for iron toxicity. D-penicillamine and succimer are antidotes for arsenic/lead/mercury, whereas trientine is the antidote for copper.

Cognitive Level: Application

Nursing Process Step: Planning

NCLEX: Physiological Integrity: Pharmacological and Parenteral Therapies

20. **Answer:** 1

Rationale: Acetone on the breath can be an indicator of overdose or poisoning with acetone, alcohol (methyl or isopropyl), phenol, or salicylates.

Cognitive Level: Application

Nursing Process Step: Assessment

NCLEX: Physiological Integrity: Pharmacological and Parenteral Therapies